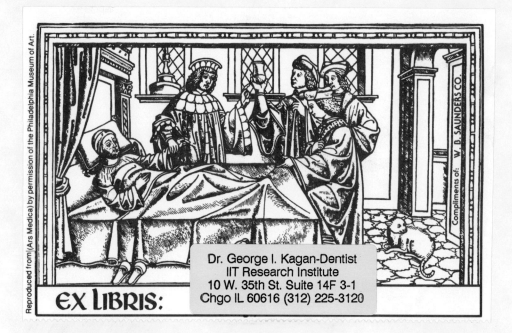

EX LIBRIS:

Dr. George I. Kagan-Dentist
IIT Research Institute
10 W. 35th St. Suite 14F 3-1
Chgo IL 60616 (312) 225-3120

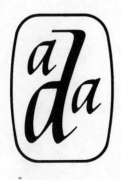

Information on the use, properties
and characteristics of dental
materials, instruments and equipment
including listings of products

DENTIST'S DESK REFERENCE: MATERIALS, INSTRUMENTS AND EQUIPMENT

First Edition

American Dental Association

PREFACE

As part of its duties, the Council on Dental Materials, Instruments and Equipment investigates and evaluates materials, instruments and equipment used in dental practice, dental technology, and oral hygiene to determine their safety and efficacy. Correspondingly, it is responsible for disseminating information to assist dentists in the selection and use or prescription of materials, instruments and equipment. Also, the Council considers methods and programs for encouraging, establishing, and supporting research on dental materials, instruments and equipment.

The Council on Dental Materials, Instruments and Equipment regularly assists, advises or consults with other councils and agencies of the American Dental Association on dental products. Products are examined either on the request of the manufacturer or distributor or on the initiative of the Council. Products are described in suitable reports in *The Journal of the American Dental Association* if they meet existing physical standards as well as standards of acceptability with respect to usefulness, safety, advertising, and labeling. They are permitted to bear either the Council's Seal of Certification or an authorized statement of Acceptance together with the Seal of Acceptance as applicable. When it is in the best interest of the public or the profession, the Council may publish reports on unacceptable dental products. Consideration of therapeutic properties or claims for such

properties is specifically assigned to the Council on Dental Therapeutics. When a material or item of dental equipment possesses or is said to possess therapeutic value, such products may be considered jointly by the Council on Dental Therapeutics and the Council on Dental Materials, Instruments and Equipment.

The Council provides the profession with reliable information on the status of recently developed dental products that are important in dental practice and in the maintenance of oral health. In evaluating new items, special emphasis is placed on safety under the conditions of use. Decisions of the Council are based on available scientific evidence and are subject to reconsideration at any time that a substantial amount of new evidence becomes available. All submissions on materials, instruments and equipment shall be in writing and directed to the Council.

The specification, certification and acceptance programs of the Association for materials, instruments and equipment are designed primarily to enable the dentist to select the most suitable products for his dental health service. These programs have been planned with the thought that the public's interest is paramount.

Dentists are advised to use certified or classified dental materials, instruments and equipment as products of good quality. Up-to-date revised lists are printed in the Reports of Councils and Bureaus section of *The Journal of the*

American Dental Association. Dentists, being responsible for the service to their patients, should specify what materials are to be used by the commercial dental laboratory in the construction of any dental appliance which they prescribe.

This book has been prepared as one of many services of the American Dental Association for its membership. It is designed to serve the dental practitioner, but will also be valuable to dental students, auxiliary dental personnel, dental laboratory technicians, as well as dental manufacturers and suppliers. This edition has a completely different design than all previous reference publications from the Council. The reader will find herein the most comprehensive and complete listing of dental materials, instruments and equipment ever printed.* With this printing the name of this book has therefore been changed to *Dentist's Desk Reference– Materials, Instruments and Equipment.*

The Council on Dental Materials, Instruments and Equipment wishes to give special recognition to its consultants, to the staff personnel of the Council, and to other agencies of the Association for assistance with this edition. The Council especially appreciates the assistance of the following:

G.J. Christensen
Provo, Utah

J.J. Crawford
Chapel Hill, North Carolina

H.W. Gilmore
Indianapolis, Indiana

M.A. Heuer
Chicago, Illinois

E.F. Huget
Washington, D.C.

G.O. Kruger
Washington, D.C.

C. Mabie
Washington, D.C.

F.M. McCarthy
Los Angeles, California

G. Myers
Ann Arbor, Michigan

R.L. Myerson
Cambridge, Massachusetts

B. Norling
San Antonio, Texas

T.J. O'Leary
Indianapolis, Indiana

M. Oringer
New York, New York

J. Powers
Ann Arbor, Michigan

L. Sadowsky
Birmingham, Alabama

C.M. Schoenfeld
Chicago, Illinois

R. Taylor
Chicago, Illinois

J.A. Tesk
Washington, D.C.

R. Voss
Alhambra, California

S. Winkler
Philadelphia, Pennsylvania

The Council welcomes continued suggestions and criticisms directed to the further improvement of future editions of *Dentist's Desk Reference* or on any other phase of the Council's programs and activities.

John W. Stanford, *Secretary*
Council on Dental Materials,
Instruments and Equipment
1981

Copies of official specifications, guidelines used in the Council's evaluation programs, and status reports are available upon request to the Council's office.

---

*This listing is basically complete as of early 1980. The Council regrets any omission of products that should have appeared in this listing.

CONTENTS

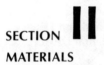

SECTION I
SAFETY

SECTION II
MATERIALS

SECTION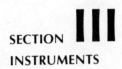

INSTRUMENTS

SECTION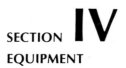

EQUIPMENT

SECTION V

ORAL HYGIENE MATERIALS AND DEVICES

Council on Dental Materials, Instruments and Equipment

Members of the Council

David E. Beaudreau, D.D.S., Washington, D.C. *Chairman of the Council*

*Alfred S. Schuchard, D.D.S., San Francisco, California. *Chairman of the Council*

Michael G. Buonocore, D.D.S., Rochester, New York.

*Gerald T. Charbeneau, D.D.S., M.S., Ann Arbor, Michigan.

Richard E. Coy, D.D.S., Edwardsville, Illinois.

Arthur W. George, D.D.S., Pittsburgh, Pennsylvania.

Karl Leinfelder, D.D.S., Chapel Hill, North Carolina.

William A. MacDonnell, D.D.S., Farmington, Connecticut.

John C. Mitchem, D.D.S., Portland, Oregon.

*Robert E. Sausen, D.D.S., Morgantown, West Virginia.

Staff of the Council

John W. Stanford, PH.D., Chicago, Illinois. *Secretary of the Council*

†Robert W. Bauer, PH.D., Chicago, Illinois. *Assistant Secretary of the Council*

P. L. Fan, PH.D., Chicago, Illinois. *Assistant Secretary of the Council*

Dorothy G. Najarian, M.S., Chicago, Illinois. *Editorial Assistant of the Council*

Atul J. Suchak, D.D.S., Chicago, Illinois. *Director, Division of Evaluation and Standards Development of the Council*

Wayne T. Wozniak, PH.D., Chicago, Illinois. *Assistant Secretary of the Council*

†Harold O. Wyckoff, Jr.,, D.D.S., Chicago, Illinois. *Assistant Secretary of the Council*

---

*Term expired at the time of going to press
†Resigned at the time of going to press

Consultants of the Council

Kamal Asgar, PH.D., Ann Arbor, Michigan (Dental Materials)

John Autian, PH.D., Memphis, Tennessee (Biological Evaluations)

Steven Bartlett, D.D.S., Charleston, South Carolina (Prosthodontics)

Gerald T. Charbeneau, D.D.S. M.S., Ann Arbor, Michigan (Dental Materials)

Carl W. Fairhurst, PH.D., Augusta, Georgia (Dental Materials)

Julian S. Gibbs, D.D.S., Nashville, Tennessee (Radiation)

William Gilmore, D.D.S., Indianapolis, Indiana (Restorative Materials)

Gilbert Glasson, D.D.S., Waterloo, Iowa (Dental Materials, Instruments and Equipment)

Robert A. Goepp, D.D.S. PH.D., Chicago, Illinois (Radiation)

William Greenfield, D.D.S., Mount Kisco, New York (Oral Surgery)

Michael A. Heuer, D.D.S. M.S., Chicago, Illinois (Dental Materials, Instruments and Equipment)

Krishan Kapur, D.D.S., Sepulveda, California (Implants)

Robert S. Kennedy, PH.D., Washington, D.C. (Dental Materials, Instruments and Equipment)

Kaare Langeland, D.D.S., Farmington, Connecticut (Biological Evaluations)

David B. Mahler, PH.D., Portland, Oregon (Dental Materials)

Lincoln R. Manson-Hing, Birmingham, Alabama (Radiation)

Frank M. McCarthy, M.D.. D.D.S., Los Angeles, California (Dental Equipment)

James Miller, D.D.S., Rockville, Maryland (Radiation)

Joseph Moffa, D.D.S. M.S., San Francisco, California (Dental Materials)

B. Keith Moore, PH.D., Indianapolis, Indiana (Dental Instruments and Equipment)

George E. Myers, D.D.S., Ann Arbor, Michigan (Dental Materials, Instruments and Equipment)

Robert J. Nelsen, D.D.S., Rockville, Maryland (Radiation)

Barry Norling, PH.D., San Antonio, Texas (Dental Materials, Instruments and Equipment)

Timothy J. O'Leary, D.D.S., Indianapolis, Indiana (Periodontology)

James E. Overberger, D.D.S. M.S., Morgantown, West Virginia (Dental Materials, Instruments and Equipment)

George C. Paffenbarger, D.D.S. D.SC., Washington, D.C. (Dental Materials)

Robert E. Patchin, D.D.S., Cleveland Ohio (Dental Instruments and Equipment)

Ralph W. Phillips, D.SC., Indianapolis, Indiana (Dental Materials)

Joseph M. Powell, D.D.S. M.S., Brooks Air Force Base, Texas (Dental Instruments and Equipment)

David T. Puderbaugh, D.D.S., Morgantown, West Virginia (Dental Materials)

Garrett Ridgley, D.D.S. M.S., Washington, D.C. (Dental Materials, Instruments and Equipment)

Sheldon W. Rosenstein, D.D.S., Chicago, Illinois (Orthodontics)

Robert E. Sausen, D.D.S., Morgantown, West Virginia (Dental Materials)

Alfred S. Schuchard, D.D.S., San Francisco, California (Dental Materials, Instruments and Equipment)

Israel Schulman, D.D.S., Washington, D.C. (Dental Materials, Instruments and Equipment)

Walter Schwartz, D.D.S., Roselle Park, New Jersey (Pedodontics)

Ralph W. Sellers, D.D.S., Brooks Air Force Base, Texas (Restorative Dentistry)

Peter Sendroy, D.D.S., Denver, Colorado (Orthodontics)

Harold J. Stanley, D.D.S., Gainesville, Florida (Biological Evaluations)

Ross Taylor, D.D.S., Chicago, Illinois (Prosthodontics)

Henry Van Hassel, D.D.S., Bellevue, Washington (Endodontics)

Robert V. Vining, D.D.S., Omaha, Nebraska (Prosthodontics)

William N. Von Der Lehr, D.D.S., New Orleans, Louisiana (Dental Materials)

Robert Wolcott, D.D.S. M.S., Los Angeles, California (Dental Materials, Instruments and Equipment)

Edward V. Zegarelli, D.D.S., New York, New York (Oral Hygiene Instruments)

IMPACT ON DENTISTRY AND THE PUBLIC—ROLE OF THE AMERICAN DENTAL ASSOCIATION

Under coverage of the Medical Device Amendments of 1976 to the Federal Food, Drug and Cosmetic Act, the term "dental device" as a medical device includes dental materials, instruments and equipment. Federal regulations, therefore, encompass a far greater range of dental products than merely materials. The agency of the American Dental Association which is responsible by its Bylaws to the profession for this area is the Council on Dental Materials, Instruments and Equipment. The following section describes the federal regulations involving the safety and efficacy of dental devices. A discussion of regulations concerning occupational safety appears later in the *Dentist's Desk Reference*.

The Council was established in 1966 to centralize the American Dental Association's activities in the field of standardization and evaluation of dental materials, instruments and equipment. With this action, the Council assumed the standardization and product evaluation programs that had been initiated by the Association in 1928 at the National Bureau of Standards. The Council is composed of seven members all of whom are active members of the American Dental Association. Members are nominated by the Board of Trustees and elected by the House of Delegates of the Association for a maximum of two three-year terms. In addition to its staff of 22, the Council has 35 consultants in various areas appointed by the Board of Trustees upon nomination by the Council.

The primary function of the Council is to provide protection for dentists in their selection of dental health care products. This is accomplished by determining the safety and effectiveness of dental products and disseminating this information to the profession. Development and improvement of materials, instruments and equipment are encouraged for use in dental practice and for improvement of the oral health of the public. The Council performs these duties primarily through the program of specification development, the Certification Program, the Acceptance Program, review of products that are advertised in the Association media or exhibited at Association meetings, a complaint reporting program, preparation of status reports, safety recommendations in clinical practice, and the preparation of the *Dentist's Desk Reference—Materials, Instruments and Equipment*.

The role of the Council, before the passage of the Medical Device Amendments of 1976 and its future role when examining the legislation, was and is principally, in the programs of specification development and evaluation by the Certification Program, the Acceptance Program and the complaint reporting program. Two of the most important sections of the legislation relate to the establishment of standards set for the premarket clearance of certain medical devices. After final classification of all available dental devices by the FDA Panel on Review and Classification of Dental Devices, the functions of which were described in the February 1977 issue of The Journal of the American Dental Association (JADA 94:353 Feb. 1977), the Council hopes to play a significant role in standardization and evaluation. At present there is every indication by the Bureau of Medical Devices that this can occur.

The Specification Program is the foundation for subsequent certification of materials, instruments and equipment. Through this program, standards are developed against which products can be tested. Currently, there are thirty four specifications with at least four additional standards under final consideration. Significant progress is being made on an additional eighteen new specifications. These specifications are being formulated by American National Standards Committee MD156 with the Council on Dental Materials, Instruments and Equipment acting as sponsor and secretariat of that Committee and working under procedures of the American National Standards Institute. Representatives from the dental industry, laboratory industry and dental schools as well as from the federal goverment, National Dental Association and American Dental Association all are members of the Standards Committee. In all, twenty organizations and associations are represented in the membership.

The Food and Drug Administration has indicated that it desires to cooperate with organizations formulating specifications in areas required by the legislation and has indicated that it desires to adopt standards developed under the American National Standards Committee MD156 and those that have been adopted by the American Dental Association. As cited in the August 12, 1976 Federal Register, seven American National Standards have already been indicated as acceptable to the Food and Drug Administration as regulatory specifications. Additional standards* indicated necessary by the Food and Drug Administration Review Panel are being submitted to the Bureau of Medical Devices. To meet this demand, American National Standards Committee MD156 initiated twelve new projects since May 1976. The Council and the Association strongly support voluntary consensus standardization programs under the procedures of the American National Standards Institute as the primary source of all needed regulatory standards.

In addition to the Specification program, the American Dental Association has a Certification Program in which a product is tested to comply with relevant specifications. Where no specifications are available, an Acceptance Program has been initiated, together with a Complaint Reporting Program and status reports, all of which will be subsequently described in detail.

With respect to the Complaint Reporting Program, it is interesting to note that the Medical Device Amendments now require every manufacturer to maintain a complaint file. The role of the Council for the future will be to coordinate complaints being received by the Food and Drug Administration and the Council to pinpoint areas deserving attention by the profession and perhaps in the Council's standardization programs.

The foregoing briefly outlines some of the Council programs which preceded the Medical Device Amendments of 1976. A more complete discussion follows later in the Dentist's Desk Reference. The Council has offered to assist in the formulation of needed standards in dentistry, to conduct the necessary evaluation of products certified as complying with regulatory

---

*The Food and Drug Administration in the February 1, 1980 issue of the Federal Register published its intended Voluntary Standards Policy for Medical Devices as well as a rule for performance standards development entitled Medical Devices: Procedures for Performance Standards Development.

standards, and to make available information not only to assist the Food and Drug Administration Dental Panel in its premarket clearance of products submitted as a result of classifications of the Dental Panel, but also to inform the dental practitioner of new products manufactured and introduced to the profession on or after May 28, 1976. The Council believes that the programs will continue as they have been favorably received by the Bureau of Medical Devices of the Federal Food and Drug Administration. The Medical Device Amendments, although they include by definition dental materials, instruments and equipment, were not aimed at dentistry. The intent of the legislation and the regulations being promulgated is aimed principally at life sustaining devices. The Council programs have and will continue to minimize the effect of regulations on products in dentistry. A discussion of the legislation follows.

MEDICAL DEVICE LEGISLATION AND THE FOOD AND DRUG ADMINISTRATION PANEL ON REVIEW OF DENTAL DEVICES

INTRODUCTION

The Medical Device Amendments of 1976, signed into law by President Gerald Ford on May 28, 1976, require the Secretary of the Department of Health, Education and Welfare to obtain advice from advisory panels of experts in the classification and scientific review of medical devices.

In anticipation of this law, the Food and Drug Administration in 1972 established thirteen device classification panels and a Diagnostic Products Advisory Committee. These panels consisted of scientific, engineering and medical experts in various medical specialties. In addition, one or more subcommittees were formed for most of the panels, and six subcommittees were appointed for diagnostic products. In August, 1976, the panels and subcommittees of the Diagnostic Products Advisory Committee were rechartered into nineteen device classification panels.

PANEL DUTIES

The Medical Device Amendments of 1976 establish three classes of regulatory control for medical devices and require the Food and Drug Administration to classify all devices intended for human use into one of three classes as follows: Class I, General Controls; Class II, Performance Standards; and Class III, Premarket Approval. To comply with these requirements, the panel reviews and evaluates available data concerning the safety and effectiveness of dental devices currently in use; advises the Commissioner of Food and Drugs regarding recommended classification of devices into one of the three regulatory categories; recommends the assignment of a priority for the application of regulatory requirements for devices classified in the standards or premarket approval category; advises on any possible risks to health associated with the use of the devices; advises on formulation of product development protocols and reviews premarket approval applications for those devices classified in the premarket approval category; reviews classification of devices to recommend changes in classification as appropriate; recommends exemption to certain devices from the applications of portions of the Act; advises on the necessity to ban a device; and responds to requests from the Agency to review and make recommendations on specific issues or problems concerning the safety and effectiveness of devices.

A complete description of the classification procedures is described in the September 13, 1977 *Federal Register* publication: 21 CFR Part 860; Department of Health, Education and Welfare, Food and Drug Administration, Medical Devices Classification Procedures. This document includes the classification (logic) scheme, the procedures for selecting panel members, and a discussion of the panel's responsibilities. The logic scheme of eighteen questions was uniformly considered by all panels, so that risk, safety, and properties of the devices could be dealt with in an organized fashion. Through use of this logic scheme, panel members determined which category was appropriate to regulate a device, and identified specific characteristics of devices that need performance standards. Consideration of the ratio of potential risks to benefits were inherent in this system. The questions were:

1. Is the device custom-made?
2. Although the device is custom-made, can standards be applied?
3. Is the device life-sustaining or life-supporting?
4. Is the device, or the diagnostic information derived from use of the device, potentially hazardous to life or good health when properly used?
5. Is the device of such a nature that (a) sufficient scientific and medical data exist from which adequate standards governing the device's safety and efficacy could now be established, and (b) the development and application of such standards would be adequate to control the device?
6. Is the device currently in use and marketed in the United States?
7. When the device is used, is it remote from the body?
8. Is the device powered by a non-manual external or internal source?
9. Will use of the device or failure of the device's power source present a potential hazard to the patient?

10. Does the device emit or inject any form of energy into the body?
11. Have the energy levels used been shown to be acceptable?
12. Will malfunction of the device result in safe energy levels?
13. Does the device use material for contact with the body which is generally acceptable or has known and acceptable properties requiring no additional controls?
14. Does the device have any known hazards, limitations, or shortcomings which can be avoided by promulgation of federal regulations applicable to the device in question?
15. If the device performs some measurement function, should the accuracy, reproducibility, or limitations of the information supplied be clearly indicated to the user by appropriate labeling, instructions, or precautions?
16. Does the device have performance characteristics which should be maintained at a satisfactory level, such level having general agreement among the user groups?
17. Is the device used with other devices in such a way that the system in which it is used can be hazardous if the system is not assembled, used, or maintained in a satisfactory fashion?
18. Is the device potentially hazardous to the fetus or the gonads when properly used?

Emphasis was placed on identification of devices that should have restrictions because of limitations, difficulties, or hazards that can be controlled by regulation (question no. 14). Eventually, these restrictions will become part of the labeling. Devices that perform measurement functions will have clearly indicated labels for the user's information on the accuracy, performance, or use considerations (question no. 15).

Also, the questions are so arranged in the logic scheme (published in the May 19, 1975 *Federal Register*, Part II, Volume 40) that the panel member is guided from one applicable question to the next by his response to the previous question. Therefore, not all eighteen questions are answered for each product.

PANEL STRUCTURE

The panel consists of members and a chairman selected by the Commissioner from among authorities knowledgeable in clinical and administrative medicine, engineering, biological and physical sciences and other related professions. In addition, industry interests are represented as non-voting members.

However, the Oral Implant Subcommittee is composed of one voting member of the panel, several consultants and an industry and consumer representative. Copies of summary minutes of Panel meetings may be obtained from the Office of the Hearing Clerk, Food and Drug Administration, 5600 Fishers Lane, Rockville, Maryland 20852.

PANEL RECOMMENDATIONS

The Medical Device Amendments of 1976 provide that the Panel shall submit to the Secretary within one year from when funds are first appropriated for the implementation of Section 513 of the "Act" their recommendations regarding all devices of a type introduced or delivered for introduction into interstate commerce for distribution before the date of enactment. The recommendations shall include (1) a summary of the reasons for the recommendation, (2) a summary of the data upon which the recommendation is based, (3) an identification of any risk to health associated with the device, (4) any needed restrictions, and (5) exemptions for Class I devices. The Dental Device Classification Panel employed the logic scheme and a supplemental data sheet as guidelines in making its recommendations.

The Dental Device Classification Panel reviewed and classified a total of 232 devices, which were placed into either the General Controls, Standards, or Premarket Approval categories. The criteria used by the Dental Panel to place devices into the General Controls category were, in the panel's opinion, sections 501, 502, 510, 518, or 520 of the Food, Drug and Cosmetic Act. These sections refer to adulterated or misbranded drugs and devices and give requirements for registration, records, and reports, and good manufacturing practices sufficient to provide an assurance of safety and effectiveness for the device to be classified. One hundred sixty-seven** devices, or approximately 72 percent of the devices classified were placed into the General Controls category.

The evaluation procedure which was used by the Dental Panel in determining whether a device should be placed into the Standards category was based on information concerning the device which made the General Controls category inadequate to provide reasonable assurance of safety and effectiveness and for which sufficient information exists to establish a performance standard to provide such assurance. Fifty-eight devices or 25 percent of the devices classified were placed into the Performance Standards category.

The Dental Device Classification Panel used several criteria in determining whether a device needed to be classified in the Premarket Approval category. One criterion was whether enough information existed to determine if General Controls or Performance Standards could adequately assure the safety or effectiveness of the device. If information was not available to show that registration, records and reports, and good manufacturing processes were adequate to control the device in Class I, or if it could not be classified as a Class II device due to lack of sufficient information for the establishment of a performance standard, it was placed in the Premarket Approval category. Another criterion which was used by the Dental Panel to determine if the Premarket Approval category was appropriate for a device was whe-

---

**The number of devices cited for classification in the three control categories may change as further reviews and considerations are made.

ther the use of the device is of substantial importance in sustaining or supporting human life or health, or presents a potential unreasonable risk of injury or illness. Seven devices, or approximately three percent of the classified devices were placed in the Premarket Approval category.

One of the duties of the Dental Panel was to identify devices classified into the Standards category which the panel believed needed to receive primary consideration due to the devices' frequency of use or potential risk to health. These devices are as follows:

1. Intraoral x-ray machines
2. Analgesia-anesthesia machines
3. Ethylene oxide sterilizers
4. Electrosurgical units and accessories
5. Compressed gas cylinders
6. Emergency oxygen and resuscitation* units
7. Jet injectors
8. Autoclave sterilizers

The Dental Device Classification Panel reviewed a study made by the Bureau of Radiological Health concerning radiation emitted from uranium-containing porcelain used in dentistry. Depleted uranium has been placed in dental porcelain for more than 40 years to give prostheses a fluorescent quality similar to tooth enamel, thereby enhancing the esthetic qualities of the porcelain. The study made by the Bureau of Radiological Health showed that the amount of radiation emitted by the depleted uranium does not pose a significant health hazard to dental patients. However, the Dental Panel recommended that due to the nature of the use of the uranium for esthetic purposes, and the undesirability of having any level of radiation, the following four steps be taken by the Food and Drug Administration: (1) The Nuclear Regulatory Commission should be petitioned to reduce the permissible level of depleted uranium to 0.03 percent by weight. (2) The Food and Drug Administration should formulate a regulation to require that depleted uranium be limited to 0.03 percent by weight. (3) A standard should be promulgated to limit the concentration of depleted uranium to 0.03 percent by weight. (4) A time limit of five years should be established to allow manufacturers of dental porcelain to find a suitable substitute for the depleted uranium.

During the classification process it was necessary for the Dental Device Classification Panel to determine which items would be considered to be implants. In order to do this, a definition for the term implant was formulated by the panel. The definition that was finally agreed upon by the Dental Panel is "A dental implant is a device that is surgically placed into or in apposition to the maxilla or mandible and which protrudes through the mucosa of the oral cavity." The rationale for acceptance of this definition was that the Dental Panel members were aware of the possibility that surgical implants could be placed in the Premarket Approval category by the proposed device legislation, and believed that restorative materials such as amalgams, gold alloys, silicates, composites and cements should not be placed in such a restrictive category due to the many years that these items have been used without significant problems.

The adoption of the dental implant definition placed one item into the Premarket Approval category: endosseous implants. Subperiosteal devices, although considered to be implants, are custom devices, and were included on the dental device list due to the Dental Panel's belief that a performance standard for the material which is used to fabricate subperiosteal implants is necessary to assure safety and effectiveness.

During the classification process, the members of the Dental Device Classification Panel were made aware of the possibility that many of the items included in the preliminary dental device list may not have been medical devices as defined in Section 201(h) of the Food, Drug and Cosmetic Act. This definition which states "A device is an article or component thereof which is (1) recognized in the Official National Formulary or the United States Pharmacopeia, (2) intended for use in diagnosis of disease or other conditions, or in the cure, mitigation, treatment, or prevention of disease in man or other animals, or (3) intended to affect the structure or any function of the body of man or other animals." Based on this definition, the Dental Panel determined that there were many items on the classification list which are used in the construction or fabrication of dental devices, but which may not be considered to be dental devices as defined by the Act. An example that was suggested is the machinery used to produce a water irrigating device. Although the machinery is essential to the construction of the irrigating device, the Food and Drug Administration is not requiring application of device regulations to the machinery. Following this line of reasoning the Dental Panel members considered all laboratory items which do not come in contact with the patient to fall outside of the definition of a medical device as stated in the Food, Drug and Cosmetic Act, although they may be necessary for the fabrication of a dental device.

A list of all the items which were recommended for deletion by the Dental Panel is available from the Bureau of Medical Devices of the Food and Drug Administration. Copies of the complete classification are also available from the same Bureau. The Food and Drug Administration and the Dental Device Classification Panel invite public comments and suggestions related to the classification activities.

PROGRAMS OF THE COUNCIL ON DENTAL MATERIALS, INSTRUMENTS AND EQUIPMENT

The Council on Dental Materials, Instruments and Equipment was established in 1966 to centralize the American Dental Association's activities in the field of standardization and evaluation of dental materials, instruments and equipment. With this action, the Council assumed the standardization and product evaluation programs for materials that had been initiated by the Association in 1928 at the National Bureau of Standards.

The Council performs its duties through a number of means, primarily through its Specification Program, Certification Program, Acceptance Program, Complaint Report Program, and Status Report Program.

SPECIFICATION PROGRAM

Formulation of Specifications

The definition of a material by means of physical and chemical properties is an old method for specifying quality. However, the dental profession did not have a specification for any of its unique restorative materials until 1926 when Dr. Wilmer Souder and his co-workers at the National Bureau of Standards formulated a specification for dental amalgam alloy.

The laboratory tests should be designed so that they will delineate satisfactory materials and rule out unsatisfactory ones. This terse dictum is difficult to carry out because the design of tests that will accomplish the foregoing commitments requires considerable imagination and the necessary research to prove that the tests are reliable and valid. By reliable it is meant that the tests can be repeated by different laboratories with satisfactory agreement in results. By valid it is meant that the laboratory testing will predict the behavior of the materials in service.

PHYSICAL AND CHEMICAL TESTS. Perhaps the first criterion should be that the properties to be delineated should have pertinence in use. The second criterion is that all laboratory tests should be designed to simulate actual service conditions as closely as possible. The laboratory test is apt to be too far removed from conditions of service. The degree of the validity of the laboratory test is determined by the degree of correlation between data obtained from laboratory tests and the behavior of the material in service. This is the single most important item in judging the worth of any laboratory test. Of course the greater the degree of correlation, the better the test.

STRUCTURAL TESTS. In addition to both laboratory tests for the materials themselves, and straight service tests, it may be desirable to assemble the material into a clinical structure or appliance. In a specification for such a material as denture base polymer, it is an advantage to process a denture as a test in the specification. One may observe some fault or discrepancy that may not be detected in symmetrical specimens as required in the tests for mechanical properties.

ABUSIVE TESTS. In the design of the tests it may be desirable to include accelerated or abusive conditions. The tests may be made abusive by exaggerating the severity and/or increasing the frequency of normal deteriorating influences.

CORRELATION OF TESTS. If one could obtain an excellent correlation among the laboratory tests, the structural tests and the service tests, then one could arrive at a nearly ideal specification.

PRINCIPLES IN FORMULATION. Georges Charpy, the renowned French engineer in 1907, set down some excellent advice for the formulation of specifications. Many decades later, the rules of this old master are axiomatic. He suggested that one avoid composition requirements and define the material by performance tests only; give a meticulous and precise description of all tests; avoid all vagueness that permits or necessitates any arbitrary decisions on the part of the personnel doing the testing; specify the relation between the precision of the testing and the precision required in the results of the tests; and state how the data are to be recorded.

LOGIC. The best testing program is one that combines both laboratory and clinical testing in a closely controlled discipline. This has been the method employed in formulating the American Dental Association specifications.

The philosophy behind the formulation of the specifications is an important factor in their usefulness. For example, should the maximum and minimum values for the various physical and chemical properties be set at the highest practical values considering the reproducibility of the test data or should the values be set on the basis of use or popularity of the available materials? The first procedure tends to specify the materials of highest quality which may not necessarily be, and often are not, those with the greatest volume of sales.

The American Dental Association believes that only the highest quality materials obtainable should be used and does not consider the price at which a product is sold as any criterion of its quality. The Association believes that this philosophy is sound and dependable from a public health standpoint, and the current specifications reflect this policy.

AUTHORITY. By authority of the House of Delegates of the American Dental Association, responsibility for the development and promulgation of American Dental Association specifications for dental materials, instruments and equipment is vested in the Council on Dental Materials, Instruments and Equipment. The Council in performing this function has been made Administrative Secretariat of American National Standards Committee MD156 for Dental Materials, Instruments and Equipment by the American National Standards Institute (ANSI). The scope of the Committee is:

1. Nomenclature, standards and specifications for dental materials except those recognized as drugs and dental radiographic film. (Dental radiographic film is under a special committee of the Council.)
2. Nomenclature, standards and specifications for dental instruments and equipment. These include all instruments, equipment and accessories used in dental practice, dental technology and oral hygiene which are offered to the public or the profession. Orthodontic, prosthetic and restorative appliances designed or developed by the dentist for an individual patient (custom devices) are excluded.

Procedure for Formulating and Revising Specifications

1. The Council on Dental Materials, Instruments and Equipment receives and con-

siders all suggestions for new specifications and revisions of existing specifications for dental materials, instruments and equipment. Any individual or group may present the suggestion and the Council welcomes correspondence in this connection.

2. The Council on Dental Materials, Instruments and Equipment may refer these suggestions to the American National Standards Committee MD156 for Dental Materials, Instruments and Equipment for which the Council serves as the Administrative Secretariat.

3. The Council as Administrative Secretariat of American National Standards Committee MD156 then determines, through the appropriate Chairman* of one of the four Groups of the Committee, if the Committee can undertake the new suggested project.

4. For projects of the Committee, Group Chairmen recommend, through the Secretary of the Committee, Subcommittee Chairmen to the Chairman of the American National Standards Committee for approval by the Committee. The Administrative Secretariat reserves the right of review. The appointment of the Subcommittee Chairman shall normally be for five years.

5. Subcommittee Chairmen canvass interested organizations or individuals having a known interest in the subject matter and also review requests for membership from other organizations and individuals.

6. Subcommittee Chairmen then establish their Subcommittees maintaining essentially a balance in all categories: Consumer (C), Producer (P), and General Interest (GI) and appoint one of the members of the duly constituted Subcommittee as its Secretary.

7. The Subcommittee as formed by its Chairman then is submitted through the

Group Chairman to the Administrative Secretariat of the American National Standards Committee for review and approval as to representation of interests. Change in membership on the Subcommittee is at the prerogative of the Subcommittee Chairman subject to review by the Group Chairman, Chairman of the American National Standards Committee and the Administrative Secretariat.

8. The Subcommittee, with the assistance of the American Dental Association, obtains information on the brands of the subject material or device that are in use, including their desirable characteristics and their shortcomings. Obtaining such information often involves personal interviews, correspondence and questionnaires sent to users and manufacturers.

9. The Subcommittee prepares a preliminary draft of the specification which enumerates the significant characteristics of the material, instrument or item of equipment, outlines methods of measuring them and proposes limiting values based upon extant knowledge. At this time any testing which may be required for checking the proposed specification requirements, methods and limits for a particular material is done by (a) the American Dental Association, (b) dental schools, (c) dental manufacturers, (d) qualified individuals or (e) a combination of the foregoing. The information so obtained is placed before the Subcommittee which prepares a revised draft of the specification.

10. The revised draft is then transmitted to the Administrative Secretariat for submission to the Standards Committee and all interested parties for criticism and comments.

11. The Subcommittee considers all comments received, revises the specification where desired, and submits it to the Standards Committee for ballot.

12. When the specification is finally approved by the Standards Committee, it is

---

*Other specific responsibilities of Group and Subcommittee Chairmen are available through the Secretariat.

American National Standards Committee MD156, Dental Materials, Instruments and Equipment.
The current membership of the American National Standards Committee MD156 for Dental Materials, Instruments and Equipment is:

Organization	Category*	Representative
Academy of General Dentistry	GI	Dr. J. Regan
American Association of Dental Schools	GI	Dr. G. Ryge
	GI	Dr. W. J. O'Brien
	GI	Prof. M. L. Swartz
American College of Dentists	C	Dr. R. J. Nelsen
American Dental Association	C	Dr. W. T. Wozniak
	C	Dr. J. W. Stanford (Secretary)
	C	Dr. N. W. Rupp
American Dental Trade Association	P	Mr. K. Austin
	P	Mr. D. L. Smith
Bureau of Radiological Health	GI	Dr. J. W. Miller
		Dr. L. C. Crabtree (Alternate)
Defense Medical Materiel Board	C	Col. W. Staehle, III
Defense Personnel Support Center	C	Mrs. G. Probst
Dental Dealers of America, Inc.	P	Mr. D. Saslow
Dental Manufacturers of America	P	Dr. J. C. Oakley
	P	Mr. D. A. Uitt
Dental Materials Group, International Association for Dental Research	C	Dr. G. T. Charbeneau
	GI	Dr. C. W. Fairhurst
	P	Mr. C. E. Ingersoll
	C	Dr. H. R. Stanley
Federation Dentaire Internationale	P	Dr. J. F. Glenn
Food and Drug Administration		Dr. R. S. Kennedy (Liaison)
		Dr. A. Acharya (Liaison)
Individual Experts	GI	Dr. D. B. Mahler
	P	Mr. J. O. Semmelman
	C	Dr. G. U. Ridgley
National Association of Dental Laboratories	GI	Mr. P. Williams
National Dental Association	C	Dr. M. G. Duncanson, Jr.
National Institute of Dental Research		Dr. T. M. Valega (Liaison)
U.S. Air Force	GI	Col. J. M. Young
U.S. Army	GI	Col. E. F. Huget
U.S. Department of Commerce	GI	Dr. G. M. Brauer
	GI	Dr. J. Tesk (Chairman)
U.S. Navy	GI	Capt. J. J. Rudolph
Veterans Administration		Dr. E. F. Irish (Liaison)

*Category: C—Consumer; P—Producer; GI—General Interest

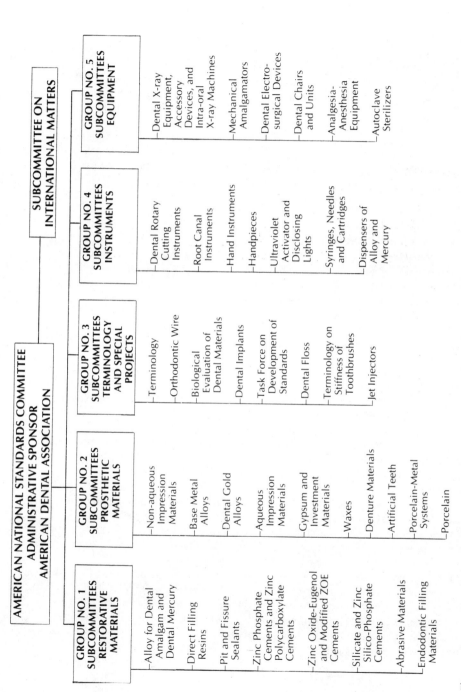

Fig. 1 Organization of American National Standards Committee MD156. The names and addresses of the members of the Subcommittees appointed for the projects listed may be found in a separate book on the "Specifications and Acceptance Programs" available upon request from the Council's office.

submitted to the Board of Standards Review of ANSI through the Administrative Secretariat of the Standards Committee, the Council on Dental Materials, Instruments and Equipment.

13. The Council on Dental Materials, Instruments and Equipment normally adopts the "American National Standard" as an American Dental Association specification showing professional acceptance and then transmits the standard to ANSI.

14. If accepted by ANSI, the specification becomes an "American National Standard."

Appeal Mechanism to be Used by Secretariat of ANSC MD156 in Development of American National Standards in Dentistry

1. In the event of the appeal of a decision or non-decision of ANSC MD156, the dissenter shall appeal in writing with documentation to the Administrative Secretariat (Council on Dental Materials, Instruments and Equipment, American Dental Association). The documentation shall include a draft proposal which would satisfy the dissenter.

2. The Administrative Secretariat shall request the Chairman of ANSC MD156 to review the statement of the dissenter and submit, in writing, an answer stating the position of the Standards Committee. The written statement of the Chairman shall be forwarded to the dissenter.

3. After review of the statement of the Chairman of ANSC MD156 by the dissenter, the Administrative Secretariat shall, if the dissenter so requests, convene an Appeal Board within sixty days, composed of at least three members.

4. The written positions of the dissenter and the Standards Committee shall be submitted to the Appeal Board. An opportunity shall be given both parties to appear before the Appeal Board if they so desire.

5. The decision of the Appeal Board shall be forwarded through the Administrative Secretariat to the Board of Standards Review of ANSI, the dissenter and the Chairman of ANSC MD156.

American Dental Association Specifications

No. 1 for Alloys for Dental Amalgam
No. 2 for Casting Investment for Dental Gold Alloy
No. 3 for Dental Impression Compound
No. 4 for Dental Inlay Casting Wax
No. 5 for Dental Casting Gold Alloy
No. 6 for Dental Mercury
No. 7 for Dental Wrought Gold Wire Alloy
No. 8 for Dental Zinc Phosphate Cement
No. 9 for Dental Silicate Cement
No. 11 for Agar Impression Material
No. 12 for Denture Base Polymers
No. 13 for Denture Cold-Curing Repair Resin
No. 14 for Dental Base Metal Casting Alloys
No. 15 for Acrylic Resin Teeth
No. 16 for Dental Impression Paste-Zinc Oxide-Eugenol Type
No. 17 for Denture Base Temporary Relining Resin
No. 18 for Alginate Impression Material
No. 19 for Elastomeric Impression Materials
No. 20 for Dental Duplicating Material
No. 21 for Dental Zinc Silico-Phosphate Cement
No. 22 for Intraoral Dental Radiographic Film
No. 23 for Dental Excavating Burs
No. 24 for Base Plate Wax
No. 25 for Dental Gypsum Products
No. 26 for Dental X-Ray Equipment
No. 27 for Direct Filling Resins
No. 28 for Endodontic Files and Reamers
No. 29 for General Specification for Hand Instruments
No. 30 for Dental Zinc Oxide-Eugenol Type Restorative Materials
No. 31 for Exposure Time Designation for Timers of Dental X-Ray Machines
No. 32 for Orthodontic Wires Not Containing Precious Metals
No. 34 for Dental Aspirating Syringes
No. 41 for Recommended Standard Practices for Biological Evaluation of Dental

Materials, Effective October,1980

No. 52 Uranium Content in Dental Porcelain and Porcelain Teeth, Effective May, 1980

Some of the Organizations Engaged in Standardization of Dental Materials, Instruments and Equipment

AMERICAN NATIONAL STANDARDS INSTITUTE (ANSI). (Formerly the American Standards Association and then the United States of America Standards Institute). The American National Standards Institute is the clearing house for standards on a national and international level. The American Dental Association submits its specifications for dental materials to ANSI for approval as American National Standard specifications. The American Dental Association is the sponsor for subsequent revisions of the specifications accepted by the American National Standards Institute and for formulation of new specifications. The Council on Dental Materials, Instruments and Equipment is assigned this responsibility. (See page xxvii for discussion of this program.)

FEDERATION DENTAIRE INTERNATIONALE (FDI). The FDI is a voluntary international federation of national dental associations and has individual supporting members. In 1953, the FDI directed its Commission on Research to explore the possibilities of creating international specifications for dental materials. The Commission appointed a subcommittee which actively prosecuted the formulation of FDI specifications for dental materials. In 1963, the status of the subcommittee was raised to that of Special Commission and in 1964 a Standing Commission (Commission on Dental Materials, Instruments, Equipment and Therapeutics) of fifteen members was created. Five of these members were technical representatives from the dental industry and were recommended by dental trade associations in the United States, Europe and Asia. The Commission was subsequently reorganized in 1979 and is now composed of eight members and has been renamed the Commission on Dental Products.

INTERNATIONAL ORGANIZATION FOR STANDARDIZATION (ISO). The ISO is an international yet non-governmental organization which has as its objective the development of world-wide international standards. The ISO members are 84 national standardization bodies (1979), the most representative one from each country. The American member is the American National Standards Institute. Annual contributions from each of these member bodies help the ISO to function. In 1979 more than 70 percent of the national standards bodies were either governmental institutions or organizations incorporated by law.

ISO International Standards are mandatory in 8 of the member bodies' countries. In 37 countries the ISO Standards are mandatory to some extent; in 20 countries they are totally voluntary. These figures reflect the influence essentially of private control in many ISO member bodies which are supported in whole or in part by government subsidies. The ISO has over 154 technical committees that prepare draft international standards in the specific fields assigned to them.

When a technical committee has reached agreement on a draft standard, the General Secretary of the ISO sends it to all member bodies for comment and suggestions which are forwarded to the pertinent technical committee. After careful appraisal, the standard is finally sent to the Council, the administrative group of the ISO, for adoption as an ISO international standard.

In 1958, the FDI contacted the International Organization for Standardization asking if they would consider FDI specifications for dental materials as ISO standards. The result of this liaison was the establishment of an ISO/TC106-Dentistry with the scope: "Standardization of terminology, methods of test and specifications applicable to materials, instruments, appliances and equipment used in all branches of dentistry." ISO/TC106 has formed seven working groups on (1) filling materials (Canada —Secretariat), (2) denture materials (U.S.A.— Secretariat), (3) terminology (France—Secretariat), (4) instruments and equipment (Germany—Secretariat), (5) classification of dental equipment (Germany—Secretariat) (deleted from work program in 1977), (6) the working position of the dentist (France—Secretariat) and (7) manual toothbrushes (United Kingdom—Secretariat). The Secretariat of ISO/TC106 is held by the British Standards Institution. The United Kingdom, Australia, Canada, Czechoslovakia, Denmark, France, Germany, India, Ireland, Italy, Netherlands, Norway, Republic of South Africa, Sweden, Switzerland, United States of America and the Union of Soviet Socialist Republics are participating members with about 21 other member countries with observer status.

Joint Working Groups between FDI and ISO were formed to avoid duplication of efforts and to complete activities initiated by the FDI before ISO/TC106 began its activities. In 1977 the Joint Working Groups were disbanded as activities were completed and all projects related to physical specifications were transferred to ISO/TC106 Working Groups. All projects related to clinical and biological activities and standards and the preparation of informative reports and/or proper methods of using materials were transferred to the Commission on Dental Products (formerly Commission on Dental Materials, Instruments, Equipment and Therapeutics).

AMERICAN SOCIETY FOR TESTING AND MATERIALS. The American Dental Association is represented on the American Society for Testing and Materials (ASTM) Committee F-4 on Medical and Surgical Materials and Devices. The Committee has as its scope the development of definitions of terms and nomenclature, methods of test, and specifications for materials for surgical implants as well as the implants themselves. The dental profession is also represented on ASTM Committee F-8 on Protective Equipment for Sports. The scope of that committee includes mouth guards.

CERTIFICATION PROGRAM

In order to improve and maintain the standards and qualities of certain materials, instruments and items of equipment used in the practice of dentistry and to promote the truthful advertising and labeling of dental products, the American Dental Association, through its Council on Dental Materials, Instruments and Equipment, maintains a program for the certification of dental materials, instruments and equipment. Under this program the manufacturer of a dental material, instrument or piece of equipment certifies that the product complies with the specifications which have been approved as official specifications of the American Dental Association and that all labels and promotional material are in compliance with the American Dental Association Advertising and Exhibiting Standards. If the product is found to comply with the specifications, its name is then placed on the List of Certified Dental Materials, Instruments and Equipment which is maintained and published periodically by the Council in *The Journal of the American Dental Association* and in *Dentist's Desk Reference.*

Procedure for Submitting a Certification

The Association's Certification Program applies only to products that are sold generally in the United States of America, and any manufacturer or distributor may certify a product. An imported product may be submitted if the certification is by the United States' distributor who will be responsible for the original certification as well as a testing program in the United States to show continuing compliance with the appropriate specification. Certifications must be accompanied by the following information and such other data as may be requested by the Council from time to time: (1) the trade name; (2) the serial or lot number; (3) the year and month of manufacture; (4) the physical properties as obtained by standard test methods with a brief description of the apparatus used in making the tests if different from that described in the specification; (5) data covering every provision of the official specification with names of the observers and the dates of the tests; and (6) specimens of all labels, guarantees and instructions that are used in connection with the product. Copies of official specifications of the American Dental Association and certification forms are available upon request from the Council office. (See page xxxii for a current listing of official specifications.)

Manufacturer's Agreement

In certifying a product, the manufacturer shall agree (1) that tests will be made regularly by the manufacturer to determine the continuing compliance of the material with the official specification; (2) that records of such tests shall be supplied as requested by the Council; (3) that test records and data for any batch of a certified product shall be made available to the Council on request; (4) that a representative of the Council, upon request, will be granted the right to inspect the testing equipment of the manufacturer; (5) that immediate notification shall be given the Council when the composition or the design of any product on the List of Certified Dental Materials, Instruments and Equipment is changed; (6) that all package inserts and promotional material shall be submitted to the Council for review to ensure compliance with the Advertising and Exhibiting Standards of the Association; (7) that in labeling and promotional material reference to the certified status of the product shall be limited to the conditions stipulated in the section entitled "Announcement and Maintenance of Certification"; (8) that no unauthorized reference will be made to the Specifications and Certification Programs of the Association in labeling, advertising or other promotional material for any of their other products which are eligible for certification; and (9) that if the certification is rejected or if acceptance of the certification is withdrawn, the manufacturer shall discontinue use of the Seal of Certification and/or any statement connecting the product with the American Dental Association within six months of the date of notification of the firm by the Council.

Testing of Products
Certified by Manufacturers

Prior to the acceptance of a manufacturer's certification for any product, it will be tested for compliance with the specification by the American Dental Association. Test samples, unless otherwise indicated in particular specifications, will be procured on the open market at the expense of the manufacturer. In the case of noble metals, any scrap remaining after the completion of the tests will be returned to the manufacturer.

Announcement and Maintenance of Certification

If a product is found to comply with an official specification of the American Dental Association, announcement of acceptance of the certification will be made by the Council and the name of the product will be placed on the List of Certified Dental Materials, Instruments and Equipment. Following such announcement, the manufacturer may appropriately indicate in promotional material and labeling that the product complies with an official specification only by displaying the Seal of Certification.

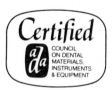

The Council may, however, permit the use of the following statement in labeling during the period from the time of receipt of a certification by the Council until such time as that certification is either accepted or rejected:

"Certification with American Dental Association pending."

The unauthorized use of either the statement or the Seal will subject the manufacturer to the usual legal responsibilities.

From time to time, the Council will publish in *The Journal of the American Dental Association* and in other appropriate publications, the List of Certified Dental Materials, Instruments and Equipment and notices of voluntary withdrawals of certified products from the List by their respective manufacturers.

If there is a change in manufacturer or distributor of a certified product the acceptance of the certification by the Council expires automatically. The product may then be resubmitted as a new certification.

Survey of Certified Products

At any time, and without notice to the manufacturer, the Council may authorize the testing of any or all products on the List of Certified Dental Materials, Instruments and Equipment. In the event that a sample fails to comply with the respective specification, the material will be removed from the List of Certified Dental Materials, Instruments and Equipment. Test samples are procured at the expense of the manufacturer as outlined in the section entitled: "Testing of Products Certified by Manufacturers."

If a product is removed from the List of Certified Dental Materials, Instruments and Equipment, the manufacturer may subsequently recertify the product provided acceptable evidence is given that the product which did not comply with the specification has been removed from the market.

Responsibility for Guarantee of Compliance

The responsibility for guaranteeing that a product complies with an official specification lies solely with the manufacturer who certified the product and not with the American Dental Association.

Promotional Material

Claims made for products in labeling, advertising, or by any other means shall be clear and accurate and shall not result in the disparagement of other useful products or useful techniques available for similar purposes. Advertisements to the dental profession or to the public shall not include misleading or unwarranted statements. Advertising and exhibiting of accepted products shall be in compliance with the Advertising and Exhibiting Standards of the American Dental Association.

Advertising and Exhibiting Standards

The American Dental Association welcomes advertising in its publications and exhibiting at its meetings because it believes that advertising and exhibiting constitute an important means of keeping the dentist informed of new and better products and services for the practice of dentistry. Such advertising and exhibiting should be attractive, factual, dignified, and calculated to provide useful product and service information.

The following standards apply uniformly to all publications and meetings of the American Dental Association in which advertising or exhibiting space is sold, namely *The Journal of the American Dental Association, ADA News, Journal of Oral Surgery,* and the Association's annual session.

Products and services not directly relevant to dentistry or dental practice will be considered on their individual merits for advertising in Association media and for exhibiting at Association meetings.

More detailed information on specific products may be found in *Accepted Dental Therapeutics* or *Dentist's Desk Reference—Materials, Instruments and Equipment.*

A. General
1. The advertisement, exhibit, or promotion shall be in keeping with the spirit and intent of all applicable legal requirements.
2. The advertisement, exhibit, or promotion shall not include unsupportable claims.
3. The advertisement, exhibit, or promotion shall be supported by suitable documentation. For products within the purview of the Council on Dental Materials, Instruments and Equipment, see section B.
4. The advertisement, exhibit, or promotion shall be acceptable for publicizing an educational course for dentists or dental auxiliaries provided that such course does not involve the teaching of or instruction in the use of a technique alone or in conjunction with a product, either of which technique or product is the subject of an unfavorable or cautionary report by an agency of the American Dental Association and provided, further, that such course is conducted by or under the auspices of the American Dental Associ-

ation, one of its constitutent or component dental societies, a national certifying board or national society for one of the specialty areas of dental practice recognized by the American Dental Association, or any dental organization specifically referred to in the *Bylaws* of the American Dental Association. The acceptability of an advertisement, exhibit, or promotion publicizing a course conducted by or under the auspices of an organization other than the aforementioned will be judged on the individual merits of such course by appropriate agencies of the American Dental Association.

5. The advertisement, exhibit, or promotion shall be unacceptable for products or services which have been adjudged worthless, dangerous, or of secret composition by official action of appropriate agencies of the American Dental Association.

6. The advertisement, exhibit, or promotion may incorporate words, phrases, or devices indicating pride or confidence in a product or service. Such promotional material shall not incorporate exaggerated claims, superlative words, or phrases which mislead or are untrue, or any printed matter which is considered to be in poor taste.

7. The advertisement, exhibit, or promotion may cite, in footnotes, references from dental and other scientific literature provided (a) the citation adequately supports the claim and (b) the citation fairly represents the body of literature on the claim made. However, direct quotations shall not be permitted.

8. The advertisement, exhibit, or promotion may include the use of a competitor's name and the description of a comparable product or service, including price, if the comparison is made in a manner that is not false or misleading.

9. The advertisement, exhibit, or promotion shall not use the name of the Association or make reference to the prior adver-

tising, exhibiting, or promotion of a product or service in any Association publication or at any Association meeting without prior written authorization from the Association, which authorization shall not be unreasonably withheld.

10. The advertisement, exhibit, or promotion used in other media shall not include claims or statements which would be unacceptable in American Dental Association media.

B. Council on Dental Materials, Instruments and Equipment

1. The advertisement, exhibit, or promotion shall be acceptable where an official American Dental Association specification exists if the certification and the claims are found to be substantiated by the Council.

2. The advertisement, exhibit, or promotion shall be acceptable if it is classified as "Acceptable" or "Provisionally Acceptable" under their evaluation programs and the claims are found to be substantiated by the Council.

3. The advertisement, exhibit, or promotion shall be permitted to use an authorized statement with reference to an evaluation program of the Council if the statement is approved by the Council.

4. The advertisement, exhibit, or promotion shall be acceptable in cases where no evaluation programs exist if the formulation for the material or construction of the device and the claims are found to be acceptable by the Council.

ACCEPTANCE PROGRAM

The Acceptance Program applies to materials, instruments and items of equipment for which evidence of safety and usefulness has been established by biological, laboratory and/or clinical evaluations where appropriate and where physical standards or specifications do not exist. Powered toothbrushes and pit and fissure sealants are examples. Products accepted under this program shall be classified as follows:

Classification of Materials, Instruments and Equipment Evaluated by the Council

After consideration of a product has been completed under the provisions of the "Acceptance Program," the Council classifies the product as Acceptable, as Provisionally Acceptable, or as Unacceptable. Products are usually classified as Acceptable for three years. Acceptance is renewable and may be reconsidered at any time. If there is a change in manufacturer or distributor of the product, the acceptance expires automatically.

ACCEPTABLE PRODUCTS. Those products classified as "Acceptable" are listed in *Dentist's Desk Reference—Materials, Instruments and Equipment* and the manufacturer or distributor may use the Seal of Acceptance and an authorized statement as specified in the sections "Announcement and Maintenance of Acceptance" and "Rules for the Use of the Seal of the Council."

PROVISIONALLY ACCEPTABLE PRODUCTS. Provisionally Acceptable products consist of those which lack sufficient evidence to justify classification as Acceptable, but for which there is reasonable evidence of safety and usefulness including clinical feasibility. These products meet the other qualifications established by the Council and are listed in the *Dentist's Desk Reference—Materials, Instruments and Equipment*. The Council may authorize the use of a suitable statement to define specifically the area of usefulness of products classified as Provisionally Acceptable. Classification in this category is reviewed each year and is not ordinarily continued for more than three years.

UNACCEPTABLE PRODUCTS. Unacceptable products are those which are dangerous to the health of the user, obsolete, markedly inferior, or useless. Such products would not meet the standards outlined in the "Provisions for Eval-

uation of Dental Materials, Instruments and Equipment."

Provisions for Evaluation of Dental Materials, Instruments and Equipment

For submission of a product to the Council, the manufacturer or distributor agrees to accept the following specific obligations. Communications with the Council shall be in writing and shall be transmitted through the Secretary of the Council. The Council feels free to use the information in these communications. The procedure for submission as well as directions for submission of specific products covered under the program may be secured upon request to the Council.

DESCRIPTION. The description of the materials used in the construction and the method of operation of a device shall be provided. With regard to submission of a dental material, the composition and use of the product shall be submitted.

SPECIMEN. A sample of the commercially available product shall be provided for examination and testing if requested by the Council. An additional sample shall be obtained on the open market at the expense of the manufacturer if requested by the Council.

SUBMISSION OF EVIDENCE. Information pertaining to composition, mechanical and physical properties, operating characteristics where applicable, safety and usefulness shall be submitted by the manufacturing firm.

NATURE OF EVIDENCE. The firm shall provide objective data with citation of sources. The data shall be based upon evaluations of the product from both the clinical and laboratory standpoint. Extended clinical experience when appropriate may be utilized as a basis for evaluation of the product.

ADDITIONAL EVIDENCE. The Association may use its own laboratory or other facilities to conduct any additional evaluation deemed necessary by the Council.

REVIEW OF PROMOTIONAL MATERIAL. The firm shall submit all package inserts and promotional material to the Council for review to ensure compliance with the Advertising and Exhibiting Standards of the Association.

MANUFACTURING STANDARDS. The firm shall provide evidence that the manufacturing and laboratory control facilities are under the supervision of qualified personnel and are adequate to ensure uniformity of products and accuracy of labeling. The firm shall permit representatives of the Council to visit factories and laboratories on request.

STANDARDS. The product shall conform to standards or specifications that may be established by the Council.

CHANGE IN COMPOSITION, NATURE AND FUNCTION. The firm shall notify the Council of any change in the composition, nature and function or use of an evaluated product.

Announcement and Maintenance of Acceptance

If a product meets the provisions for evaluation and is accepted as safe and useful for the purpose intended, announcement of classification as "Acceptable" or "Provisionally Acceptable" is made by the Council. Following such announcement, the manufacturer may, when authorized by the Council, appropriately indicate this classification in promotional material and labeling by inclusion of an appropriate statement indicating the area or areas of usefulness of the product. A manufacturer of a product classified as "Acceptable" may also use the Council's Seal of Acceptance.

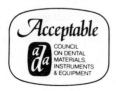

In the event that acceptance of a product is withdrawn, all use of the above classification in connection with the product must be discon-

tinued within six months of the date of notification of the firm by the Council.

Responsibility

The responsibility of providing substantiation of claims for safety and efficacy or claims of compliance with an official standard shall reside with the manufacturer and not with the American Dental Association.

Promotional Material

Claims made for products in labeling, advertising, or by any other means shall be clear and accurate and shall not result in the disparagement of other useful products or useful techniques available for similar purposes. Advertisements to the dental profession or to the public shall not include misleading or unwarranted statements. Advertising and exhibiting of accepted products shall be in compliance with the Advertising and Exhibiting Standards of the American Dental Association (See page xxxvi).

Government Regulations

Materials, devices, labeling, promotional, and related material shall conform to all applicable laws and government regulations.

Product Areas Under Acceptance Programs

The following product areas are presently covered by Council Acceptance Programs:

1. Accessory Devices for X-Ray Machines
2. Alloys for Cast Dental Restorative and Prosthetic Devices
3. Autoclave Sterilizers, Effective June, 1981
4. Carboxylate Cements
5. Dental Electrosurgical Devices
6. Dental X-Ray Equipment
7. Denture Adherents
8. Dispensers for Dental Amalgam Alloys and Mercury, Effective June, 1981
9. Glass Ionomer Cements, Effective August, 1980
10. Mechanical Denture Cleaning Devices
11. Nitrous Oxide/Oxygen Scavenging Equipment
12. Nitrous Oxide/Oxygen Sedation Machines and Devices
13. Nitrous Oxide/Oxygen Waste Gas Monitoring Equipment

14. Oral Irrigating Devices
15. Orthodontic Bracket Attachment Materials
16. Pit and Fissure Sealants
17. Powered Oral Hygiene Devices
18. Rapid Processing Devices for Dental Radiographic Film
19. Resilient Reliner Materials
20. Treatment Reliner Materials
21. Ultrasonic Scaling Devices
22. Ultraviolet Radiation Emitting Devices

Copies of guidelines for submission of any of these products for consideration are available upon request to the Council office.

Directions for Submission of Products Under the Acceptance Program

All submissions and other information sent to the Council's office unless otherwise indicated, should be in triplicate as it is usually necessary to forward copies to Council's consultants for review. Only complete submissions will be accepted by the Council; partial submissions will be returned.

A manufacturer is advised that the review process for classification of a product is complex. Typically, notification of the classification status of a product can be expected three months after the date of receipt of the complete submission by the Council. More time may be required for the classification process if additional information or clarification is requested.

A. Unless otherwise indicated, provide the Council with at least one original trade package item produced for market. The Council agrees to return subject item within six months if requested.
B. Provide the Council with three copies of all informative and descriptive material, directions for use, cautions, and so forth.
C. Provide the Council with three copies of a submission that contains the following:
   1. Name and use of item.
   2. Number of patent relating to product.
   3. Composition, physical, and chemical properties of dental materials.
   4. Materials used in construction and method of operation of a device.
   5. Evidence of safety and usefulness of product based on in vitro, biological, and clinical evaluations.

   Evidence of safety and usefulness of the product may be in the form of published reports or unpublished information obtained from appropriate scientific studies using in vitro, biological, and clinical observations. Biological evaluations should be in compliance with American Dental Association Document No. 41 for Biological Evaluation of Dental Materials.

   Evidence should be both sufficient in quantity and adequate in quality to permit sound conclusions. This requirement is especially important because most clinical studies involve subjective interpretations on the part of both the observer and the patient.

   To provide a sufficient quantity of data, not only should the number of clinical cases available for observation in a single study be adequate, but reports of additional investigations by independent groups are usually required.

   To obtain evidence that is adequate in quality, it is usually necessary in a study to use controls or comparison products under the same conditions of use as the test products. Double-blind studies are desirable whenever possible.
   6. A description of quality control processes routinely performed on the subject product.
   7. Names of owners, officers of the firm, or other individuals who are authorized to furnish information and represent the firm to the Council.
   8. Names and qualifications of scientific personnel responsible for formulation and testing of item or product.
   9. All other information required by the Guidelines for a specific Acceptance Program.
D. All advertising and promotional material for the product must conform with the Association's Advertising and Exhibiting Standards.

The manufacturer or distributor shall, therefore, agree to submit promotional material to the Council for review to ensure compliance with these Advertising and Exhibiting Standards.

Arrangement of a Submission to the Council

The following arrangement for a submission to the Council on Dental Materials, Instruments and Equipment should be used as a guide in preparing and structuring a submission. Each submission must include a summary report, no more than five pages in length, covering all information on safety and efficacy of the material, instrument or item of equipment. Each submission must also be indexed.

COVER

1. Name and address of applicant.
2. Name and use of products.
3. Number of patent(s) relating to product.
4. Name of owner, officers of the firm, or others who are authorized to furnish information to the Council and represent the firm to the Council.

5. Names and qualifications of scientific personnel responsible for formulation and testing of item or product.

TEXT

1. *Table of contents of entire submission.
2. *Comprehensive summary of all information on safety and effectiveness of material or device.
3. *Statement of composition, properties, or components.
   a. Complete listing of the composition, physical and chemical properties of a dental material.
   b. Materials used in construction and principles of operation of a dental device.
4. *In vitro evaluations.†
5. *Biological evaluations.†
6. *Clinical evaluations.†
7. *Instructions on labeling, packaging, operating, and installation.

---

*Indicates tabs.
†Extended details of in vitro, biological, and clinical studies should be included in the Appendix to the Submission.

CLASSIFICATION PROCESS OF THE COUNCIL ON DENTAL MATERIALS, INSTRUMENTS AND EQUIPMENT (CDMIE)

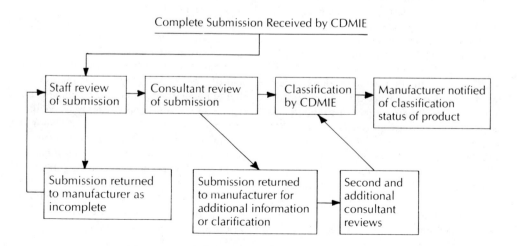

Complete Submission Received by CDMIE

8. *Promotional material.
9. *Description of quality control processes.
10. *Comprehensive bibliography.
11. *Copies of most significant articles.
12. *Appendices—evaluation forms, individual case histories, detailed descriptions of test evaluation methods, and so forth.

Information required by the Guidelines for a specific Acceptance Program should be placed in the appropriate section(s) of the submission.

If a submission is too large, it should be divided into two or more volumes.

COMPLAINT REPORT PROGRAM

The Council on Dental Materials, Instruments and Equipment of the American Dental Association conducts a program for receiving reports of complaints about dental materials, instruments and equipment that may be unsatisfactory or are suspected of being defective. All dental practitioners are invited to participate in this program.

Specifically, the Council is accepting complaints on materials, instruments and equipment that may have been found to be harmful, defective, deteriorated or otherwise unsuitable for use. This may include equipment that is unsatisfactory because of malfunction, design, or defects attributable to faulty material, workmanship or performance.

Complaints about suspected defective or unsatisfactory dental products should be carefully reviewed by the dentist involved and should include only items that are considered inherently injurious or unsatisfactory and are potentially hazardous to the patient or to the dentist and his office assistants. Complaints involving idiosyncrasies or sensitivities of individuals should be ruled out and not reported.

The following information should be provided when filing a complaint to the Council on Dental Materials, Instruments and Equipment.

- Identification of item
- Manufacturer
- Date purchased
- Serial/model number or manufacturer's lot/control number
- Source of supply and from whom it was purchased
- Specific complaint, defect, or malfunction
- Total number of episodes, incidents, or reactions–number of severe
- Hospitalization, if it was required–and the length
- Name and telephone number of dentist and physician most familiar with incident
- Other pertinent undesirable characteristics or performance features

A suitable form for reporting complaints to the Council office is included with *Dentist's Desk Reference*.

The Council will evaluate all complaints and may require additional information as well as procurement of samples to be subjected to laboratory testing by the manufacturers or by the Association. Therefore, it may be necessary to request samples, photographs, and supporting information from the dentist and the consulting physician involved. If complaints are confirmed, the Council will advise the dentist involved and notify the profession through Association media.

In some cases the Complaint Reporting Program has led to a recertification of products or changes in composition and quality control of products. Also the directions for handling products have been changed. In other cases the manufacturer has agreed to repair or replace the product. Dental dealers have been requested to assist in service calls and replacement of parts. This program formalized one that had already been going on for many years—that of receiving complaints and helping a dentist on an informal one-to-one basis. While the program was principally aimed at determining technical complaints or defects in instruments and equipment, or improper performance of materials, the primary impetus to initiating a formal complaint program was to provide a central neutral collecting point for complaints on dental materials, equipment and instruments.

STATUS REPORT PROGRAM

The Council develops status reports on existing and new dental products to assist the dentist in evaluating their application and usefulness. These reports summarize the existing information and, depending upon the amount and quality of the available evidence, may make certain recommendations. Their primary purpose is to acquaint the dentist with the extant knowledge on materials, instruments and equipment.

This program usually precedes formal acceptance of a specific generic area of product by the Council and is an expeditious means of informing the profession of new developments.

The contents and in some cases the conclusions of a few of the more than 70 Council status reports formulated during the past ten years are briefly reviewed. These reports are based on questions received by the Council on specific areas of products, questions on techniques of use, requests for recommendations on how to handle products and recognized applications, along with constant reviews of new literature and new products recently introduced.

A Council member, consultant or staff member may prepare the article for subsequent review by a specialty committee, formed at the suggestion of the Council, to give the Council the opinion and direction from those with expertise in a specific product area. Other specialists are also consulted and when the report has been revised it is then submitted to the Council for review and revision before final adoption. After adoption the reports are then submitted to the Editor of The Journal of the American Dental Association for publication in the section on "Reports of Councils and Bureaus," the only official area through which the Council can report to the members of the profession. The extensive reviews given the articles before submission for publication insure that the reports reflect the Council's opinion and not that of one investigator.

Council reports are divided into at least four areas: informative reports on generic areas, recommendations for proper use or handling of products and/or techniques, do's and don'ts on handling products, and official specifications of the Association along with lists of accepted or certified products.

Examples of reports which have been published along with brief summaries are presented below to give an idea of the available material. A complete listing of Council publications including status reports may be found on page 349.

INFORMATIVE REPORTS: First is the area of informative reports related to generic product areas. Examples of these reports cover products or techniques such as pit and fissure sealants, base metal crown and bridge alloys, newer silver amalgam alloys, newer polymers used in dentistry—cyanoacrylates, and the BIS-GMA resins —the matrix resin primarily used in composite restorative materials, and dental endosseous implants.

Pit and fissure sealants, if they present a seal, are considered by the Council as part of preventive measures but are not preventive materials, since there is no active ingredient such as fluoride reacting in situ to prevent caries. The effectiveness of such materials, therefore, may be only that they provide physical barriers or seals. The Council recognizes the short-term benefits shown by such materials but continues to believe that questions of long-term use and effectiveness have not been completely answered and, therefore, the decision to use and the placement of such products should continue at present to be a clinical judgment of the dentist.

The report on base-metal crown and bridge alloys reviews the needs to substitute base metal alloys for gold-based alloys. It also reviews the alloys available and the specific recommendations for handling such alloys as they cannot be handled in the same manner as the conventional gold-based alloys. In addition, the report contains the specific recommendations to be followed in handling beryllium-containing base-metal alloys. The report concludes that base-metal alloys for crown and bridge and porcelain veneering applications are useful additions to the dental materials available to the dentist. These alloys possess a combination of high sag resistance, low specific gravity, and low cost; this can be of potential clinical advantage. The overall manipulation of the alloys is significantly different from that for conventional gold-based alloys, and the manufacturer's recommendations must be followed explicitly to minimize technique sensitivity. Further research is needed on porcelain-alloy treatment variables and their effect on porcelain bond strength; on effects of variations in technique parameters on corrosion; and on burnishability and the accuracy of the finished castings. Such recommendations for future research projects are another important aspect of the Council's informative reports.

Another topic reviewed was the newer alloys for dental amalgam. Should high copper-containing alloys or conventional alloys be used? The report published by the Council in September 1975 updates the status of silver amalgam as a dental restorative material. It includes a brief history of the evolution of silver amalgam as relates to current properties, a review of the metallography of amalgam as relates to ongoing modifications, a description of the size and shape of particles in the alloy systems, and suggested uses of the new forms of silver amalgam.

Another subject covered by a Council informative report involved the newer polymers used in dentistry. Two recent reports published in this area cover cyanoacrylics and BIS-GMA resins used for coating and cementing. The report on cyanoacrylics concludes that such materials, on the basis of current knowledge, cannot be recommended for routine use in dentistry. The biodegradable characteristic with loss of properties, along with the potential toxic response to the degradation products dictates the need for additional long-term biologic and clinical evaluations. When these cyanoacrylates are used, care must be exercised that the liquid does not contact skin because the hardened film is difficult to remove. The second report on the BIS-GMA resins used for coating and cementing concludes that the use of these resins for cementing restorations is controversial. Additional research is needed in this area. The Council does not recommend the use of BIS-GMA resins in unprepared areas of cervical erosion. Restorations will not be retained on dentinal surfaces unless traditional retentive preparations are made.

RECOMMENDATIONS AND GUIDELINES: The second type of Council report encompasses recommendations and/or guidelines for the proper use of products or handling of certain techniques. The following are examples of such reports: guidelines for electrical safety in the dental office, recommendations in mercury hygiene, noise control in the dental operatory, recommendations in radiographic practices, precious metal scrap: what it is and how to handle it, and guidelines on the use of ultraviolet radiation in dentistry. One involves mercury hygiene. Much concern has been expressed about the materials and methods used in dental office construction to reduce the potential of mercury contamination. Impervious and seamless work and floor areas with edges lipped to confine spills have been universally recommended. Even so, many decorators continue to install rugs on floors of dental operatories. Carpeting is not recommended, as decontamination in the event of spills is not possible.

The degree of mercury hygiene observed by dental personnel in the offices is the determining factor influencing vapor levels. Consequently, efforts to establish guidelines for proper mercury hygiene must center on the few minutes during proportioning of the mercury and alloy and mixing of the amalgam mechanically. The guidelines published originally in February 1974 and revised in March 1978 concentrated on that area and have been updated in another area of the Dentist's Desk Reference.

Another area deals with radiographic practices. The most recent summary of Council recommendations was published in March 1978. The recommendations cover protection of the patient during radiographic procedures, protection of office personnel, modernization of x-ray equipment, use of fast-speed film, and the frequency of radiographic examinations. In this connection, the American Dental Association has consistently stated that the use of x-radiation for diagnostic purposes should be made only after careful consideration of both the dental and the general health needs of the patient. The primary deciding factor is the total welfare of the patient. The nature and extent of the diagnosis for required patient care constitute the only rational basis for determining the frequency of need for dental radiographic examination. The Council does not agree with a routine requirement of postoperative radiographs to show proof of service rendered. In other words, diagnostic radiography should be limited to those instances in which the dentist anticipates that the information he is likely to obtain will contribute materially to proper diagnosis and prevention of disease.

Lastly, the guidelines on the use of ultraviolet radiation in dentistry were published in April 1976. Several dental procedures, recently developed and currently in use, involve the use of limited amounts and specific wavelengths of ultraviolet radiation in the oral cavity. The guidelines include a discussion of the ultraviolet spectrum, the possible hazards from various areas of the spectrum, the useful area of the spectrum in dentistry, contraindications to the use of ultraviolet radiation in dentistry, and a series of precautions to be followed when using ultraviolet radiation in dentistry.

DO'S AND DON'TS: A third type of status report, which is succinctly called the do's and don'ts, is the newest area. One of the do's and don'ts reports concerns the handling of composite restorative materials. It contains brief statements regarding the time from the planning of treatment through the finishing of the restoration into the subsequent recall appointments. A second report in this area contains do's and don'ts for obtaining successful base metal alloy restorations and a third contains do's and don'ts concerning porcelain-fused-to-metal systems.

OFFICIAL SPECIFICATIONS AND LISTS OF PRODUCTS: The Council publishes new official specifications as well as all revisions of existing specifications. Periodically, lists of certified and/or accepted products are published in *The Journal of the American Dental Association.*

The Status Report Program, including all of the aforementioned divisions, should probably be increased as another role of the Council in view of the Federal Legislation to provide up-to-date information on recent developments in products. Again, such reports have already been used by the Food and Drug Administration Panel on Review of Dental Devices in arriving at a number of classifications.

SECTION I

Safety

SAFETY IN THE DENTAL OFFICE

This chapter contains information on potential hazards from materials, instruments and equipment which may be encountered in the dental office. All effects are dependent upon the quantity of exposure, the longevity of the exposure, and individual variability. The potential risk of a particular hazard can be minimized if caution is taken in the handling of these items. Also, following recommended office procedures and using common sense further enhances the safety of office personnel.

Practical limitations preclude a comprehensive listing of all potential hazards and precautions. Additional information can be obtained from the manufacturers or suppliers of the specific items of concern. Accepted environmental standards are included whenever possible. Major concerns on the effect of long term exposure to some materials have prompted the federal government to initiate safety standards. The Occupational Safety and Health Adminis-

tration (OSHA) has the responsibility for establishing and enforcing standards either directly or through state agencies. OSHA recommendations as well as safe levels of exposure to toxic materials are generally developed by the National Institute for Occupational Safety and Health (NIOSH). OSHA standards may or may not be similar to NIOSH recommendations for environmental exposure limits. The safety standards listed in this chapter are based on 1980 OSHA standards. NIOSH recommendations are used when OSHA standards are not available. Other recommendations such as from the National Fire Protection Association and the American Conference of Government Industrial Hygienists are listed as applicable. At times these recommendations may be cited in addition to governmental standards.

Further information and assistance in establishing safety practices may be obtained from:
   1. state health or labor agencies;

3

2. constituent (state) and component (local) dental societies, some of which may already have established safety programs;
3. federal health and labor agencies; and
4. the American Dental Association.

ELECTRICITY

Electricity is one of the most versatile energy forms used. At the same time, the safe use of electricity requires carefully designed equipment and an understanding of the potential hazards inherent in this usually invisible, powerful energy source.

The most widely used utility electricity is two-wire 120 volt alternating current (AC). The two-wire system has one energized or hot wire, most often with black insulation although red, blue, brown, or another dark color, except green, may be used. Green insulated wire is reserved for a separate ground (green-ground). The other power circuit wire is white and is the "neutral" wire. Appliances must be connected between the hot wire and neutral to receive power.

The neutral wire is grounded where power comes into the building but is also connected to the transformer on the utility pole or in the transformer vault where grounding is available. Grounding is necessary to establish a voltage reference for the utility.

The round connector on a three prong/three hole system is the ground system within a building. The ground system is wired usually with green insulated wire, although bare copper wire may sometimes be used in older installations.

The purpose of using the three-wire grounded appliance circuit is to provide an electrically conductive path of very low resistance which will absorb any dangerous electrical current surge which an equipment failure may produce and which will turn off the current source by burning out the fuse or opening the circuit breaker. The ground path is of very low resistance and is capable of conveying almost all the current away from the appliance even if a person is also providing a path to ground at the same time.

Hazards:
1. Shock
2. Fire
3. Physical injury due to reaction
   a. If the current passing over and through a person is 5 ma and sustained, it can cause involuntary muscle contraction. A victim holding an object and becoming a pathway for such a current will be unable to release the source of the electric current. Continuous current above the "let go" value can lead to fatigue, collapse and ultimately death.
   b. Currents over 50 ma can cause ventricular fibrillation and death. Larger currents can produce serious burns to skin and muscle and damage to nerves even if fibrillation does not occur.

Sources:
1. Shock or physical injury can be caused by the person contacting a grounded object and a faulty or poorly designed appliance that is connected to a source of electricity. The risk is increased when the skin is wet because the resistance to current flow is decreased.
2. Fire can result from a number of factors.
   a. Lightning
   b. Failure of electrical insulation
   c. Overloaded circuits or poor wire joints causing overheating of current carrying parts

In selecting electrical systems and appliances, the following features should be sought to minimize potential hazards.

Insulation: Electrically energized parts are insulated so that they cannot touch grounded metal and cannot be touched by people. This insulation serves not only to prevent leakage currents, but also guides the electrical current in its intended path so that it can perform useful work. The most visible of this insulation is the rubber or plastic coating on wires and cords.

Guarding: The metal or plastic housing of an

electrical appliance guards and, thus, prevents contact with the internal live parts. The insulated cord also serves as a guarding component.

Isolation: Most electrical systems in the United States and Canada are grounded at some point (on 120 volt systems, usually the white wire). Contact with a live or hot part of the system and a grounded object, such as a cold water pipe, will provide a path for current to flow and therefore be a hazard. However, if a transformer is provided to isolate both wires of the supply circuit from ground, there is no path for current flow even if contact is made between one side of the isolated circuit and a grounded object. Isolation is used in some dental appliances and is required in the supply circuits to hospital operating rooms.

Ground Fault Protection: Electronic devices are available that automatically disconnect the electrical supply if it detects a leakage current in excess of some predetermined value, usually 5 ma. This leakage current may be either from a live part to a grounded part inside an electrical device, in the electrical wiring, or through the body. The electronic circuit acts so quickly that, even if the current is through the body, the contacts are opened before the current-time relationship reaches dangerous levels. The ground fault circuit interrupter continuously monitors the supply line that it protects. It will not protect against electric shock if the contact is between two sides of the supply line, unless enough leakage current flows to ground to permit tripping. The permanently installed design cannot be used on certain types of circuits (the protectors come with warnings about this problem). For example, ground fault interrupters cannot be installed on some circuits with a low (below shock level) leakage current within the building wiring; the sensitivity of the protectors will prevent their use unless the wiring faults are corrected.

Ground fault circuit interrupters, however, will provide shock hazard protection under most normal shock situations in the dental office, and the portable ones can be used without any changes in wiring, receptacles, and so

forth. Because such devices will provide protection only if they are designed and calibrated properly, only Underwriters Laboratories (UL)-listed ground fault circuit interrupters should be used. This type of system should be utilized in areas where the potential for shock is high, especially in wet areas.

Low Voltage: Transformers or batteries can reduce the voltage. The voltage reduction in conjunction with the normal high body resistance prevents hazardous currents from flowing, even if both sides of the low voltage circuit are contacted simultaneously. Examples of this protection method are telephones, doorbells, and most battery-operated appliances.

Grounding: Connection of the exposed metal frame of an electric appliance to ground by a low impedance path will allow a momentary high current flow and cause the fuse or circuit to open. This may occur when an electrically energized part touches the frame, perhaps as a result of insulation failure. Since electric current tends to flow through the path of least resistance, most of the current will flow through the path from the metal frame directly to the ground. Only a small fraction of the current will flow through a person touching the appliance. Grounding, therefore, provides protection by opening an additional circuit under high current conditions, utilizing a fuse or circuit breaker to stop current flow, and directing the current away from the body.

Double Insulation: Incorporation of a second system of insulation in the product (so that if either system fails, the remaining system will provide protection) is the basis of double insulation. Many electric tools and gardening appliances are double-insulated.

FIRE PROTECTION

Fire is a real concern in the dental environment. Of the many causes of fire, electrical problems (described in the previous section), gases stored in or near the dental office, and

ELECTRICITY

Do:

1. Check the grounding of outlet receptacles. Although this will not demonstrate the resistance of the ground, it will indicate which should be tested by an electrician.

2. Check periodically the grounding of appliances. Put one probe of the continuity meter or ohm meter on the metal frame of the appliance and one on the grounding pin of the plug. Flex the cord at the plug to be sure the connection is not broken and continuity is only by intermittent contact of one or two wire strands. Although this test will not indicate whether the current path is capable of carrying the high currents present when there is a short circuit, it is the best method readily available today.

3. Purchase equipment listed by Underwriters Laboratories.

4. Identify control boxes and panels as to use and voltage; keep free from obstructions, and maintain a minimum clearance.

5. Make certain all switch and junction box covers are in place.

6. Examine all cords. If the insulation is cut, worn, frayed, or cracked, have the cord replaced with one of the same type and size. Especially check the points where the cord enters the equipment or the attachment plug.

7. When replacing cords with a grounding conductor (green insulation) be sure a cord with a grounding conductor is used as a replacement. Be sure that proper connections are made at both the plug and appliance. Connection of the green connector to other than the grounding pin of the plug can result in an immediate and lethal shock hazard: so, too, can an incorrect connection inside the appliance.

8. Check plugs for damaged or cracked bodies, bent blades, missing grounding pins, and a missing insulating disk on plugs with front screw-wiring terminals. Replace faulty or questionable plugs. Be sure the green conductor of the cord, if any, is connected to the grounding pin. Be sure strain relief is provided to prevent a pull on the cord from being transmitted to the connections.

9. Check wall and floor receptacle outlets for cracked insulation. If plugs fit loosely, have the receptacle changed. A loose fit can result in overheating and high impedance in the grounding path of grounding-type receptacles.

10. Check the physical condition of enclosures that guard and support parts of appliances. If any damage or overheating is evident, have the appliance checked for safety by a qualified electrician or repairman who is familiar with the product, or return it to the factory for repair. Some permanently installed appliances, such as dental units, have removable access panels that permit examination of interior parts and wiring. Open such panels only after the fuse has been pulled or the circuit breaker that protects the circuit has been opened. There are live parts inside the appliance even when the integral appliance switch is off.

11. Ground permanently installed equipment by connecting the metal frame of the equipment to a grounded cold water pipe. This should be done by a qualified electrician, because the size of the grounding wire will depend on the size of the circuit supplying the equipment.
12. Place cords in locations which allow dissipation of heat into the surrounding air; care should be taken to avoid placing cords adjacent to hot surfaces.
13. Equip each room with a fire extinguisher of the A-B-C type.

Don't:

1. Attempt electrical wiring and repair unless you are qualified.
2. Ground equipment not intended for grounding.
3. Drape electrical cords on any protrusions.
4. Break off the grounding pin of a three-prong appliance plug for any reason, including using the plug in a two-hole receptacle. Receptacles not properly grounded should be replaced by a grounding type. If the receptacles cannot be replaced, use a grounding adapter. The adapter may or may not provide a ground path for fault and leakage currents (tests will help determine this) but at least it will provide some means of grounding the appliance.
5. Run cords under rugs or where wear can occur.
6. Operate high current devices on low capacity extensions. If labeled in terms of watts, the current (amperes) can be determined by dividing the watt figure by 120. If the quotient is in excess of 10, the device or group of devices should not be operated on a common, flat lamp cord extension. This precaution will help minimize the risk of fire.
7. Overload circuits; breakage of circuit at the fuse or breaker indicates current leakage or overload, and these faults should be corrected. Fuses or circuit breakers should not be replaced with a device of greater ampere rating unless rewiring has been done.
8. Use bulbs in excess of the recommended size in lighting equipment.

---

ignitable liquids are the most common sources of concern.

GASES

Hazards:

1. Inhalation anesthetics
   a. Nitrous oxide, in combination with oxygen and in the presence of a combustible material and a source of ignition, is extremely susceptible to explosion and fire.
   b. Other inhalation anesthetics, when mixed in certain proportions with oxygen and air, may be explosive.

2. Other flammable gases

Sources:

1. Nitrous oxide and oxygen can be ignited in the presence of a combustible material such as hair, oils, oil-base lubricants, skin lotions, clothing, linens, paper, rubber, alcohol, acetone, some plastics, teflon manifolds, and oil or grease contaminated gas lines. Sources of ignition include heat from open flames, burning tobacco and electric heating coils, as well as electricity from defective electric equipment.
2. Static electricity can ignite certain volatile agents.

GASES

Do:

1. Follow recommendations of applicable standards.

   a. Nitrous oxide systems should be installed according to the Standard for Nonflammable Medical Gas Systems NFPA No. 56F, 1974, Boston, National Fire Protection Association, 1974, 28p. NFPA recommendations include installation and monitoring information. Installation instructions include materials to be used, warning systems to be included, and location and storage of gas supplies.

   b. Cylinder valve outlets should comply with the American National Standard for Compressed Gas Cylinder Valve Outlet and Inlet Connections (ANSI B57.1-1965; CSA B96-1965).

2. Have equipment installed by a competent supplier of gaseous equipment.

3. Use all metal manifolds or a suitable replacement material.

4. Periodically test equipment for leakage or mislabeling. Record the results of inspections of this type.

5. Install pressure warning systems (both audible and visible alarms).

6. Turn off valves at cylinder prior to leaving the office for the day.

7. Securely lock cylinders in an upright position in a room used only for the storage of gases.

8. Vent gas storage areas to the outside.

9. Protect cylinders, gas lines and line outlets from abnormal mechanical shock or tampering.

10. Properly label all cylinders and lines.

11. Separate cylinders of oxygen and fuel gases by a partition five feet high and having a one half hour fire rating.

12. Locate containers and first stage regulating equipment for propane and liquified petroleum gas outside the building except when portable systems are used.

13. Incorporate excess flow valves for liquified petroleum gas and propane into the fuel system.

14. Check for and replace defective valves, cylinders, or connections.

Don't:

1. Allow oils, greases, organic lubricants or other materials of an organic nature to contact oxygen or nitrous oxide under pressure.

2. Create sparks or open flames near cylinders or gas lines (including electrosurgical units).

3. Use oxygen as a compressed air source.

4. Use manifolds coated with flammable material.

5. Use a labeling system which is accessible to tampering.

LIQUIDS

A number of the liquids used in dentistry are either flammable or combustible. Flammable liquids have a flash point below 140° F (60° C). Table I classifies the liquids used in the dental environment according to their boiling and flash points.

Storage of these materials requires strong, durable containers or tanks. Table II lists the types and capacities of containers recommended for each class of flammable and combustible liquid.

Hazards:

1. Fire or explosion.

2. Leaks in storage containers or tanks leading to greater susceptibility to fires and the spreading of flames.

Sources:
1. Storage of flammable and combustible liquids in an area near a source of heat, spark or open flame.

Table I.
Characteristics of Flammable and Combustible Liquids*

Class	Boiling Point	Flash Point
FLAMMABLE		
IA ethyl ether	<100°F (37.8°C)	<73°F (22.8° C)
IB acetone benzene ethyl alcohol gasoline isopropyl alcohol methanol methyl ethyl ketone toluene	≥100°F (37.8°C)	<73°F (22.8°C)
IC	——	≥73°F (22.8°C) <100°F (37.8°C)
II mineral spirits Stoddard's solvent	——	≥100°F (37.8°C) <140°F (60°C)
COMBUSTIBLE		
III fuel oil #6	——	≥140°F (60°C)

*From Dental Laboratory OSHA Manual, Northfield, Illinois, Illinois Dental Laboratory Association, 1974.

Table II.

Containers for Flammable and Combustible Liquids*

Container Type	Flammable Liquids by Class				Combustible Liquids Class III
	IA	IB	IC	II	
Glass or approved plastic	1 pt.	1 qt.	1 gal.	1 gal.	1 gal.
Metal (except DOT drums)	1 gal.	5 gal.	5 gal.	5 gal.	5 gal.
Safety cans (SC)	2 gal.	5 gal.	5 gal.	5 gal.	5 gal.
Metal drums (DOT spec)	60 gal.	60 gal.	60 gal.	60 gal.	60 gal.

DOT = drums are those meeting the specifications of The Department of Transportation

SC = container not greater than 5 gal. in capacity with a spring closing lid, flash arrestor, and ability to release intended pressure when exposed to fire.

*From Dental Laboratory OSHA Manual, Northfield, Illinois, Illinois Dental Laboratory Association, 1974.

LIQUIDS

Do:

1. Store flammable and combustible liquids in an appropriately labeled and tested storage cabinet.
2. Use storage cabinets designed to limit the internal temperature to no more than 325° F (162.78° C) when subjected to a ten minute fire test.
3. Transfer flammable and combustible liquids in areas physically separated from other activities in the building either by adequate distance or by barriers having adequate fire resistance.
4. Provide adequate ventilation (several exchanges/hour).
5. Have fire control devices available at locations where these liquids are stored or utilized. The devices should include a type B extinguisher but the A-B-C type is recommended.

Don't:

1. Store more than 60 gallons of flammable or 120 gallons of combustible liquid in a storage cabinet.
2. Allow sources of ignition in the storage or work areas or in the path of the vapor. "No smoking" signs should be posted.

X RADIATION

Hazards:

1. Evident somatic effects; e.g. erythema of the skin, destruction or necrosis of tissues, or retardation of growth in children.
2. Late somatic effects; e.g. leukemia, cancers and life shortening.
3. Genetic effects (effects exhibited by descendents of exposed persons).

Sources:

Radiographic machines including conventional extraoral source, curved surface tomography (panoramic machine), intraoral source, cephalometric machines.

X RADIATION

Do:

1. Use professional judgment to determine the frequency and extent of each radiographic examination. Determine the minimum number of film exposures that will produce the desired diagnostic information.

2. Select radiographic film on the basis of the maximum emulsion sensitivity (film speed) consistent with the image resolution (sharpness) required for the diagnostic task. Only film of an American National Standards Institute Speed Group "D" rating or faster should be used.

3. Make certain the x-ray machine contains a minimum total filtration consistent with federal and state requirements. In general, total filtration should be equivalent to 1.5 mm aluminum up to 70 kilovolt (peak) and 2.5 mm for equipment operating above 70 kV (p). (More detailed information can be obtained from the Bureau of Radiological Health and state public health departments.) The filtration should be located in the useful beam as near the x-ray source (focal spot of the tube) as is practicable. Higher beam energy (kVp) allows decreased exposure; however, image contrast is reduced as energy increases, especially above 90 kVp. Therefore, the maximum beam energy compatible with adequate image contrast should be used.

4. Use shielded open-end cylinders or rectangular-collimating devices in conjunction with the long-cone technique. The combination of these devices and techniques will reduce the amount of scatter radiation reaching the patient's skin. All scat-

tered radiation should be eliminated or contained, except for that occasioned by the passage of x-rays through the tissues to reach the film.

5. Expose the x-ray film properly. Film exposures should be established for optimal density, using complete development. Films should be processed under the film manufacturer's recommended conditions with proper processing equipment. Image development should be extended to produce the maximum film density for the different x-ray exposures used without inducing significant chemical fog. Overexposure corrected by underdevelopment subjects the patient and office personnel to unnecessary radiation and may result in loss of diagnostic information in the resulting radiographic image.

6. Use leaded aprons on all patients to prevent unnecessary radiation of the gonads and thyroid glands.

7. Use film holders, bite tabs, or other methods to position the film during exposure.

8. Stand at least six feet from the patient and outside the path of the useful beam when exposures are being made unless protective shielding is provided for the operator. Work loads of more than 30 milliampere minutes per week may require the use of an adequately shielded screen. Information on shielding design, including determination of barrier requirements, can be obtained from "Dental X-ray Protection NCRP Report No. 35," National Council on Radiation Protection and Measurements, Washington, D.C., 1970.

9. Have state radiological health personnel or other qualified experts per-

iodically conduct radiation protection surveys (including personnel monitoring quality control) of the dental office so that adequate measures can be taken to protect the health and safety of all patients and occupationally exposed personnel at all times.

10. Continue education in all aspects of radiology.

Don't:

1. Exceed the minimum coverage of tissue area (and volume) exposed to the primary x-ray beam (for each film) necessary to meet diagnostic requirements and clinical feasibility. When a cylindrically collimated x-ray beam is used, the beam striking the face should not be more than 2.75 inches (7 cm) when the source-to-skin distance is greater than 7 inches (18 cm). The beam should not exceed 2.38 inches (6 cm) if the source-to-skin distance is less than 7 inches (18 cm). Further restriction of the beam to reduce patient radiation exposure is preferred and can be obtained by smaller collimation such as rectangular collimation circumscribed by the aforementioned circular limits.

2. Hold a film in place for a patient.

ULTRAVIOLET RADIATION

Hazards:

1. Surface erythema and eye irritations: Mucous membranes which line the oral cavity and comprise the conjunctiva of the eye do not have a hornified layer like normal skin and therefore do not filter ultraviolet light readily.

2. A long term alteration effect on cells and viruses normally present in the oral cavity: Studies suggest that an oncogenic potential may be effected by transformation of a virus to the oncogenic form, an increase of the susceptibility of cells to invasion by ultraviolet-irradiated virus, or activation of a latent virus already present within the cell.

Sources:

Most dental sources currently available have a long ultraviolet light spectrum (320-400 nm). This includes:

1. Photopolymerization of ultraviolet-sensitive compounds for restorative dentistry, orthodontics, and pit and fissure sealants.

2. Plaque control programs.

3. Specialized intraoral photography.

Safety Standards:

The following are current NIOSH recommendations.

1. Maximum exposure incident on unprotected skin or eyes is (based on machine output or measurement data):
   a. 1.0 mW/cm^2 for periods greater than 1,000 seconds.
   b. 100 mWsec/cm^2 for periods less than 1,000 seconds (Electromagnetic radiation energy is attenuated with distance. The energy at a given distance will vary inversely with the square of the distance. In addition, low wave length energy is partially absorbed by elements in the atmosphere).

2. Workers and/or patients giving a positive medical history of conditions exacerbated or aggravated by exposure to sunlight should be restricted from ultraviolet radiation exposure.

3. Employees exposed to ultraviolet radiation must be apprised of hazards, precautions, and symptoms of overexposure.

4. All sources, work areas, housings and containers must carry a warning label.

5. Protection of the eyes and skin is necessary.

ULTRAVIOLET RADIATION

Do:
1. Follow NIOSH recommendations.
2. Minimize exposure; use only the amount and type of ultraviolet radiation necessary to accomplish the clinical procedure.
3. Take a complete medical history to rule out medical conditions or drugs which might be affected by ultraviolet radiation. Medical conditions that are known to be sensitive are systemic lupus erythematosa, xeroderma pigmentosa, and erythropoietic porphyria. Drugs such as dimethylchlortetracycline (Declomycin) or 8-methoxypsoralen may cause the patient to be hypersensitive to ultraviolet radiation.
4. Restrict ultraviolet radiation used in the oral cavity to the area of clinical treatment to minimize unnecessary primary and scatter radiation to adjacent structures and tissues. The use of a rubber dam and light confining devices on the ultraviolet source are two mechanisms of confining exposure.
5. The dentist, chairside assistant, and the patient should use protective glasses if their eyes are directly exposed to ultraviolet radiation during the use of ultraviolet activator devices. Ordinary glasses might not give adequate protection. The supplier of the ultraviolet device should be contacted for lenses that will offer effective protection.
6. Protect skin surfaces through the use of clothing, ultraviolet absorbing creams containing benzophenones or p-amino benzoic acid, or barrier creams containing titanium dioxide or zinc oxide.
7. Frequently inspect ultraviolet sources and keep them in good condition. Follow the manufacturer's recommended maintenance schedule. Damaged devices should not be used until repaired.
8. Read and follow carefully the manufacturer's instructions.

RADIO WAVES

Hazards:
1. Arrhythmia of unshielded pacemakers.

Sources:
1. Using the following instrumentation on patients with unshielded cardiac pacemakers:
   a. Ultrasonic scalers
   b. Powered toothbrushes
   c. Induction casting machines
   d. Electrosurgical devices

Safety Standards:
According to OSHA standards, the radiation protection guide should be 10 mW/cm^2 as averaged over any possible 0.1 hour period for normal environmental conditions and for incident electromagnetic energy of frequencies from 10 MHz to 100 GHz. This means the power density is 10 mW/cm^2 for periods of 0.1 hour or more and the energy density is 1 mW-hr/cm^2 during any 0.1 hour period. This guide applies whether the radiation is continuous or intermittent.

RADIO WAVES

Do:
1. Avoid using the above listed devices near people with cardiac pacemakers.
2. Consult the patient's cardiologist if the device must be used near individuals with pacemakers.

Don't:
1. Use the above listed devices in the vicinity of an individual with an unshielded pacemaker.

NOISE

Noise above ambient levels in any environmental situation poses a potential health hazard. With the advent of new dental instrumentation and equipment, the potential for auditory problems has become an especially important consideration in the dental profession. Factors influencing the risk of acoustical trauma are age and physical condition of the individual, frequency of vibration (measured in cycles per second), intensity or loudness (measured in decibels) of the equipment, length of exposure time and interval between exposures. Of major concern are the effects of the low torque, ultra high-speed cutting instruments and their frequencies of audible vibration.

To measure the frequencies of equipment such as dental handpieces, manufacturers usually conduct sound analysis studies. These investigations are carried out under ideal analysis conditions with new equipment operating at optimum rotation speeds. New free-running roller bearing handpieces at recommended air pressures record 68 to 97 decibels (dB); Mid-west American reports the recordings for air-bearing handpieces to be approximately 10 dB lower. These recordings can be affected by the distance and position of the handpiece in relation to the recording device. A decibel level drop of 8 to 12 dB has been recorded when handpieces are subjected to cutting torque. Accepted decibel ratings are: safe range, 0 to 70 dB; moderate risk range, 80 to 100 dB; and high risk range, 110 to 130 dB.

Hazards:
1. Temporary threshold shift (loss of hearing sensitivity) due to short loud noise periods.
2. Threshold change in the higher frequency range [4,000 to 6,000 Hertz (cycles per second)].

Sources:
Handpiece wear, bur concentricity, misuse, poor maintenance, and individual operatory design can influence the frequencies and decibel readings (loudness) for individual handpieces.

Safety Standards:
NIOSH recommendations include the following.
1. 85 dBA adjusted for 8 hour exposure.
2. An audiometric testing program should be instituted. A baseline audiogram should be taken at the start of employment and every sixth year thereafter with checkup audiograms every two years.
3. When noise intensity is above the recommended level, engineering controls should be used to reduce exposure.
4. Personal protective equipment (ear protectors) should be utilized by individuals exposed to noise above the recommended level and are required for noise exceeding 115 dBA.
5. Personnel exposed to noise shall be appraised of hazards, symptoms, and proper conditions and precautions.
6. Noise monitoring and audiograms shall be retained by employers.

NOISE

Do:

1. Use optimum maintenance procedures for rotary equipment including methods of decreasing wear deterioration and utilization of concentric burs.
2. Reduce the ambient noise level in the operatory by soundproofing, acoustical ceilings, baffle drapes, resilient floors, and/or location of the compressor and other noise-making equipment.
3. Protect personnel through the use of ear plugs (cotton with petroleum jelly, defibered soft glass, or plastic plugs, capable of 20 to 35 dB reduction).
4. Have an otologic examination and an audiometric evaluation to assess the present condition. Noise levels in each individual office should be studied with monitoring periods of more than a week. An audiometric evaluation should be made after a typical workday and again at the beginning of the next day to observe temporary threshold shift and apparent recovery. Annual tests of hearing should be taken.

INFECTIONS

Hazards:
1. Hepatitis B
2. Syphilis
3. Herpetic paronychia (herpetic whitlow)
4. Upper respiratory tract infection
5. Tuberculosis

Sources:
1. Direct contact with infected patient.
2. Exposure to infected blood and tissue fluids, contaminated environmental surfaces such as switches or counter tops, contaminated equipment, or contaminated clothing.
3. Exposure to contaminated aerosol and splatter.
4. Accidental needle stick following injection into an infected patient.
5. Contaminated waterlines of equipment: for example, handpieces and ultrasonic units.

INFECTIONS

Do:

1. Take a careful medical history to identify patients who have pharyngitis, syphilis, tuberculosis, or hepatitis.
2. Require additional diagnostic testing on patients suspected as carriers of disease. For example:
   a. Hepatitis B—Test blood serum by radioimmunoassay, enzyme immunoassay and reverse passive hemagglutination.
   b. Syphilis—Venereal Disease Research Laboratory (VDRL) serologic test.
   c. Tuberculosis—bacteriologic testing.
3. Sterilize all instruments and equipment used intraorally. Sterilization can be performed by:
   a. Dry heat at 160°C for 60 minutes.
   b. Autoclaving using steam at 121°C and 15 psi for 30 minutes.
   c. Chemical vapor (alcohol-ketone-formaldehyde) at 127°C and 20 to 25 psi for 20 minutes.
   d. Ethylene oxide (10 percent in CO_2) at 55 to 69°C for 8 to 10 hours.

4. Use disinfection techniques when sterilization is not possible. Possible methods of disinfection are:
   a. Boiling water at 100°C for 30 minutes.
   b. Activated 2 percent glutaraldehyde for 10 minutes (10 hours if instruments have been used on a patient known to be infected with tuberculosis or another spore-forming microorganism).
   Instruments and equipment not damaged by aqueous solutions can be treated by:
   c. 1 percent solution of sodium hypochlorite (approximately 1:5 dilution of commercially available liquid chlorine bleach) for 10 minutes.
   d. 1 to 2 percent solution of formaldehyde for 20 to 30 minutes.
5. Clean surfaces contaminated with blood or saliva after each patient. Cleaning can be assisted by quaternary ammonium compounds, 90 percent isopropyl or 70 percent ethyl alcohol.
6. Wear masks and gloves when a risk of contamination, either by inhalation, ingestion, or transmission, exists: for example, when treating patients known to have an acute or chronic systemic infection or when working with dental personnel known to be carriers of chronic infections such as hepatitis B.
7. Wear protective eyeglasses in instances when aerosol and splatter are created.
8. Minimize talking, coughing, and sneezing.
9. Instruct patients to rinse with a mouthwash or water, or brush teeth prior to treatment.
10. Use a rubber dam.
11. Use a high velocity evacuation system with the aspirator tip placed adjacent to the work area.
12. Rinse the work area by alternating air and water spray rather than using the combined air-water spray.
13. Use rubber polishing points or prophylaxis cups rather than brushes for polishing.
14. Clean prosthetic devices prior to grinding or polishing.
15. Use shields and blower evacuation systems when polishing or grinding prosthetic appliances.

The following procedures are methods for reducing contamination that would require alteration of equipment or extra time by dental personnel. They may not be necessary in regular practice, but could be incorporated into a practice in which patients are known to be infectious.

16. Use disposable equipment and covers when possible. Areas of special consideration include the instrument tray, lamp handle, tray pull handle, radiographic equipment, and so forth. Disposable covers can reduce cleaning and disinfecting time between high risk patients.
17. Flush the waterlines of the dental unit and ultrasonic scalers for at least two minutes before and after use on patients. After long periods of inactivity, such as after weekends or holidays, longer flushing may be necessary.
18. At the beginning and end of each day of practice, flush the dental unit with a germicide, such as a 1:4 dilution of iodophor detergent for 5 minutes; a 2 percent activated alka-

line glutaraldehyde for 10 minutes; or 50 ppm chlorine solution (approximately 1:1,000 dilution of commercially available liquid chlorine bleach) for 10 minutes. This requires installation of a quick disconnect valve and may not be possible with all units.
19. Periodically check waterlines for contamination. This may be done by plating a 0.1 ml water sample on an agar blood plate and incubating it for 48 hours at 37°C. If more than ten colonies are formed, the waterlines should be flushed as previously described.
20. Replace dense waterline filters with fine wire screen filters.
21. Remove water retraction valves. This valve is located in series with the waterline and inside the dental unit.

Don't:

1. Use quaternary ammonium compounds as disinfectants.

ACID ETCH SOLUTIONS

Solutions used for acid etch techniques associated with placement of composites, sealants, and orthodontic brackets are mostly phosphoric acid solutions although other acids are sometimes used. Being acidic, the solutions should be handled with care.

Hazards:

1. Acid burns and possibly sloughing of tissue.
2. Eye damage.
3. Irritation of the respiratory system.

Sources:

1. Skin or tissue contact with acid etch solutions from:
   a. spills
   b. misapplication
   c. absorbent materials used in acid etch procedures
   d. residual films on outside surfaces of containers.
2. Inhalation of airborne droplets.

Safety Standards:

The maximum concentration of airborne droplets of phosphoric acid is 1 mg/m^3 of air, according to OSHA standards.

ACID ETCH SOLUTIONS

Do:

1. Avoid skin or soft tissue contact with acid etch solutions.
2. Handle acid soaked material with forceps or gloves.
3. Avoid eye contact with acid etch solutions and airborne acid droplets.
4. Have soda or a commercial acid spill cleanup kit available in case of spills.
5. In case of skin contact, rinse with a large amount of running water; seek medical help as necessary.
6. In case of eye contact, rinse with a large amount of water; seek medical help immediately.
7. Use high vacuum evacuators to minimize aerosol dispersion while rinsing after acid etching.

Don't:

1. Handle acid soaked absorbent material with unprotected hands.
2. Allow skin or soft tissues to contact acid etch solutions directly.
3. Use acid etch solutions without eye protection.

ASBESTOS

Asbestos is the generic term for a number of hydrated silicate minerals which, under crushing or other processing procedures, separate into flexible fibers. There are many such minerals, including chrysotile, asmosite, crocidolite, anthophyllite, tremolite, and actinolite; most asbestos is classified as chrysotile.

Asbestos has a number of dental applications. It is used as a lining material for casting rings and crucibles, in some soldering investments, in filters used to prepare drugs, and in the structural fabrication of dental offices such as insulation, counter tops and flooring tile. Primarily, it is used as a binder in periodontal dressings.

Hazards:
1. Airborne asbestos causes:
   a. pulmonary asbestosis and fibrosis
   b. lung cancer (recent epidemiologic studies have indicated a greater incidence of lung cancer in smokers exposed to airborne asbestos than in nonsmokers.)
   c. pleural and peritoneal mesotheliomas
2. Parenteral administration of asbestos in animals can result in:
   a. local malignancies
   b. malignant mesothelioma
   c. dissemination of fibers in lymph nodes, spleen, kidneys, and brain.

Sources:
1. Airborne fibers or dust particles released into the air during processing techniques: It is interesting to note that there appears to be no health danger of inhaling asbestos from periodontal dressings once they are mixed and applied.
2. Parenteral injection of drugs containing asbestos: A number of drug solutions are prepared using filters containing asbestos. Such filters may release asbestos particles into the solutions and thus may be injected into the patient.

Safety Standards:
Standards established by OSHA limit airborne fibers of asbestos to the following maximum concentrations.
1. 2 fibers (longer than 5 um)/cm^3 of air over an 8 hour, time weighted average.
2. 10 fibers/cm^3 at ceiling height.

NIOSH recommends the following maximum airborne concentrations of asbestos.
1. 0.1 fiber/cm^3
2. 0.5 fibers/cm^3 at ceiling height.

ASBESTOS

Do:
1. Store, handle, apply, remove, cut and otherwise work asbestos in a wet state to reduce the emission of airborne asbestos.
2. Use kaolin type material for casting ring lining.
3. Add traps to sewage lines to prevent the release of fibers to community sewage lines.
4. Avoid the use of asbestos-containing soldering investments.
5. Use periodontal dressings that do not contain asbestos.
6. Wear a face mask when handling any asbestos-containing material capable of generating an aerosol.

Don't:
1. Use asbestos-containing periodontal packs.
2. Sand or drill asbestos-containing counter tops.

BERYLLIUM

Hazards:
1. Contact dermatitis with eventual ulceration and inflammation
2. Corneal burns
3. Granulomatous formations leading to fibrous

replacement of the functioning tissues. This causes:

a. Respiratory tract—inflammation of the nasal mucosa and pharynx, tracheobronchial involvement, cough, chest pains and weakness, pulmonary dysfunction, pneumonitis (secondary effects of cyanosis and digital clubbing).

b. Circulatory system—secondary effects of right heart enlargement, congestive heart failure and enlargement of the liver and spleen.

c. Liver—changes in serum proteins and liver function.

d. Kidney—changes in uric acid and urinary calcium with appearance of kidney stones.

Sources:

Beryllium dust and fumes arise from the melting, grinding and milling of some base metal alloys.

Safety Standards:

The following are current NIOSH recommendations.

1. Maximum airborne concentrations of beryllium:
   a. 2μgm beryllium/m^3 time weighted average for 8 hour day.
   b. 25μgm beryllium/m^3 peak concentration based on 30 minute sample.
2. Medical history and physical exams are required prior to employment and annually thereafter. All records shall be retained and be accessible to HEW & DOL physicians and medical consultants and those physicians designated and authorized by employees.
3. Adequate local exhaust ventilation should be provided for all operations such as grinding, polishing and finishing where beryllium-containing alloys are handled and dusts and fumes may be generated.
4. Approved respirators must be used whenever local exhaust ventilation is not operating or until it can be installed in the laboratory.
5. Adequate general ventilation should be provided for casting areas. Although beryllium fumes normally are not generated during the casting of base-metal alloys, casting should not be performed in confined areas.
6. Precautionary labeling shall be applied to containers of beryllium or its compounds when exposure to dusts, fumes, powders or

---

BERYLLIUM

Do:

1. Follow Safety Standards.
2. Make certain that the manufacturers of beryllium-containing alloys alert the laboratory purchaser, by appropriate labels, of the beryllium content and need for appropriate handling safeguards.
3. Be aware of any laboratory warning of the presence of beryllium in the completed fixed or removable partial denture so that appropriate ventilation safeguards may be used if any adjustment of the casting is required.
4. When grinding a beryllium alloy at chairside, use a washed field technique and high velocity evacuation. Wear a face mask and gloves. Wash the appliance thoroughly with soap and water upon completion.
5. Use high velocity ventilation in close proximity to the high speed grinding operation in dental laboratories. Use high efficiency particulate filters (HEPA) to decontaminate exhaust ventilation air. Dispose of wastes in sealed bags.

Don't:

1. Grind or polish beryllium containing compounds intraorally.
2. Eat, drink or smoke in contaminated areas.

liquids appear likely.

7. Warning signs shall be placed in visible locations and on equipment when exposure to beryllium is likely.
8. Each week, clean protective clothing or its equivalent should be provided to each employee working with beryllium-containing alloys.
9. Dust removal from clothing and the cleaning of machinery should be accomplished by power suction methods and not by air hoses.
10. Every employee exposed should be apprised of the hazard and informed of the proper handling procedures for beryllium containing alloys.
11. Disposal of any wastes, storage of materials or contaminated clothing shall be carried out in sealed bags.
12. Food preparation and eating shall not be done in beryllium contaminated areas.
13. Locker and toilet facilities shall be separated from contaminated or potentially contaminated areas.
14. Periodic sampling of the breathing zone is required. A record of the results shall be retained.

HALOGEN CONTAINING ORGANIC LIQUIDS

The halogen containing organic liquids used in dental offices primarily include chloroform and carbon tetrachloride as well as some solvents and cleaners.

Hazards:

1. Contact dermatitis
2. Burns
3. Dizziness
4. Central nervous system depression
5. Nausea
6. Liver and kidney damage
7. Possible fire hazard (See "Liquids" under Fire Protection)
8. Poisonous decomposition products on heating

HALOGEN CONTAINING ORGANIC LIQUIDS

Do:

1. Work in well ventilated areas. Ventilation should have several exchanges of air per hour. The system should be vented to the outside if contaminant concentrations are high.
2. Use forceps or gloves to handle contaminated gauze or brushes.
3. Keep bottles tightly closed when not in use.
4. Store bottles on flat, sturdy surfaces.
5. Avoid inhalation of organic halogen vapors.
6. Keep liquids away from heat or open flames.
7. Educate office personnel on the handling and hazards of organic halogens.
8. Make certain that all office personnel have periodic medical examinations including tests on liver and kidney functions.

Don't:

1. Use halogen containing organic liquids in areas without adequate ventilation.
2. Directly contact materials containing organic halogen compounds.
3. Warm, heat, or burn organic halogen liquids.
4. Touch liquids with bare hands.
5. Eat, drink, or smoke in the vicinity of containers of organic halogen liquids.

Sources:

1. Skin contact during chlor percha obturation, rough polishing with chloroform, or using carbon tetrachloride as a wax solvent.
2. Inhalation of volatile vapors.

Safety Standards:

OSHA has set the following limits as maximum air concentrations of fumes from halogen containing organic liquids.

	ppm	mg/m³ air
Carbon tetrachloride	10	75
Chloroform	50	245
Methylene chloride	500	1740
1,1,1 Trichloroethylene	350	1900

MERCURY

Hazards:

1. Fine tremor observable in handwriting or other fine movements eventually progressing to convulsions
2. Loss of appetite
3. Nausea and diarrhea
4. Sensitivity to mercury
5. Depression, fatigue, increased irritability, moodiness
6. Birth defects in offspring
7. Pneumonitis
8. Nephritis
9. Nervous excitability
10. Insomnia
11. Headache
12. Swollen glands and tongue
13. Ulceration of oral mucosa
14. Dark pigmentation of marginal gingiva and loosening of teeth

Sources:

1. Direct contact or handling of mercury or mercury containing compounds.
2. Inhalation of vapors from mercury or mercury containing substances.
3. Exposure to contaminated office spaces caused by:
   a. Accidental spills
   b. Leaky or contaminated amalgamator capsules
   c. Wringing excess mercury from the amalgam mass
   d. Vaporization of mercury from contaminated instruments placed in sterilizers
   e. Amalgam condensation, especially with ultrasonic compactors
   f. Scrap amalgam improperly stored
   g. Organic mercurial disinfectants
   h. Milling old amalgam restorations
   i. Contaminated amalgamators

Safety Standards:

1. OSHA: 0.1 mg/m³ at the ceiling
2. NIOSH: 0.05 mg/m³ in the breathing zone for 8 hours per day, 40 hours per week.
3. American Association of Governmental and Industrial Hygienists: 0.15 mg/m³ for 15 minutes, limited to 4 hours of an 8 hour work day and at intervals of 60 minutes.

MERCURY

Do:

1. Alert all personnel involved in handling mercury to the potential hazards of mercury and mercury vapor and the necessity for observing good mercury hygiene practices.
2. Work in well ventilated spaces. Ventilation should include fresh air exchange and outside exhaust. Any filters placed in line, such as air conditioning filters, may act as mercury reservoirs and should be replaced periodically.
3. Periodically monitor the office for atmospheric mercury. The established threshold limit value is 0.05 mg/m³ based on a time weighted average. Personal monitoring is preferred to area monitoring, although the physical characteristics of most dental offices and work assignments may not lend themselves to personal monitoring.

a. Area monitoring conducted by a positive air flow absorber system or dosimeter system designed to minimize the effect of air currents with a sensitivity of $15\mu g/m^3$ is recommended. (Sources of such equipment have been gathered and are available upon request to the Council office.) Positive flow systems should use a flow rate of 1 liter per minute for one or more hours. The mercury exposure data should be reported as a time-weighted average for an eight hour period.

b. Contact the state health or labor departments concerning surveys of dental offices.

4. Perform urinalyses for mercury yearly on all dental office personnel. This should be performed on a 24-hour urine specimen or first morning urine voiding. The maximum allowable level according to OSHA is 0.15 mg mercury per liter. Generally, the normal level is 0.015 mg mercury per liter.

5. Store mercury in unbreakable, tightly sealed containers away from any source of heat.

6. Salvage all amalgam scrap and store under HgX solution in a tightly closed container.

7. Design and maintain work areas and equipment to limit the possibility of mercury contamination.

a. Flooring should be a continuous seamless sheet carried up the walls for at least 10 cm. Avoid carpeting dental operatories.

b. Areas of mercury use should be impervious and have lipped surfaces so as to confine and facilitate recovery of spilled mercury or excess amalgam.

c. Capsules should be tightly closed during amalgamation. Rubber "O" rings can be used as gaskets between the two sections.

d. Capsules should be checked periodically for leakage. One method involves wrapping black electrical tape around the capsule. After amalgamation, capsule leakage will appear as droplets of mercury on the adhesive. Care must be taken to avoid firmly attaching the tape to both sections of the capsule which might prevent the normal reaction of the capsule during trituration.

e. Amalgamator arms and capsule should be completely enclosed during trituration.

f. Amalgamators should be recalibrated periodically to assure proper speed.

g. Mercury dispensers should be cleaned periodically and orifices checked for residual mercury.

h. Mercury dispensers should be handled with care and checked periodically for leakage as some leak spontaneously.

8. Handle amalgam with extreme caution.

a. Use a no touch technique of handling amalgam. Use a low mercury: alloy ratio (preferably 1:1) to eliminate the necessity of squeezing the amalgam mass to express excess mercury. Wear nonporous gloves when handling mercury or amalgam and frequently clean skin exposed to mercury.

b. Reassemble amalgamator capsules, both reusable and disposable, immediately upon dispensing the amalgam mass. The used amalgam capsule is highly contaminated and is a significant source of mercury vapor if left opened.

c. Use water spray and high volume evacuation when removing old or finishing new dental amalgam restorations. The exhaust for such systems should be outside the office.

d. Use a face mask to avoid breathing amalgam dust.

9. Clean up any spilled mercury immediately by using one of the following techniques.

a. Narrow bore tubing connected (via a wash bottle trap) to a low volume aspirator of the dental unit.

b. Strips of adhesive tape to clean up small spills.

c. Sulfur powder dusting for droplets which cannot be reached. It must be remembered that this is only a film coating of the mercury and will be effective only while the mercury droplets remain undisturbed.

10. Place contaminated disposable materials in polyethylene bags and seal before disposal.

Don't:

1. Heat mercury or amalgam.
2. Use mercury containing solutions.
3. Use ultrasonic condensors.
4. Directly contact or handle mercury.
5. Carpet operatories.
6. Eat, drink, or smoke in the dental operatory.

NITROUS OXIDE

Nitrous oxide is reportedly being utilized by 35 percent of the dental profession. The dental profession considers this drug an essential part of the armamentarium for the control of pain and anxiety in dental patients.

Until recently, most reports linking nitrous oxide to adverse effects were studies using laboratory animals or studies in which nitrous oxide was used in conjunction with halogenated anesthetics. A recent mail survey study,[1] however, appears to demonstrate some correlation between adverse health effects and heavy use of nitrous oxide. The limitations of such data are realized, but the data does confirm an earlier preliminary study. Therefore, it would seem reasonable to attempt to achieve in the dental suite the lowest level of nitrous oxide possible.

These recommendations are not intended to curtail or limit the use of nitrous oxide. It is believed that nitrous oxide is important and an essential adjunct to the practice of modern dentistry.

Hazards:

1. Spontaneous abortion in female assistants and wives of dentists. (In the studies reported thus far, the sample did not include an adequate number of female dentists to enable a report of incidence.)
2. Congenital abnormalities, primarily musculoskeletal defects in offspring of females directly exposed.
3. Cancer of the cervix in females directly exposed.
4. Loss of functional capabilities, including audio-visual performance, dexterity and behavioral performance.
5. Liver disease.
6. Renal disease, primarily renal lithiasis in males and urogenital infections in females.
7. General and nonspecific neurologic disease, generally numbness, tingling, and muscle weakness.

Sources:

1. Leakage from anesthesia/analgesia machines caused by worn connectors; deformed fittings; loose fittings; loose, defective or missing gaskets and seals; worn or defective bags and breathing hoses; or improper design of system.
2. Leakage from scavenging devices.
3. Improper disposal of waste gases including improper location of waste gas exhaust caus-

ing the waste gas to reenter the dental suite by way of the window, adjacent operatory, air conditioning system, or high speed evacuation system.

4. Leakage around exhalation valve.
5. Leakage around nasal mask.
6. From patient's mouth.

Safety Standards:

The following are current NIOSH recommendations for nitrous oxide.

1. Occupational exposure to nitrous oxide, when used as the sole anesthetic agent, shall be controlled so that no worker is exposed to time-weighted average concentrations greater than 25 ppm during anesthetic administration. Available data indicate that with current controlled technology, exposure levels of 50 ppm and less for nitrous oxide are attainable for dental offices.

2. As soon as practicable after promulgation of a standard for occupational exposure to waste anesthetic gases, anesthetic delivery systems shall be equipped for scavenging.

3. Medical surveillance shall be made available to all employees subject to occupational exposure to waste anesthetic gases.

   Comprehensive preplacement medical and occupational histories shall be obtained and maintained in each employee's medical records, with special attention given to the outcome of pregnancies of the employee or spouse, and to hepatic, renal, and hematopoietic systems which may be affected by agents used as anesthetic gases. This information should be updated at least yearly and at any other time considered appropriate by the responsible physician.

   The preplacement and annual physical examination of employees exposed to anesthetic gases are recommended and, when performed, the results shall be maintained in the employee's permanent medical records.

   Employees shall be advised of potential undesirable effects of exposure to waste anesthetic gases such as spontaneous abortions, congenital anomalies in their children, and effects on the liver and kidneys.

Any abnormal outcome of the pregnancies of the employees or of the spouses of employees exposed to anesthetic gases shall be documented as part of the employee's medical records, and records shall be maintained for the period of employment plus 20 years. This medical information shall be available to the designated medical representatives of the Secretary of Health, Education, and Welfare, of the Secretary of Labor, of the employees or former employee, and of the employer.

4. Containers of gaseous and volatile anesthetic agents shall carry labels.

5. On assignment and at least annually thereafter, each worker shall be informed of the possible health effects of exposure to waste anesthetic gases. This information shall emphasize the potential risks to workers of reproductive age and to their unborn children. Each worker shall be instructed as to the availability of such information, which shall be kept on file and shall be accessible to the worker in each place of employment where a potential exposure to waste anesthetic gases exists.

6. A monitoring program shall be supervised by an eligible individual with sampling and monitoring techniques or by a professional industrial hygienist. The agent to be monitored and the method chosen will depend on the frequency of the agent's use, availability of sampling and analysis instrumentation, and on whether the facility chooses to initiate its own monitoring program or take advantage of commercial service.

7. Records of all collected air samples shall be maintained including date of sample, sampling methods, sampling location, analytical method, and measured concentrations. If waste anesthetic gas levels are found above the environmental limits prescribed, corrective actions shall be taken and recorded. Results of environmental measurements shall be made available to exposed employees on request. Air sampling results and results of leak tests shall be maintained for at least 20 years. Medical records shall be kept for the

duration of employment plus 20 years after an employee's termination of employment or termination of work of a self-employed person.

As of this writing, no action has been taken by OSHA with respect to acceptance and enforcement of NIOSH recommendations.

NITROUS OXIDE

Do:

1. Attempt to maintain less than 50 ppm nitrous oxide in the dental office.
2. Follow NIOSH recommended guidelines.
3. Monitor office for nitrous oxide at the time nitrous oxide equipment is installed and at four month intervals thereafter.
4. Institute a scavenging program. Select scavenging equipment that meets or exceeds the guidelines of the American Dental Association Council on Dental Materials, Instruments and Equipment. This will help ensure the effective and safe utilization of nitrous oxide sedation/anesthetic equipment. Each installation must be customized to meet the proposed standards and existing local and state codes.
5. Check nitrous oxide machine, lines, hoses and mask for leakage.
6. Maintain adequate ventilation. The maximum circulation and venting to the outside should be achieved with a minimum of recirculation. The particulars of the situation can be worked out with local air conditioning engineers. Well functioning air conditioning and heating units that provide fresh air dilution will aid in the dispersal of the gas from the operatory and decrease the trace concentrations about the dentist and dental assistants.
7. Check to make sure air ventilation systems are functioning properly.
8. Use high speed evacuation systems vented to the outside.
9. Minimize talking with the patient and, if possible, use a rubber dam.
10. Use an air sweep fan which blows across the patient and increases mixing of air with nitrous oxide adjacent to operators.
11. Modify the air conditioning system to be of the nonrecirculating type.
12. Exhaust waste gas away from windows, ventilators, air conditioning inlets, or other areas which might provide entrance back into the office. A roof exhaust, for example, might solve the problem.
13. Check the fit of the face mask.
14. Maintain and service equipment regularly.
15. Employ a method of nitrous oxide/oxygen administration which does not allow admixture of room air. Such a technique requires increased nitrous oxide concentrations and flow rates from the machine to reach the desired alveolar air concentration.

ORGANIC CHEMICALS

Organic chemicals used in dentistry include: alcohols, ketones, esters; aromatics such as benzene and toluene; ethers; most solvents and thinners; formaldehyde; ethylene oxide; and monomers such as methyl methacrylate and dimethacrylates.

Hazards:

1. Fire (See "Liquids" under Fire Protection)
2. Contact dermatitis
3. Sensitization
4. Irritation to mucous membranes
5. Headaches
6. Drowsiness
7. Respiratory problems
8. Unconsciousness
9. Possible mutagenesis

Sources:

1. Skin contact with chemicals such as cavity varnishes, composites, pit and fissure sealants, polyether impression materials, brush cleaners or denture base materials. Contact can be caused by spillage, contaminated clothing, or using bare hands.
2. Inhalation of volatile vapors such as methyl methacrylate from denture base liquids; sealants; ether from varnishes; and ethyl acetate from cleaners.
3. Inhalation of or contact with fumes from sterilizers.

Safety Standards:

OSHA has set the following limits as maximum air concentrations of organic chemicals.

	ppm	mg/m^3 air
Acetone	1000	2400
Benzene	10	32
Ethyl acetate	400	1400
Ethyl alcohol	1000	1900
Ethyl ether	400	1200
Ethylene oxide	50	90
Formaldehyde	3	8
Isopropyl alcohol	400	984
Methyl alcohol	200	260
Methyl ethyl ketone	200	590
Methyl methacrylate	100	410
Toluene	200	750

ORGANIC CHEMICALS

Do:

1. Work in well ventilated areas. Ventilation should include several exchanges of air per hour and be vented to the outside if contaminant concentrations are high.
2. Use forceps or gloves when handling contaminated gauze or brushes.
3. Keep bottles tightly closed when not in use.
4. Store bottles on flat sturdy surfaces.
5. Avoid inhalation of volatile vapors.
6. Educate office personnel on proper handling and hazards of organic chemicals.
7. Clean outside surfaces of containers after using to avoid residual drops from contacting the next user.
8. Obtain from the manufacturers or suppliers information on precautions and proper handling of the materials.
9. Be certain that all office personnel have periodic medical examinations including tests on respiratory, liver and kidney functions.
10. Contact the local environmental safety agency on methods of disposing of these materials.
11. Have a commercially available flammable solvent cleanup kit in case of spills.

Don't:

1. Use organic chemicals in areas without adequate ventilation.
2. Allow skin to contact materials containing organic liquids or monomers. Never touch materials with bare hands.
3. Leave containers of materials uncovered.
4. Use or place materials near an open flame.
5. Eat, drink or smoke in the vicinity of these materials.

PHOTOGRAPHIC CHEMICALS

Hazards:
1. Contact dermatitis
2. Irritation of eyes, nose, throat, and respiratory system from volatile vapors and fine particulates of chemicals.
3. Damage of radiographs due to contamination.

Sources:
1. Skin contact with photographic chemicals and solutions from:
   a. handling solutions and bottles
   b. spills
   c. processing
   d. preparing solutions
2. Inhalation of volatile vapors from:
   a. inadequate ventilation
   b. uncovered tanks
   c. spilled chemicals
   d. preparation of solutions
   e. warm temperature of solutions
3. Inhalation of fine particulates of dry photographic chemicals.

Safety Standards:
OSHA standards for maximum allowable concentrations of air contaminants include:

	ppm	mg/m^3 air
Acetic acid	10	25
Hydroquinone	—	2

PHOTOGRAPHIC CHEMICALS

Do:
1. Minimize agitation of dry powder during mixing of solution.
2. Avoid skin contact with photographic chemicals and solutions; wear rubber gloves if necessary.
3. Insure good general room ventilation, consisting of at least ten air exchanges per hour in the workroom. Venting to the outside is desirable if there are high levels of air contamination.
4. Use local exhausts for chemical solutions containing volatile components.
5. Clean up splashed or spilled chemicals immediately.
6. Wash off chemicals, if contacted, with large amounts of water and a pH balanced soap such as pHisoderm.
7. Regularly launder clothing which may come in contact with photographic solutions.
8. Store photographic solutions in tightly covered containers.
9. Store dry photographic chemicals in airtight containers.

Don't:
1. Allow skin to come in direct contact with photographic chemicals.
2. Use photographic chemicals in inadequately ventilated areas.
3. Use uncovered tanks for storage of photographic solutions.
4. Use uncovered containers for storage of dry photographic chemicals.
5. Eat, drink, or smoke in the photographic darkroom.

PICKLING SOLUTIONS

Pickling solutions are strongly acidic and contain metal ions after use. The components may be volatile.

Hazards:
1. Burning and charring of skin.

2. Irritation of skin and mucous membranes.
3. Irreparable damage to eyes.
4. Irritation to respiratory system.
5. Pulmonary irritation.

Sources:
1. Skin contact with acidic solution from:
   a. splattering of solution in use
   b. spilling of solution
   c. airborne droplets on agitation
2. Inhalation of volatile components or airborne droplets.

Safety Standards:
Standards established by OSHA limit airborne droplets of pickling solution components to the following maximum concentrations.

	ppm	mg/m^3 air
Hydrogen chloride	5	7
Sulfuric acid	0.3	1
Potassium dichromate (as chromic acid)	—	0.1

PICKLING SOLUTIONS

Do:
1. Wear safety goggles for eye protection when pickling.
2. Avoid splattering of solution; avoid putting hot objects into solution.
3. Insert object into solution slowly to avoid splashing.
4. Store solution containers on sturdy surfaces to prevent spilling.
5. Rinse the prosthesis after pickling.
6. Have available soda or a commercial acid spill cleanup kit in case of spills.
7. In case of skin contact, rinse with a large amount of running water; seek medical attention as necessary.
8. In case of eye contact, rinse with a large amount of running water; seek medical help immediately.
9. Use pickling solutions in well ventilated areas. Ventilation should include several exchanges of air per hour, vented to the outside if necessary.
10. Minimize the formation of airborne droplets. Avoid agitating the solution vigorously.
11. Educate office personnel in the handling and hazards of pickling solutions.
12. Make sure all office personnel have periodic medical evaluations including examinations of the eyes, skin and respiratory system.
13. Store pickling solutions in glass containers.
14. Contact local environmental safety agencies on methods of disposal of used pickling solutions.

Don't:
1. Use pickling solutions without adequate eye protection.
2. Use in areas without adequate ventilation.
3. Leave pickling solutions uncovered.
4. Store pickling solutions near table edges or on unsteady surfaces.
5. Hold the object for pickling with bare hands.
6. Pickle without the use of forceps.
7. Heat solutions prior to the addition of the casting.
8. Insert hot objects into pickling solutions.
9. Agitate solutions vigorously.

PLASTER AND OTHER GYPSUM PRODUCTS

Plaster, other gypsum products and investment powders are sources of fine airborne particulate matter. These fine dust particles are composed mainly of silica and calcium sulfate. Gypsum investments may release gaseous decomposition products (SO_2) during burnout processes.

Hazards:
1. Irritation and impairment of respiratory system
2. Silicosis
3. Irritation of eyes
4. Damage to eyes by flying airborne projectiles during trimming and cutting of models

Sources:
1. Agitation of dry powders on weighing and mixing
2. Cutting and trimming of models
3. Burnout of investments

Safety Standards:
Current OSHA standards include the following.
1. In units of million particles/ft^3, the maximum allowable concentration of silica (crystalline) can be calculated by either of the following formulas:

$$\frac{250}{\% \ SiO_2 + 5} \quad or \quad \frac{10 \ mg/m^3}{\% \ SiO_2 + 2} \quad \begin{array}{l} respirable \\ free \ SiO_2. \end{array}$$

2. The maximum allowable concentration of sulfur dioxide is 5 ppm or 13 mg/m^3 of air.

PLASTER AND OTHER GYPSUM PRODUCTS

Do:
1. Use plasters and other gypsum products in areas equipped with an exhaust system.
2. Use eye protection (goggles) while handling powders or trimming models.
3. Cut and trim models and investments only in areas equipped with an exhaust system.
4. Burnout investments only in areas with an exhaust system.
5. Minimize agitation of powder during handling.
6. Be certain that all office personnel have periodic medical examinations including an eye examination and tests of respiratory function.

Don't:
1. Use in areas without an exhaust system.
2. Burnout in unventilated areas.
3. Use these powders without eye protection.

Literature References

1. Cohen, E. N., et al. Occupational disease in dentistry and chronic exposure to trace anesthetic gases. JADA 101:21 July 1980.

Materials

AMALGAM AND MERCURY

DENTAL AMALGAM

Alloys for dental amalgam consist principally of silver and tin, with smaller amounts of copper, often zinc, and sometimes mercury or other metals which may alter substantially the physical properties of the material and require different manipulative techniques. When mixed in a manner so as to wet the surfaces of the alloy particles with mercury, a plastic mass is formed that can be condensed into a prepared cavity to form a dental restoration.

COMPOSITION AND PROPERTIES: Throughout the years, clinicians have selected dental amalgam alloys on the basis of one or more of the following factors: (1) particle size, (2) presence or absence of zinc, (3) particle shape, (4) alloy composition and (5) general manipulative characteristics. There has been a general trend towards smaller-sized particles; consequently, the coarser cut filings are no longer available. Reduction of particle size has provided certain advantages in handling characteristics. Neither the presence nor absence of zinc has been shown to be specifically advantageous in amal-gam restoration longevity. However, it is well documented that moisture contamination of zinc-containing alloys during their mixing or insertion results in an undesirable excessive delayed expansion and excessive corrosion of the amalgam.[1,2] On the other hand, it is known that moisture contamination even of a zinc-free alloy is injurious to certain physical properties and, therefore, dentists should not be led into a false sense of security by selecting a zinc-free alloy. Moisture contamination of any alloy should be avoided.

Prior to 1961, amalgam alloy particles had been limited to irregular shapes (Fig. 1) with rather rough surfaces having some microcracks due to the method of cutting the particles from a cast ingot. Since that time spherical (Fig. 2A) or spheroidal (Fig. 2B) particles, formed by atomizing the molten metal, have been available.[3] These spherical particles have smoother surfaces with no microcracks, and this together with the particle shape permits an acceptable plasticity with low mercury:alloy ratios.[4]

The innovation of spherical particles has allowed a significant departure[5] from established alloy formation (Table I). An increased amount of copper beyond the maximum formerly permitted by the American Dental Association Specification No. 1, when used in the spherical form of alloy, has been shown to effect a change in the phase composition. (Fig. 3). Merely increasing the copper content of lathe-cut alloys above the 6 percent level of the specification has damaging effects on the alloy. With the lathe-cut alloys, because of the size of the ingot, solidification is slow and copper reacts completely with the tin forming Cu_6Sn_5 in the original ingot. Therefore, no more copper is available to react with tin-mercury (γ_2) phase which will be formed during the amalgamation (Table II). With spherical alloys, however, solidification of the molten metal into individual spherical particles is much faster; copper and tin can only form Cu_3Sn. This compound of copper-tin, which is concentrated near the particle surface, is capable of reacting with more

tin of the tin-mercury phase (γ_2) to form Cu_6Sn_5 and eliminate the tin-mercury γ_2 phase which is the weakest and most corrosion prone phase of dental amalgam.[6,7] (Table II) Clinically, this phase change is reflected in reduced margin breakdown on crevicing.[8] Such alloys have been termed "dispersed phase," and may be mixtures of lathe-cut and spherical (Fig. 4) or may be totally spherical with a single composition.[9]

A property which is measurable in the laboratory has been shown to have a positive correlation with this improved margin integrity; alloys with lower "creep" values, along with higher compressive strength, result in less margin breakdown.[8] Lower creep values are generally associated with the higher copper content in the spherical particles.

General manipulative characteristics are influenced by a number of factors already cited

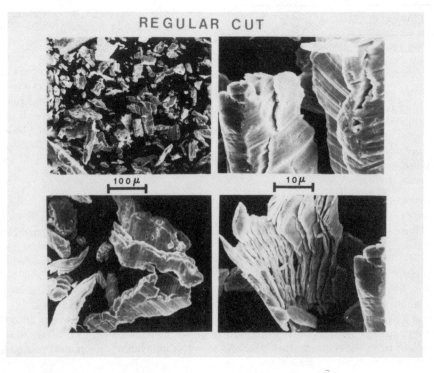

REGULAR CUT

100μ   10μ

Fig. 1   Amalgam alloy particles irregular in shape with some microcracks.

including particle size, shape, and alloy formulation as well as the heat treatment or "annealling" given the alloy, the mercury-alloy ratio and the amount of trituration.

Thus, the dentist can choose among three forms of dental amalgam alloy: (1) the conventional lathe-cut, (2) the conventional spherical, and (3) the high copper content or dispersed phase admixture of lathe-cut and spherical or dispersed phase single composition.

Uses: Dental amalgam is used in all Classes of restorations, I through V, with very limited use for Classes III and IV, in both the primary and permanent dentitions. It is also used to build a core, usually in conjunction with some form of pin retention, upon which preparation for a gold casting is made. In endodontics, amalgam is used as a retrograde filling material for the apical end of a treated tooth.

Directions for Use: The mercury-alloy ratio is important in that these materials constitute the reactants of amalgam and the ratio influences the ease of trituration or wetting of the alloy particles with mercury as well as the plasticity of the amalgam mass. A ratio which is considered by the manufacturer to be optimum is expressed as a simple alloy/mercury proportion where the alloy is given as one, thus 1/1 or

Table I.

Particle Shape and Composition of Some Current Dental Amalgam Alloys

	Silver	Tin	Copper	Zinc
†DISPERSALLOY				
Spherical Particle	72	—	28	—
Irregular Particle	68-69	27-28	2-4	0-1
†PHASEALLOY				
Spherical Particle	70	0.2-0.3	28-29	—
Irregular Particle	68-69	27-28	2-4	0-1
††TYTIN				
Spherical Particle	60	27	13	—
††ARISTALOY C R				
Irregular Shaped				
Spheroids	60	27	13	—
††SYBRALOY				
Spherical Particle	40	30	30	—
†OPTALOY II				
Spherical Particle	67	25.5	7.5	—
Irregular Particle	76	22.75	1.25	—
†MICRO II				
Spherical Particle	65	26	9	—
Irregular Particle	72	26.75	1.25	—
†††CONVENTIONAL ALLOYS	68-72	26-28	2-4	0-2

†Admix type. Spherical particle of Ag-Cu mixed with lathe-cut of Ag-Sn.
††All particles have the same composition with high copper.
†††All particles have the same composition with low copper.

1/1.2, and so forth.

A mechanical method for triturating the prescribed ratio is fully specified by the alloy manufacturer and should be followed. Condensation whether by hand or mechanical means should be carried out without delay. Condensation of remaining increments should not be attempted whenever coherence of these to the already condensed mass becomes at all difficult to attain. This stage should be anticipated and a new incremental mass of amalgam mixed. The rate of hardening varies greatly among alloys complying with the specification. Comments are made by dentists that some alloys produce amalgam that has prolonged hardening times and others provide insufficient time to adequately condense or carve. At present, no carving test appears to give reliable quantitative data. A cohesiveness test has been shown to provide a basis for judgment of the setting characteristics of various dental amalgams. Alloys that have characteristics described by the manufacturer as "regular set," "fast set" and/or "slow set" are becoming available. The convenience and ultimate possibility for the dentist to gain intimate adaptation of the dental amalgam to the walls and margins of the prepared cavity are to some degree controlled by these setting characteristics.

LIMITATIONS OF USE: Dental amalgam withstands higher compressive forces than tensile forces.

Table II.
Some Phases in Dental Amalgam

Alloy	Amalgam		
CONVENTIONAL	Residual alloy particles (silver-tin)	Ag_3Sn	(Gamma)
(Based on	Reaction product (silver-mercury)	Ag_2Hg_3	(Gamma 1)
silver-tin)	Reaction product (tin-mercury)	$Sn_{7-8}Hg$	(Gamma 2)
Ag_3-Sn	Copper-Tin	Cu_3Sn	(Delta)
HIGH COPPER CONTENT*	Residual alloy particles (silver-tin)	Ag_3Sn	(Gamma)
Admixture of Conventional	Reaction product (silver-mercury)	Ag_2Hg_3	(Gamma 1)
and Silver-Copper	Residual alloy particles (silver-copper)	Eutectic	
Alloy Eutectic		composition	
(or near eutectic		or near	
composition)			
	Copper-Tin	Cu_6Sn_5	(Epsilon)
Unicomposition	Residual particles (silver-tin-copper)		
(Silver-Tin-Copper)	Reaction product (silver-mercury)	Ag_2Hg_3	(Gamma 1)
	Copper-Tin	Cu_3Sn	(Delta)
	Copper-Tin	Cu_6Sn_5	(Epsilon)

*Note: No Gamma 2 is formed in either alloy with high copper content unless excess residual mercury is present.

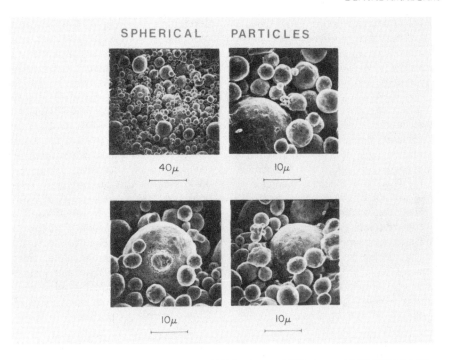

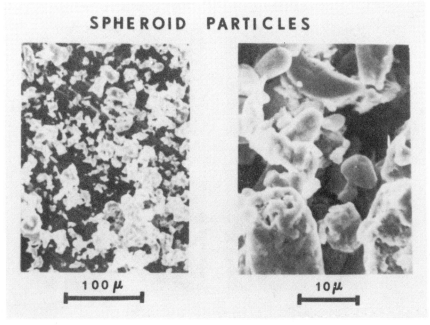

Fig. 2 (A) Spherical alloy particles with no microcracks.   (B) Spheroid alloy particles irregular in shape with no microcracks but with projections on surface.

Thus, the use of amalgam in thin cross-sections where it will be subject to bending should be avoided. A bulk of amalgam is required for strength. When such bulk in the restoration cannot be attained, a gold casting may be indicated.

EVALUATION PROGRAM: The original American Dental Association Specification No. 1 for Alloy for Dental Amalgam was the outgrowth of a cooperative research program with the National Bureau of Standards. Since its inception in 1930, three revisions have been made. These changes reflect the continual improvement in physical properties and, of particular recent interest, the clinically meaningful characteristic of creep.[8]

The alloys for dental amalgam covered by the specification are composed essentially of silver and tin and may be in a powder or tablet form, either for bulk dispensing or in sealed capsules containing pre-weighed portions of alloy and mercury. Although copper, zinc, gold and/or mercury may be present in amounts less than the silver and tin content, other elements may be included provided the manufacturer submits the composition of the alloy and the results from adequate clinical and biological investigations to show its safety when used in the mouth.

An alloy used in making the amalgam that contains zinc in excess of 0.01 percent is designated as "zinc-containing." Printed instructions must include the precautionary statement in bold type, "The alloy contains zinc and the amalgam made therefrom will show excessive corrosion and expansion if moisture is introduced during mixing and condensing."

When mixed according to the manufacturer's suggested optimum ratio and instructions for mechanical trituration the alloy and mercury should form a smooth plastic amalgam mass. These instructions should include: (1) the

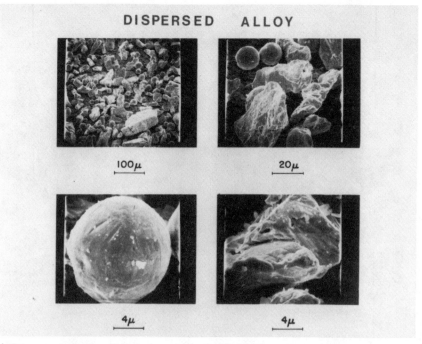

DISPERSED   ALLOY

100μ   20μ

4μ   4μ

Fig. 3 Admixture type of alloy. Spherical particles are silver-copper eutectic; the irregular shaped type is basically a silver-tin alloy.

model of mechanical amalgamator and speed in cycles per second, (2) size, weight and type of capsule and pestle, and (3) times required for mixing the various amounts of alloy specified. All three factors affect the trituration.

Reproducibility of the alloy tablet mass or weight should not vary by more than 1.5 percent of that stated by the manufacturer. This same percentage variation or tolerance is also specified for the pre-proportioned capsules of alloy and mercury.

Physical tests in the specification include inspection for foreign material, compressive strength, and dimensional change during hardening in addition to the test for creep previously described. The presence of foreign matter from packaging machines or other sources can affect the success of a restoration and is to be avoided. A compressive strength determination at one hour indicates not only that a setting reaction does take place to produce in time a mass cap-

able of withstanding certain oral functions, but also the *rate* of that reaction. Dimensional changes that occur during hardening are of importance from the standpoint of assuring appropriate interfaces of tooth and restoration, and as an indicator of the stresses involved at those areas. A slightly expanding *or* contracting amalgam ($\pm$ 20 um/cm) appears to be acceptable for clinical use.

AVAILABLE PRODUCTS

Argentum Hi-Copper Spherical Blend; Micro Fine Cut; Micro Non-Zinc; Hammond Dental Mfg. Co.

ARISTALOY, Baker Dental Dept. of Engelhard Industries, Engelhard Minerals & Chemicals Corp.

ARISTALOY CR, Baker Dental Dept. of Engelhard Industries, Engelhard Minerals & Chemicals Corp.

ARISTALOY MS, Baker Dental Dept. of Engel-

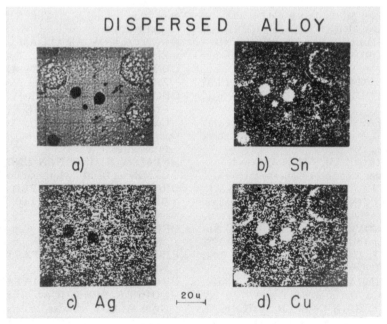

Fig. 4 Electron probe analysis of dispersed type alloy. (a) The areas analyzed, (b) x-ray map of tin, (c) x-ray map of silver, (d) x-ray map of copper. White areas indicate presence of the element analyzed. Parts (b) and (d) show that tin is compounded with copper.

hard Industries, Engelhard Minerals & Chemicals Corp.

ARISTOCRAT ALLOY, Healthco, Inc.

Aristocrat Corrosion Resistant, Healthco, Inc.

ARISTOCRAT CR NON-ZINC; Powder, Pellets, Healthco, Inc.

BLUE RIBBON MICRO CUT; 68%; Rugby Laboratories, Inc.

CAULK FINE CUT; FINE CUT NON-ZINC, L. D. Caulk Co., Div. of Dentsply International, Inc.

Caulk Micro Alloy Micro II Alloy, L. D. Caulk Co., Div. of Dentsply International, Inc.

CAULK SPHERICAL ALLOY, L. D. Caulk Co., Div. of Dentsply International, Inc.

CRESILVER, Crescent Dental Mfg. Co.

CUPRALLOY, ZINC, Pellets, Star Dental Mfg. Co., Inc.

DISPERSALLOY, ZINC, Johnson & Johnson Dental Products Co.

EASE ALLOY, L. D. Caulk Co., Div. of Dentsply International, Inc.

FELLOWSHIP, Moyco Industries, Inc.

H & M SPECIAL, Hauser & Miller

HAMMOND'S ARGENTUM SPHERICAL BLEND HIGH COPPER AMALGAM ALLOY, Powder, Pellets, Hammond Dental

HAMMOND ARGENTUM SPHERICAL BLEND FILLING ALLOY; MICRO NON-ZINC; MICRO FINE CUT, Hammond Dental Mfg. Co.

IMPROVED 72% FINE CUT; MICRO CUT; 72% FINE CUT (NON–ZINC), Henry Schein, Inc.

INDILOY FAST SET AMALGAM ALLOY, NON ZINC; Powder, Tablets, Capsules, Shofu Dental Corp.

INDILOY REGULAR SET AMALGAM ALLOY, Powder, Capsules, Shofu Dental Corp.

INDILOY REGULAR SET AMALGAM ALLOY, NON-ZINC Powder, Tablets, Capsules, Shofu Dental Corp.

KENT IMPROVED FINE CUT FILLING ALLOY 72%; IMPROVED NON-ZINC 72% FINE CUT; IMPROVED FINE CUT 68%; MICRO CUT, Stratford-Cookson Co.

KERR SPHERALOY, ZINC; ZINC FREE, Kerr Mfg. Co., Div. of Syborn Corp.

LEE ALLOY, HIGH COPPER SPHERICAL BLEND AMALGAM WITH ZINC, Powder, Pellets, Capsules, Lee Pharmaceuticals

LINC ALLOY, FINE GRAINED, Lincoln Dental Supply Co.

LUSTRALOY, REGULAR; MICRO FINE; EXTRA FINE, Pfingst & Co., Inc.

MICRO II ZINC; NON-ZINC, L. D. Caulk Co., Div. of Dentsply International, Inc.

MINIMAX 178; 178 NON-ZINC; 178 FINE CUT; WHITE GOLD AND PLATINUM, Minimax Co.

Minimax Alloy #178 Pellets (6 grain), Minimax Co.

MOSER MDM AMALGAMATABLE HIGH COPPER SPHERICAL BLEND AMALGAM ALLOY WITH ZINC, Powder, Pellets, Moser Dental Co.

MOSER MDM AMALGAMATABLE HIGH COPPER SPHERICAL BLEND Disposable Capsules, Powder, Pellets, Moser Dental Mfg. Co.

MOSER MDM REGULAR CUT; MICRO CUT SILVER ALLOY; FINE CUT; FINE CUT NON-ZINC; SPECIAL FOR McSHIRLEY & DENTOMAT; MICRO CUT BIMODAL; MICRO CUT BIMODAL NON-ZINC; SPHERICAL: SPHERICAL BLEND, Moser Dental Mfg. Co.

NEW TRUE DENTALLOY, S. S. White Div., Pennwalt Corp.

New True Dentalloy, No Zinc, S. S. White Div., Pennwalt Corp.

ODONTALLOY AMALGAM ALLOY, NO-ZINC, Powder, Pellets, Imex Trading Co.

ODONTALLOY AMALGAM ALLOY, WITH ZINC, Powder, Pellets, Imex Trading Co.

ODONTOGRAPHIC "IMPROVED"; EXTRA FINE CUT; MICRO FINE CUT, Pfingst & Co., Inc.

Optaloy Alloy, L. D. Caulk Co., Div. of Dentsply International, Inc.

OPTALOY II ZINC; NON-ZINC, L. D. Caulk Co., Div. of Dentsply International, Inc.

OROSPHERE HIGH COPPER SPHERICAL BLEND AMALGAM ALLOY, Powder, Pellets, Pentron Corp.

OROSPHERE, NO ZINC, Capsules, Pentron Corp.

PHASEALLOY ZINC, FAST SETTING, Phasealloy, Inc.

PROALLOY AMALGAMATABLE HIGH COPPER SPHERICAL BLEND AMALGAM ALLOY, Powder, Pellets, Professional Products

PROALLOY FINE CUT; FINE CUT NON-ZINC; SUPERFINE; SUPERFINE NON-ZINC; SPHERICAL BLEND; SPECIAL

FOR McSHIRLEY & DENTOMAT, Professional Products Co.

ROYAL ALLOY; ROYAL SUPER FAST SETTING, Jelinek Alloy Div., Sterndent Corp.

SAFCO AMALGAMATABLE HIGH COPPER SPHERICAL BLEND ALLOY; Powder, Pellets, Safco Dental Supply Co.

SAFCO SILVER ALLOY, Safco Dental Supply Co.

SAFCO 69 FINE CUT; NON-ZINC FINE CUT; REGULAR CUT ZINC; SPHERICAL ALLOY NON-ZINC, Safco Dental Supply Co.

S-C REGULAR MEDIUM; SPECIAL MEDIUM, Stratford-Cookson Co.

70% SILVER FILLING ALLOY, Pure Lab Co. of America

SHOFU SPHERICAL ALLOY; NON-ZINC, Shofu Dental Corp.

SILVER CREST ALLOY ZINC; PREMIUM ALLOY ZINC; NON-ZINC, Colwell Co.

SILVER CROWN FINE CUT NO. 2; FINE CUT NON-ZINC; MEDIUM; NON-ZINC; NO. 5 FINE CUT; NO. 6 NON-ZINC FINE CUT; SUPER-FINE ALLOY 8; SUPER-FINE NON-ZINC 9; SUPREME ALLOY NO. 10; NO. 11 NON-ZINC; SPHERICAL ALLOY NO. 12; No. 13 NON-ZINC, General Refineries, Inc.

SILVERLOY F.C. NO. 20 FOR PROPORTIONER, Crescent Dental Mfg. Co.

SILVERMAN'S EX-CEL, Silverman's

SPEYER, Speyer Smelting & Refining Co.

STANDALLOY AG 68% NON-ZINC, Williams Gold Refining Co., Inc.

SUPERDENT DISPERSED PHASE ALLOY, NO-ZINC, Powder, Pellets, Darby Dental Supply Co.

SUPERDENT DISPERSED PHASE ALLOY, WITH ZINC, Powder, Pellets, Darby Dental Supply Co.

SUTERLOY AMALGAMATABLE HIGH COPPER, SPHERICAL BLEND AMALGAM ALLOY, Powder, Pellets, Disposable Capsules, Chico Dental Specialties

SUTERALOY MICRO CUT ZINC; NON-ZINC; FINE CUT ZINC; NON-ZINC; SPHERICAL BLEND; SPECIAL FOR McSHIRLEY AND DENTOMAT, Chico Dental Specialties

SYBRALOY, Kerr Mfg. Co., Div. of Sybron Corp.

TERNALLOY AMALGAM ALLOY, NON-ZINC, Powder, Pellets, Darby Dental

TRUE DENTALLOY, ZINC FREE, S. S. White

Div., Pennwalt Corp.

Twentieth Century, L. D. Caulk Co., Div. of Dentsply International, Inc.

TYTIN, S. S. White Div., Pennwalt Corp.

UNITEK DISPERSED PHASE ALLOY, Powder, Pellets, Disposable Capsules, Unitek Corp.

UNITEK DISPERSED PHASE ALLOY WITH ZINC, Powder, Pellets, Disposable Capsules, Unitek Corp.

UNITEK HI-COPPER SPHERICAL BLEND ALLOY, Powder, Pellets, Disposable Capsules, Unitek Corp.

UNITEK HI-COPPER SPHERICAL BLEND ALLOY WITH ZINC, Powder, Pellets, Disposable Capsules, Unitek Corp.

UNITEK MICRO-CUT SILVER ALLOY, Powder, Pellets, Disposable Capsules, Unitek Corp.

UNITEK MICRO-CUT SILVER ALLOY WITH ZINC, Powder, Pellets, Disposable Capsules, Unitek Corp.

VELVALLOY; NON-ZINC, S. S. White Div., Pennwalt Corp.

WHITE BEAUTY FINE CUT; REGULAR, Lang Dental Mfg. Co., Inc.

DENTAL MERCURY

Mercury emits small amounts of vapor under normal atmospheric conditions, but this vaporization stops as soon as the mercury reacts with an amalgam alloy, forming mercury compounds. The toxic effect of mercury vapor in dental practice has been a subject of investigation for a number of years and has not been shown to be significant when good mercury hygiene, described in Chapter 1, Safety in the Dental Office, is observed.[10-14]

EVALUATION PROGRAM: Although many terms are used in an attempt to designate the quality of mercury, the only standards that are defined are U.S.P., A.C.S., and the American Dental Association Specification No. 6 for Dental Mercury. A mercury designated U.S.P. must conform to the specification given in the *United States Pharmacopeia*. Mercury conforming to either of these standards is suitable for mixing with a dental amalgam alloy.

The term "chemically pure," whether used in connection with mercury or other chemicals, is

DENTAL AMALGAM AND DENTAL MERCURY

Do:

1. Compress adequately.
2. Select alloys with low "creep" values.
3. Use the alloy:mercury ratio suggested by the manufacturer.
4. Use the proper capsule and pestle and mixing time for the mechanical amalgamator suggested for triturating a given alloy.
5. Familiarize yourself with clinical characteristics of the alloy selected.
6. Anticipate the need for using multiple mixes for large or complex restorations.
7. Use a clean mercury having a shiny, mirror-like surface.
8. Exercise all of the necessary precautions to minimize mercury hazards.
9. Use sufficient trituration for "dispersed phase" alloys by selecting appropriate amalgamation procedures.

Don't:

1. Be misled into believing that moisture contamination of a zinc-free alloy will *not* result in an inferior amalgam.
2. Substitute capsule-pestle combinations designated for a "slow-speed" amalgamator in "high-speed" units, or vice versa.
3. Use alloys or mixing procedures requiring high quantities of mercury for trituration and the subsequent need for removing excess mercury with a "squeeze cloth" or other means.
4. Use dental amalgam in thin cross sections.

not defined by legal or by generally accepted standards. Such terms as "distilled," "double-distilled," "triple-distilled," and "redistilled" are without meaning in reference to purity because the degree of purification obtained by distillation varies with the raw materials and the methods of distillation.

The purity of dental mercury in the American Dental Association Specification is defined by the surface appearance, the residue after pouring and the nonvolatile residues. The tests for surface appearance and pouring residue can determine the presence of 0.001 percent or more of base metal impurities. The addition of 0.001 percent of copper, zinc, tin, lead, bismuth, cadmium, arsenic or antimony causes an immediate change in the appearance of the surface of mercury. The mercury loses the mirror-like appearance and a film or "skin" forms on the surface. The contaminated mercury wets the glass container and the container cannot be completely emptied. The effect is very pronounced and can be detected in each case. However, the addition of 0.001 percent of silver or gold does not cause a change in the appearance of mercury.

This simple test can be used as a limiting test for all base metal impurities and any dentist can determine whether mercury contains minute amounts of base metals by a glance at the surface. If the mercury has a mirror-like surface, it is pure enough for use in dental amalgams. Repeated exposure to air may cause surface dulling. If the surface is dull and appears to be covered with a film, the mercury should be filtered through chamois skin or clean cloth.

Available Products

AMALCAP, H.D. Justi Co., Div. of Williams Gold Refining Co., Inc.

AMC DENTAL MERCURY, Associated Mercury Products

AMERICAN MERCURY, Pure Lab Co. of America

ARGENTUM, Hammond Dental Mfg. Co.

BALLARD's, Quicksilver Products, Inc.

BELMONT DENTAL MERCURY, Belmont Smelting & Refining Works, Inc.

BETHLEHEM INSTRUMENT MERCURY, Bethlehem Apparatus Co., Inc.

Centra Chemically Pure Triple Distilled Quality Mercury, Doric Corp.

CHEMICALLY PURE, Stratford-Cookson Co.

CROWN, General Refineries, Inc.

DENTAL MERCURY, Mercury Distributors, Inc.

DFG DENTAL MERCURY, D.F. Goldsmith Chemicals & Metals Corp.

HDS MERCURY, Highlander Dental Supply

HEALTHCO DENTAL MERCURY, Healthco, Inc.

MERCURY PURIFIED REDISTILLED CODE 1280, Mallinckrodt Chemical Works

MOSER MDM, Moser Dental Mfg. Co.

MOWREY MERCURY, W.E. Mowrey Co.

MOYCO, Moyco Industries, Inc.

ODONTOGRAPHIC, Pfingst & Co., Inc.

PRO MERCURY, Professional Products Co.

SAFCO MERCURY, Safco Dental Supply Co.

SCHEIN MERCURY TRIPLE DISTILLED, Henry Schein, Inc.

SHOFU MERCURY, Shofu Dental Corp.

SPECTROPURE, Baker Dental Dept. of Engelhard Industries, Engelhard Minerals & Chemicals Corp.

SPEYER, Speyer Smelting & Refining Co.

STAR TRIPLE DISTILLED MERCURY, Star Dental Mfg. Co., Inc.

TRIPLE DISTILLED MERCURY, Eastern Smelting & Refining Corp.

TRIPLE DISTILLED MERCURY CP, Oceanic Chemical Co., Inc.

TWENTIETH CENTURY, L.D. Caulk Co., Div. of Dentsply International, Inc.

VERATEX MERCURY, Veratex Corp.

LITERATURE REFERENCES

1. Schoonover, I. C.; Souder, W.; and Beall, J. R. Excessive expansion of dental amalgam. JADA 29:1825 Oct. 1942.

2. Van Gunst, I. C. S., and Hertog, H. J. P. M. On the relation between delayed expansion of amalgam and the composition of amalgam alloys. Br. Dent. J. 103:428 Dec. 1957.

3. Demaree, N. C., and Taylor, D. F. Properties of dental amalgams made from spherical alloy particles. J. Dent. Res. 41:890 July-Aug.1962.

4. Eden, G. T., and Waterstrat, R.M. Effects of packing pressures on the properties of spherical alloy amalgams. JADA 74:1024 Apr. 1967.

5. Innes, D. B. K., and Youdelis, W. V. Dispersion strengthened amalgams. J. Can. Dent. Assoc. 29:587 Sept. 1963.

6. Asgar, K., and Sutfin, L. Brittle fracture of dental amalgam. J. Dent. Res. 44:977 Sept.-Oct. 1965.

7. Guthrow, C. E., Jr.; Johnson, L. B., Jr.; and Lawless, K. R. Electrochemical studies of the corrosion of dental amalgams. IADR Program and Abstracts of Papers. Abstract 280, p. 108, 1965.

8. Mahler, D. B., et al. Marginal fractures vs. mechanical properties of amalgam. J. Dent. Res. 49:1452 Dec.1970.

9. Asgar, K. Amalgam alloy with a single composition behavior similar to Dispersalloy. J. Dent. Res. 53 (Special Issue):60, 1974.

10. Lippman, D. S. Mercurial poisoning and sensitivity from copper and silver amalgam fillings. Dent. Abs.7:465 Aug. 1962.

11. Engelman, M.A. Mercury allergy resulting from amalgam restorations. JADA 66:122 Jan. 1963.

12. Souder, W., and Sweeney, W. T. Is mercury poisonous in dental amalgam restorations? Dent. Cosmos 74:1145 Dec. 1931.

13. Meyer, A. Mercury poisoning: a potential hazard to dental personnel. Dent. Prog. 2:190 Apr. 1962.

14. Airaksinen, S. Risk of exposure of dental staff to mercurial poisoning. Dent. Abs. 6:620 Oct. 1961.

RESTORATIVE RESINS

One of the newest and most rapidly changing classes of dental materials is the restorative resins. Introduced at the close of World War II and challenged by research and clinical trial, these materials have become the most commonly used tooth colored materials. Included in the class are the unfilled resins, the composite or filled resins, and pit and fissure sealants.

The unfilled resins were the forerunners of composite resins.[1,2] Shortcomings of the unfilled resins, notably low hardness, thermal dimensional changes, and poor abrasion resistance, prompted the development of epoxy and, more recently, composite resins. The main difference between the unfilled and composite resins is the presence of a high percentage of inorganic filler material in the structure of composite restorations. The addition of filler particles to resins results in a lower coefficient of thermal expansion, reduced polymerization shrinkage, higher compressive and tensile strengths, greater stiffness, lower water sorption, and increased resistance to abrasion. The composite products currently being marketed are very similar to the experimental materials developed by R. L. Bowen of the American

Dental Association Research Division at the National Bureau of Standards.[1-3]

UNFILLED TOOTH RESTORATIVE RESINS

Esthetic qualities and low solubility were the major attractions of unfilled resins, which were introduced in the late 1940's. Initially there were heat cured materials that were cemented as inlays and slab mixed resins that were used with doughy consistencies. The polymerization and low stiffness resulted in a high failure rate, the result being poor adaption of the restoration and recurrent caries. An early clinical study reported, at the end of three years, over 10 percent of the 289 resin restorations had recurrent caries while no decay was associated with the 115 silicate restorations that were used as controls.[4]

COMPOSITION AND PROPERTIES: The unfilled resins consist of a powder and a liquid. The principal component of the powder is poly

Table I.
Some Physical Properties of Unfilled and Composite Tooth Restorative Resins*

Material	Compressive Strength MN/m² (PSI)	Tensile Strength MN/m² (PSI)	Modulus of Elasticity MN/m² (PSI × 10⁶)	Volumetric Shrinkage on Hardening %	Coefficient of Thermal Expansion in/in/°C
Poly (methyl methacrylate)	71.7 (10,400)	22.8 (3,300)	2,340 (0.34)	5.2	92
Typical composite	223 (32,400)	37.9 (5,500)	13,600 (1.97)	1.2	31
Range of composites	200-241 (29,000-35,000)	34.5-47.6 (5,000-6,000)	11,700-16,500 (1.7-2.4)	1.2-2.1	27-39

*Data from Dennison and Craig[16]

(methyl methacrylate) in the form of beads or grindings.[5] The powder also contains the initiator, benzoyl peroxide (0.3 to 3.1 percent). The polymer beads are assorted by size to enhance mixing. The colors are produced by combining beads containing metallic oxides with clear beads. The numbers of colors are unlimited and produce an excellent initial result.

The liquid is the monomer with the main composition being methyl methacrylate. Some liquids contain cross-linking agents such as ethylene dimethacrylate in the amount of 5 percent or more and a small amount of inhibitor (e.g. the monomethyl ether of hydroquinone) 0.006 percent.

In 1952, fluid exchange at the margins of the resin restorations was reported to be associated with recurrent caries around the restoration.[6] Marginal percolation is caused by the difference in thermal coefficients of expansion between the unfilled resin and the tooth. Unfilled resins were found to have a coefficient of expansion as high as 127 ppm per degree Celsius when the specimens were made without pressure and tested in salt water.[7]

The temperature changes cause spaces to develop at the interface of the poorly adapted restoration. The poor adaption and resultant leakage are associated with marginal, deep dark stains around the resin restoration. This problem of discoloration led to the use of products catalyzed with p-toluene sulfinic acid or other derivatives of sulfinic acid. Color change initi-

ally occurred with these products because benzoyl peroxide (tertiary amine system) was used to react to form free radicals and to initiate the polymerization.

Uses: The unfilled resins are limited to small cavities not subjected to stress, particularly Class III and Class V problems. They are used also to cover small enamel defects or white spots on the labial surfaces of incisor teeth.

Directions for Use: The unfilled resins can only be inserted with minimal pressure because of the low viscosity of the mix.[8,9] There are two methods for inserting unfilled resins.

(1) In the flow technique, a standard mix of unfilled resin is made and flowed into the cavity form with a brush. The resin is retained until the polymerization is completed.

(2) The bead technique involves adding the resin, in increments, to the cavity form, waiting between applications until the polymerization is completed and the resin is hardened. Three to four portions are needed for the larger cervical restorations; excessive material is used to offset the 6 to 8 percent volume of contraction during polymerization.[10]

Laboratory and in vivo studies with temperature cycling have documented that the unfilled resins, with proper technique, can develop and maintain acceptable adaptation to tooth structure.[11] With acid etching and the described insertion methods, the microleakage is minimal and comparable to other restorative materials.

UNFILLED TOOTH RESTORATIVE RESINS

Do:

1. Only place the mix in an extremely dry and clean cavity preparation.
2. Use an unfilled resin with a short polymerization cycle (5 to 6 minutes from start of mix).
3. Secure the matrix with little pressure.
4. Place an excess of material for finishing.
5. Use in a conservative, retentive cavity form that has acid etched enamel.
6. Finish the resin with conventional burs, discs, strips and pumice.

Don't:

1. Move the matrix during polymerization.

COMPOSITE RESTORATIVE MATERIALS

COMPOSITION AND PROPERTIES: Dental composite restorative materials consist of an organic polymeric matrix, commonly the BIS-GMA resin system,[5,12] reinforced with a fine dispersion of an inorganic filler such as quartz, glass, or lithium-aluminum silicate.[13] The filler is coupled chemically to the organic matrix by a silane coating on the filler particles. There are two main types of composites based on the method of polymerization: chemically polymerized and ultraviolet radiation polymerized.

Chemically Polymerized Composites: The organic components of the polymeric matrix, ranging from 15 to 30 percent by weight, consist of BIS-GMA as the primary monomer and triethyleneglycol-dimethacrylate, Bis-phenol-A-dimethacrylate, and methacrylic acid as the diluents. The polymerization process is catalyzed by benzoyl peroxide using dihydroxyethyl-p-toluidine as the accelerator. Inhibitors such as p-methoxyphenol are added to prolong the storage life of the resin and ultraviolet stabilizers including phenyl-salicylate-glycidyl methacrylate or 1-hydroxy-4-dodecyl-benzophenone are incorporated into the system to minimize any color change of the restoration. Dyes and pigments, usually metal oxides or sulfides, are used to color match the restoration to the tooth, mask yellowing, and impart fluorescence.

The filler or inorganic components vary in concentration between 70 and 85 percent by weight. The filler blend and viscosity of the resin are responsible for the handling and finishing characteristics of the materials. Among the most commonly used fillers are lithium-aluminum silicate, barium glass, quartz, and barium-aluminum-silicate glass.[13] They are used in many shapes with the sizes ranging from 1 to 40 microns. The smaller particle sizes normally improve manipulation and finishing. A reduction of the high coefficient of thermal expansion is especially enhanced by low-expanding fillers.[1,4,14,15] Such composites shrink less on hardening, are stronger and stiffer, are more resistant to abrasion, and have a much lower coefficient of thermal expansion than the usual unfilled tooth restorative resins.[2,3,13,15-19] (See Table I)

Silane coupling agents such as gamma-methacryloxypropyl-trimethoxysilane are used to improve bonding between the resin matrix and the filler and to prevent the penetration of moisture.

For the dental patient, the above advantages may mean restorations with better margin integrity, showing less margin stain and secondary caries, less stain within the restorative material itself, and better maintenance of anatomic form in comparison with the unfilled resins.

An understanding by dentists and their assistants of the basic properties of the composite resins and their manipulative characteristics should result in greater success and longevity of the resulting restorations.

Ultraviolet Radiation Polymerized Composites: Ultraviolet radiation polymerized systems differ from the chemically polymerized systems in the nature of the catalyst. The catalyst used in the ultraviolet polymerized systems is usually an ultraviolet-sensitive benzoin derivative dissolved in the organic components of the system. Benzoin-methyl-ether is an example of such a catalyst.

Special devices designed to emit ultraviolet radiation in the 320 to 365 nm range are used to photopolymerize composite resins. The devices are shielded and equipped with proper filters so that radiation below 320 nm and any stray unfiltered radiation are essentially eliminated.

The ultraviolet device may be a part of the composite system (Nuva system) or it may be available separately (Cavitron Quick-Lite). The manufacturer's instructions should be followed and the safety precautions for using ultraviolet radiation should be strictly observed. (See chapter on Safety in the Dental Office.)

USES: Principally, composite resins are used for Class III and Class V restorations. They have limited use in Class I restorations in premolars and selected Class IV restorations where esthetics is of primary importance.[20] Clinical studies have reported a three year comparison of Class II amalgam and composite restorations.[21,22] The composites did not hold up well in the Class II design, failing at a high rate from the lack of abrasion resistance and marginal integrity.

Composite resins are also being promoted for a number of other uses including covering enamel defects, repairing fractured incisors, repairing cervical erosion, attaching orthodontic brackets, cementing orthodontic bands, splinting teeth, and cementing certain types of cast restorations.

Composite resin has been suggested as a substitute for amalgam in a pin-retained core to be covered with a gold, porcelain-fused-to-gold, or porcelain crown in the restoration of a mutilated tooth.[23]

DIRECTIONS FOR USE: *Bonding:* The strength of the bond between a resin restoration and the walls of the cavity preparation must be at least 49 kg/cm^2 (700 psi) to counteract the estimated tensile force that develops during the hardening of the resin;[10] otherwise, the bond may be too weak to hold. The weakness of the bond is another reason why the polymerization shrinkage must be as low as possible. The bond will also be under considerable stress during temperature changes if the thermal expansion of the filling material and tooth are appreciably different.

Since the advent of composite resin restorative materials, there has been increased research on bonding material to the prepared tooth surfaces. Enhanced bonding is achieved through the use of bonding or coupling agents and by acid etching the enamel around a cavity preparation. Many of the commercially available composite restorative materials are packaged with a supply of bonding agent and acid etchant. One coupling agent that has shown promise is a surface-active comonomer which is the addition reaction product of N-phenylglycine and glycidyl methacrylate (NPG-GMA). Trial tests showed that this agent, when applied to dentin or enamel, caused a significant improvement in bonding.[24]

Acid etching of enamel permits bonding agents and composite materials to penetrate into the etch induced micro-irregularities on the enamel surface to form interlocking tags.

Phosphoric acid solutions of different strengths are used as etchants. Common etchants are 37 and 50 percent phosphoric acid solutions, the latter sometimes buffered with zinc oxide.

It is generally recognized that use of a bonding agent following acid etchings of enamel increases resistance to marginal leakage in thermal cycling and increases the retention of the restoration.

Pulp Protection: Exposed dentin should be protected prior to acid etching to avoid pulpal reaction.

Even when acid etching is not employed, a suitable liner or base should be used in the prepared cavity because the pulpal response to a composite resin material is of the same order as that found associated with silicate cement.

Polymerization of composites may be impaired by certain liners and bases, such as those containing eugenol. Manufacturer's recommendations should be followed in the choice of a base or liner.

Surface Finish: Using the matrix strip gives the smoothest surface texture to the composite resin.[19,25,26] Polishing with abrasives is, however, usually required. Not only is the finished restoration surface dependent upon the particle size (grit) of the abrasive instrument but also upon the hardness of the abrasive itself. (See Table II.) The effect of polishing does not appear to extend over a period longer than 4 to 6 months due to abrasion of the surface.[26] "Glaze" materials in the form of unfilled resins or filled resins with a low percentage of fine inorganic particles are marketed for coating composite restorations to improve their surface smoothness. The value of such materials over a period of time is currently being investigated. The film thickness in which some coatings are applied effects a negligible surface change after removal of the air inhibited layer.[27]

EVALUATION PROGRAM: The Council on Dental Materials, Instruments and Equipment has a Certification Program for unfilled and composite or filled resin restorative materials. All of the composite resins recognized in this program contain a high percentage of inorganic filler particles which are bonded to the resin by means of a primer.

Table II.
Surface Roughness of Composite Resins*

Instrumentation	Microinches
1. Waterproof disk–xx fine (Moore)	14
2. Zirconium silicate disk (3M)	14
3. Diamond disk–6 microns†	15
4. Diamond disk–9 microns†	16
5. Waterproof disk–x fine (Moore)	16
6. White polishing point–46P (Chayes)	16
7. Cuttle disk–fine (Moore)	20
8. Carbide finishing bur–Jet (Midwest)	22
9. Waterproof disk–fine (Moore)	24
10. Aluminum oxide disk (3M)	28
11. Sand disk–fine (Moore)	30
12. "Composite" point (Shofu)	34
13. Sulci disks–Burlew (Jelenko)	36
14. Silex and Tin Oxide slurries–with rubber cup	48
15. Diamond point–flame (Den-tel-ez)	48
16. Mounted point–47 (Chayes)	50
17. Diamond disk (Den-tel-ez)	68
18. Diamond point–SF 3/4A (Densco)	75
19. Diamond point–flame (Star)	88
20. Diamond point–flame (3M)	94
21. Diamond point–SF 1/8A (Densco)	96

*Data furnished by Dr. J. B. Dennison, University of Michigan.
†Experimental.

COMPOSITIVE RESTORATIVE MATERIALS

Treatment Planning

Do:

1. Use in anterior teeth where esthetics is important.
2. Limit their use in posterior teeth to Class I and Class V restorations where esthetics is important.
3. Use composites in Class IV problems when full coverage cannot be used.
4. Recognize that attrition and wear occurs in time when the restoration is subjected to those forces.
5. Recognize the possibility of staining or discoloration of the margins of the body of the restoration.
6. Select the color (where indicated) before rubber dam application.

Don't:

1. Use on the distal aspect of canines (except in rare instances).
2. Use in areas where the material is required to support centric stops.

Preparation of the Cavity

Do:

1. Use rubber dam isolation.
2. Prepare a cavity design with the internal retentive form.

3. Use adequate pulpal protection.
4. Minimize tooth tissue loss, internally and externally.
5. Enter the carious lesion through the lingual aspect whenever feasible (Class III).
6. Maintain the labial plate of enamel when possible (or lingual plate if labial approach is dictated by position of the Class III carious lesion).
7. Permit the extent of caries, convenience, and need for retention to dictate outline form.
8. Use a suitable base, where necessary, to cover all exposed dentin prior to acid etching.
9. Use acid etching as a means of enhancing the bond of resin to enamel. All the enamel surfaces contacted by the resin should be etched.

Don't:

1. Use eugenol liners or bases in contact with the resin.
2. Use eugenol, phenol, or other benzene-ring-containing medicaments.
3. Use a film-forming cavity varnish for pulp protection.
4. Use high rotary speeds to complete the entire preparation (low speed and hand instrumentation are usually indicated to refine conservative preparations).

Manipulation of the Materials

Do:

1. Proportion the materials according to the manufacturer's instructions.
2. Mix according to the manufacturer's instructions.
3. Have everything in readiness before mixing is begun.

Don't:

1. Prolong the working of the chemically initiated composite material once mixing is begun.
2. Mix with a metallic instrument.

Insertion of the Materials

Do:

1. Use a pretested matrix for Classes III, IV and V cavities.
2. Stabilize the matrix after placement of the composite (wedging is usually helpful for Class III cavities).
3. Gain complete filling of the preparation with a minimum incorporation of air voids (a syringe is useful).
4. Remove gross excess of inserted material before matrix is finally stabilized.

Don't:

1. Lubricate matrix strips.
2. Delay the placement of the chemically initiated composite material after mixing.
3. Overfill to great excess.

Finishing of the Restoration

Do:

1. Remove excess material in contour and overextension.
2. Maintain glossy surface imparted by matrix when contour is correct.
3. Adjust contour and remove overextension of material as required.
4. Adjust for all occlusal contacts when required.
5. Recognize the outline form as established by the cavosurface margins of the preparation.
6. Finish with rotary instruments at conventional speeds.

Don't:

1. Attempt to "polish" the restoration by usual metallic or unfilled resin techniques.
2. Finish adjacent enamel surfaces, inadvertently changing contour.
3. Use high speed instrumentation for finishing (except possibly for gross excess removal).

AVAILABLE PRODUCTS

ADAPTIC RADIOPAQUE DENTAL RE-STORATIVE, Johnson and Johnson Dental Products Company

Adaptic Dental Restorative; Adaptic Bonding Agent; Glaze; Universal Tints, Johnson and Johnson Dental Products Company

Bonfil, L. D. Caulk Co., Div. of Dentsply International, Inc.

Caulk Uni-Strips, L. D. Caulk Co., Div. of Dentsply International, Inc.

Cervident, S. S. White Dental Products International Div., Pennwalt Corp.

COMPODENT II, Teledyne Dental Products

Composite Polish, Teledyne Dental Products

Compatit Type II, W. H. Byron

CONCISE RADIOPAQUE COMPOSITE, 3M Company

Control Etch, Den-Mat, Inc.

Core Paste, Den-Mat, Inc.

Dencoa Compofil Type II, Wallace A. Erickson

Ease, Mid-America Dental Products

Enamalite, Enamalite 500, Lee Pharmaceuticals

Enamel Etching Liquid, Teledyne Dental Products

Epoxydent Type II, Lee Pharmaceuticals

Epoxylight HL-72; Epoxylite CBA 9080, Lee Pharmaceuticals

Exact; Exact Coreform; S. S. White Div., Pennwalt Corp.

Finite, Lee Pharmaceuticals

FINNESSE DIRECT FILLING RESIN TYPE I, L. D. Caulk Co., Div. of Dentsply International, Inc.

FOTOFIL DENTAL RESTORATIVE, Johnson and Johnson Dental Products

Healthco Composite Type II, Healthco Corporation

HL-72 Type II, Lee Pharmaceuticals

INCISAL, Den-Mat, Inc.

Incisal Edge, Healthco Co.

Isosit, Vivadent

Kadon, L. D. Caulk Co., Div. of Dentsply International, Inc.

KERR SIMULATE, Kerr Mfg. Co., Div. of Sybron Corp.

Lee-Fill, Lee Pharmaceuticals

Mix Kit, The Lorvic Corporation

NEW RESTODENT, TYPE II, Lee Pharmaceuticals

NIMETIC, ESPE Dental Products

Nuva-Fil P.A., L. D. Caulk Co., Div. of Dentsply International, Inc.

Poly-Fil, American Consolidated Mfg. Co., Inc.

Portrait, Lorvic Corp.

Posite, American Consolidated Mfg. Co., Inc.

Powderlite, S. S. White Dental Products International Div., Pennwalt Corp.

Prestige, Type II, Lee Pharmaceuticals

Profile, Type II, S. S. White Dental Products International Div., Pennwalt Corp.

Prosthodent, Lee Pharmaceuticals

Protecto, Lee Pharmaceuticals

Replica, Hoyt Laboratories

Restodent, Lee Pharmaceuticals

Silar, Type I, 3M Company

SMILE TYPE II, Kerr Mfg. Co., Div. of Sybron Corp.

SPECTRABOND, Den-Mat, Inc.

SUPER C, AMCO

Temple, Premier Dental Products Co.

Uni-Bond, Den-Mat, Inc.

Uviofil, Type II, ESPE

VERITÉ COMPOSITE RESTORATIVE MATERIAL, Unitek Corp.

VERITÉ-M MICROFILL COMPOSITE RESTORATIVE MATERIAL, Unitek Corp.

VYTOL COMPOSITE, L. D. Caulk Div. of Dentsply International, Inc.

Yellow Duralay Powder, Charles Development Co.

PIT AND FISSURE SEALANTS

Although the fluorides have provided for a major reduction in caries, their cariostatic effect through communal water supply, dietary supplements, or topical application in a variety of ways has been preferential for smooth surfaces of enamel. Protection of enamel faults—pits and fissures—from dental caries remains a high priority in preventive dentistry. For over a decade, the obturation or sealing of pits and fissures using some form of resin has received considerable attention.

Most pit and fissure sealants are similar to the resins used in formulating composite restorative materials and contain bisphenol A-glycidyl methacrylate (BIS-GMA) and methyacrylates or dimethacrylates. Polymerization results by either mixing in two component systems or by the use of ultraviolet light in one component systems. Such products, when properly used to seal enamel pits and fissures, provide a barrier to some of the causative factors of dental decay and, therefore, contribute to the prevention of occlusal caries. However, such a benefit results only when the sealant has been retained in the pits and fissures of the occlusal surfaces. For this reason, treated surfaces should be examined at not more than six-month intervals following the date of application. Further, lost sealant should be replaced to ensure maximum benefit of the treatment procedure. Tints or white opacifying agents are sometimes incorporated into the sealants to aid in checking for retention.

The clinical procedures involved in sealant applications are (1) cleaning of the pits and fissures through prophylaxis, (2) acid etching of the enamel to promote resin bonding, and (3) resin placement. Prophylaxis before conditioning and sealant placement does not remove debris from the pits and fissures. Shallow fissures may be filled with the sealant, but deep, constrictive fissures are not. Residual materials in the fissures, air entrapment and fissure geometry contribute to limiting sealant penetration.

EVALUATION PROGRAM: The Council on Dental Materials, Instruments and Equipment has an Acceptance Program for Pit and Fissure Sealants.

AVAILABLE PRODUCTS

CONCISE BRAND WHITE SEALANT, 3M Company
CONCISE ENAMEL BOND, 3M Company
DELTON, Johnson and Johnson Dental Products Co.
EPOXYLITE 9075, Lee Pharmaceuticals
KERR PIT & FISSURE SEALANT, Kerr Mfg. Co., Div. of Sybron Corp.
Lee-Seal, Lee Pharmaceuticals
NUVA-COTE, L. D. Caulk Co., Div. of Dentsply International, Inc.
NUVA-SEAL P.A., L. D. Caulk Co., Div. of Dentsply International, Inc.

LITERATURE REFERENCES

1. Bowen, R. L. Dental filling material comprising vinyl-silane treated fused silica and a binder consisting of the reaction product of bisphenol and glycidyl acrylate. U.S. Patent 3,006,112 Nov. 27, 1962.

2. Bowen, R. L. Properties of silica-reinforced polymer for dental restorations. JADA 66:57 Jan. 1963.

3. Bowen, R. L. Effect of particle shape and size distribution in a reinforced polymer. JADA 69: 481 Oct. 1964.

4. Hedegard, B. Cold-polymerizing resins. Acta Odontol. Scand. 13, Supplement 17, 1955.

5. Phillips, R. W. The science of dental materials, ed. 7, Philadelphia, W. B. Saunders Co., 1973.

6. Nelsen, R. J., et al. Fluid exchange at the margins of dental restorations. JADA 44:288 Mar. 1952.

7. von Dreudenstein, T.S. Thermische volumenanderung und randschluss von fullengen aus schnellhartendem. Kunstsoff Deut. Zahnartztl. Zchr. 8:143, 1953.

8. Nealon, F. G. Acrylic restorations: operative nonpressure procedure. J. Prosthet. Dent. 2:513 July 1952.

9. Fusayama, T., et al. Comparison of the technics for direct acrylic fillings. Bul Tokyo Med.-Den. U. 2:235, 1956.

10. Bowen, R. L. Adhesive bonding of various materials to hard tooth tissues. VI. Forces developing indirect-filling materials during hardening. JADA 74:439 Feb. 1967.

11. McCurdy, C. R. Jr., et al. A comparison of in vivo and in vitro microleakage of dental restorations. JADA 88:592 Mar. 1974.

12. Guide to dental materials and devices. ed.7, Chicago, American Dental Association, 1974.

13. Macchi, R. L., and Craig, R. G. Physical and mechanical properties of composite restorative materials. JADA 78:328 Feb. 1969.

14. McLean, J. W. Anterior filling materials in Europe. Dent. Prog. 2:181 Apr. 1962.

15. Stanford, J. W. The current status of restorative resins. Dent. Clin. N. Am. 15:57 Jan. 1971.

16. Dennison, J. B., and Craig, R. G. Physical properties and finished surface texture of composite restorative resins. JADA 85:101 July 1972.

17. Phillips, R. W.; Swartz, M. L.; and Norman, R. D. Materials for the practicing dentist. St. Louis, C. V. Mosby Co., 1969, Chapter 11.

18. Peterson, E. A.; Phillips, R. W.; and Swartz, M. L. A comparison of the physical properties of four restorative resins. JADA 73:1324 Dec. 1966.

19. Gotfredsen, C. Physical properties of a plastic filling material. Acta Odontol. Scand. 27:595 No. 6, 1969.

20. Council on Dental Materials and Devices: Recommended standard practices for clinical evaluation of dental materials and devices. JADA 84:388 Feb. 1972.

21. Leinfelder, K. F., et al. Clinical evaluation of composite resins as anterior and posterior restorative materials. J. Prosthet. Dent. 33:407 Apr. 1975.

22. Phillips, R. W., et al. Observations on a composite resin for Class II restorations: Three year report. J. Prosthet. Dent. 30:891 Dec. 1973.

23. Spalten, R. G. Composite resins to restore mutilated teeth. J. Prosthet. Dent. 25:323 Mar. 1971.

24. Bowen, R. L. Adhesive bonding of various materials to hard tooth tissues II. Bonding to dentin promoted by a surface-active comonomer. J. Dent. Res. 44:895 Sept.-Oct. 1965.

25. Chandler, H. H.; Bowen, R. L.; and Paffenbarger, G. C. Method for finishing composite restorative materials. JADA 83:344 Aug. 1971.

26. Johnson, L. N.; Jordan, R. E.; and Lynn, J. A. Effect of various finishing devices on resin surfaces. JADA 83:321 Aug. 1971.

27. Calatrava, L. A. Clinical evaluation of two glazing agents for composite resin surfaces with and without polymer coatings. Oper. Dent. 1:137, 1976.

METALS AND ALLOYS

COHESIVE GOLDS

Pure gold in leaf or foil-form has been used for the restoration of carious teeth for more than 500 years. The mechanical and biological advantages of restorations fabricated from well compacted gold have never been contested seriously. However, because of the time and skill required for replacement of a direct gold restoration where indicated, the use of cohesive gold in modern clinical practice has been supplanted by the use of cast alloys, amalgam and composite resins.

Uses: Cohesive gold is used primarily for Class I, Class III and Class V restorations with limited use in Class IV restorations and in Class II restorations in premolars.

Cohesive golds are used also to repair planned holes following cementation of cast full crown restorations, repair perforated castings and reinforce semirigid connectors.

Directions for Use: Cohesive and direct filling golds are supplied in three forms: foil, crystalline or mat, and powdered or sintered. Pure gold, as well as that alloyed with calcium, can be cold welded to itself. The materials, therefore, can be used interchangeably within the same cavity.

The handling characteristics of cohesive golds differ dramatically. The high mass per unit volume and spreading quality of powdered gold facilitates the condensation of the restoration.[1-4]

To maintain cohesiveness, all direct filling golds must be free from contaminants such as saliva, moisture and lubricants.

Limitations of Use: These forms of cohesive gold, when properly condensed, appear to possess comparable strength, hardness, density and abrasion resistance.[5-8] Unlike cast gold alloys, direct filling golds exhibit neither high hardness nor high strength. Therefore, the use of compacted gold should be limited to areas where strength is not a critical requirement.

53

COHESIVE GOLDS

Do:

1. Avoid exposure to atmospheric gases and moisture during storage.
2. Maintain high standards of cleanliness with respect to work areas and instruments.
3. Use an ethyl alcohol or acetone-free methanol flame or electric heater for annealing.

Don't:

1. Handle material roughly or unnecessarily.
2. Use annealing heat sources that yield deposits of carbon or sulfur or chlorine-containing compounds.

AVAILABLE PRODUCTS

Williams Cylinders, Williams Gold Refining Co., Inc.

Williams Electroloy RV, Williams Gold Refining Co., Inc.

Williams Mat Foil, Williams Gold Refining Co., Inc.

Williams Morgan Hasting Goldent, Williams Gold Refining Co., Inc.

Williams Mat Gold, Williams Gold Refining Co., Inc.

Williams Pure Gold Foil, Williams Gold Refining Co., Inc.

Williams Ropes, Williams Gold Refining Co., Inc.

GOLD CASTING ALLOYS

The development of gold casting alloys commenced after disclosure of a lost-wax dental casting technique and machine by Dr. William H. Taggart in 1907. Today, a variety of suitable gold alloys is available for use in restorative procedures.

USES: Gold casting alloys are used for inlays of all classes as well as individual partial and full coverage restorations. Fixed partial denture and removable partial denture frameworks are also made with these alloys. Additional uses of casting gold alloys include the fabrication of posts and cores for the restoration of endodontically involved teeth and construction of surgical and periodontal splints.

DIRECTIONS FOR USE: Rigid criteria for selection of casting golds do not exist. However, the user must be cognizant of the fact that gold alloys are classified according to their hardness as determined by their resistance to indentation. The alloys fall into four groups: soft (Type I Inlay), medium (Type II Inlay), hard (Type III Crown-and-Bridge), and extra hard (Type IV Partial Denture). Hardness is used to classify the types because, in general, other mechanical properties correlate with hardness.

For most practical purposes a satisfactory gold casting alloy can be defined mechanically by its values for hardness and elongation. The relationship between hardness and elongation is much less definite than the relationship between hardness and elastic limit, or between hardness and tensile strength. In general, however, the soft alloys exhibit higher elongation than the hard alloys, as might be expected. The classification makes possible the rational selection and use of alloys on the basis of properties in relation to functional requirements imposed by the clinical situation.

Compositional ranges of the four types of gold casting alloys are given in Table I.

The minimum requirement for gold and metals of the platinum group varies from 83 percent for the soft alloys, Type I, to 75 percent for the extra hard alloys, Type IV. More base metal is required in the hard alloys but the noble metal content is kept high enough to provide tarnish and corrosion resistance.[9]

The properties of fine grain alloys are superior to those of coarse grain materials.[10,11] Grain refinement increases tensile strength and elongation by about 30 percent. A hundredfold in-

Table I.
Range of Percentage Composition of Dental Casting Gold Alloys

Type of alloy	Component					
	Gold	Silver	Copper	Palladium	Platinum	Zinc
I	80.2-95.8	2.4-12.0	1.6- 6.2	0.0- 3.6	0.0-1.0	0.0-1.2
II	73.0-83.0	6.9-14.5	5.8-10.5	0.0- 5.6	0.0-4.2	0.0-1.4
III	71.0-79.8	5.2-13.4	7.1-12.6	0.0- 6.5	0.0-1.5	0.0-2.0
IV	62.4-71.9	8.0-17.4	8.6-15.4	0.0-10.1	0.2-8.2	0.0-2.7

crease in the number of grains per unit volume may be obtained by the addition of approximately 50 ppm of ruthenium or iridium.

The mechanics of hardening in dental gold alloys has been found to be an order-disorder reaction and the precipitation of a silver rich phase.[12] Many of the dental gold alloys can be hardened by appropriate heat treatment. The alloys that contain large amounts of gold and metals of the platinum group (Types I and II)

GOLD CASTING ALLOYS

Do:
1. Select an alloy on the basis of anticipated mechanical requirements.
2. Use the correct casting technique and equipment.
3. Clean used gold alloys by melting on a charcoal block before reuse.
4. Add new gold alloys to reused gold alloys to restore the zinc content.
5. Employ prescribed heat treatment procedures to ensure development of optimum mechanical properties of age hardenable alloys.

Don't:
1. Cast mixtures of scrap dental gold alloys.
2. Add coinage alloy or other metals to dental casting gold alloys.

---

have a low hardness and respond very little to heat treatment. Hard and extra hard alloys (Types III and IV) can be softened by quenching after holding at about 700°C (1,295°F) for ten minutes. Subsequent hardening is attained by cooling uniformly from 450°C to 250°C (842°F to 482°F) in 30 minutes. Greater strength and hardness are developed under this treatment, but with a consequent loss in ductility. In the softening and hardening of any specific alloy, the recommendation of the manufacturer should be followed.

Reported values for the linear shrinkage of gold and its alloys range from 1.0 to almost 2.2 percent.[13-18] The reason for the relatively large spread in values may be the variation in size and shape of the specimen upon which shrinkage was measured, the composition of the alloys and the casting technique. No single values, therefore, can be given for the casting shrinkage of gold and its alloys unless these three variables are defined precisely; then the determined linear shrinkage would apply to those precisely controlled conditions only. However, a value of 1.5±0.2 percent is considered to be satisfactory only for practical castings. Auxiliary laboratory materials as well as mold burnout and casting procedures play prominent roles in establishing the clinical accuracy of cast gold restorations.

LIMITATIONS OF USE: Where esthetics is of primary importance, and the display of gold is undesirable, use of a cast gold restoration may be contraindicated. Often, however, problems with esthetics can be minimized or overcome completely by skillful and conservative tooth preparation.

EVALUATION PROGRAM: To further international standardization in dental materials, the American Dental Association adopted the Federation Dentaire Internationale Specification for Dental Casting Gold Alloy in 1965. The requirements for dental gold casting alloys have been incorporated as Specification No. 5 in the American Dental Association's program on dental materials, instruments and equipment.

AVAILABLE PRODUCTS

TYPE I, SOFT
VICKERS HARDNESS NUMBER 59-90

ADERER "A" SOFT, J. Aderer, Inc.
BAKER INLAY SOFT, Baker Dental Dept. of Engelhard Industries, Engelhard Minerals & Chemicals Corp.
CODESCO PREMIUM, Codesco, Inc.
DEGULOR A., Degussa, Inc.
LEFF LIGHT INLAY, Leff Dental Golds
MOWREY S-1; S-M; 22K, W. E. Mowrey Co.
NEY-ORO A-A, J. M. Ney Co.
NOBLE 1, Noble Metals & Alloys Co., Inc.
Paladin I, Sterngold Div. of Sterndent Corp.
PENTRON I CASTING GOLD, Pentron Corp.
RX JENERIC A, Rx Jeneric Gold Co., Inc.
S-1 CASTING GOLD, I.L.G.S.
STERNGOLD S., Sterndent Corp.
VERIBEST 22 Kt INLAY, A. Szabo Co., Inc.
WILKINSON 2S, Wilkinson Co.
WILLIAMS HARMONY LINE SOFT, Williams Gold Refining Co., Inc.

TYPE II, MEDIUM
VICKERS HARDNESS NUMBER 90-120

ADERER "B" MEDIUM, J. Aderer, Inc.
AMERICAN GOLD "M" INLAY MEDIUM, American Gold Co.
AMERICAN GOLD "M-H" INLAY, American Gold Co.
BAKER INLAY MEDIUM, Baker Dental Dept. of Engelhard Industries, Engelhard Minerals & Chemicals Corp.
CODESCO PREMIUM, Codesco, Inc.

CODESCO INLAY MEDIUM, Codesco, Inc.
CROWN NO. 1; KNAPP NO. 2; T, General Refineries, Inc.
Crown No. 2, General Refineries, Inc.
DG#1, Heraeus Dental Gold Corp.
DEGULOR B, Degussa, Inc.
DENT GOLD NO. 1, A. Szabo Co., Inc.
D-INLAY CASTING GOLD, I.L.G.S.
HOWMEDICA A-2, Howmedica, Inc., Dental Div.
INLAY II B, Direct Dental Sales & Supplies, Inc.
JELENKO MODULAY; PLATINCAST; 820 MEDIUM HARD, J. F. Jelenko & Co., Pennwalt Corp.
JENSEN JB GOLD, Jensen Industries, Inc.
LEFF MEDIUM SOFT, Leff Dental Golds
LIBRA II INLAY AND CROWN, Libra Gold Co.
MOWREY B INLAY; NO. 91; S-2; T, W. E. Mowrey Co.
NEY-ORO A-1, J. M. Ney Co.
NOBLE 2, Noble Metals & Alloys Co., Inc.
Paladin II, Sterndent Corp.
Pentron II Casting Gold, Pentron Corp.
PENTRON III CASTING GOLD, Pentron Corp.
RX JENERIC B, Rx Jeneric Gold Co., Inc.
STERNGOLD 1, Sterndent Corp.
Sterngold 10, Sterndent Corp.
TICONIUM TG2, Ticonium Co.
WILKINSON 8M; 76, Wilkinson Co.
WILLIAMS HARMONY LINE MEDIUM, Williams Gold Refining Co., Inc.

TYPE III, HARD
VICKERS HARDNESS NUMBER 120-150

ADERER "C"; BRIDGE; DRESSEL, J. Aderer, Inc.
AMERICAN GOLD "B" BRIDGE, American Gold Co.
AMERICAN GOLD "T" BRIDGE HARD, American Gold Co.
Aurora, Aztec, Sterndent Corp.
BAKER INLAY HARD, Baker Dental Dept. of Engelhard Industries, Engelhard Minerals & Chemicals Corp.
BRIDGE III-C, Direct Dental Sales & Supplies, Inc.
CODESCO PREMIUM, Codesco, Inc.
CODESCO BRIDGE HARD, Codesco, Inc.
CROWN KNAPP NO. 3; NO. 9; SUPREME; TT, General Refineries, Inc.

DEGULOR C, Degussa, Inc.
DENT GOLD NO. 2, A. Szabo Co., Inc.
Dent Gold Type 8, A. Szabo Co., Inc.
Econocast, Pentron Corp.
Horizon, Sterndent Corp.
HOWMEDICA A-5, Howmedica, Inc., Dental Div.
HOWMEDICA A-6, Howmedica, Inc., Dental Div.
JELENKO DUROCAST; FIRMILAY; J-9; NO. 13, J. F. Jelenko & Co., Pennwalt Corp.
JENSEN JC GOLD, Jensen Industries, Inc.
LEFF "C," Leff Dental Golds
LIBRA III CROWN AND BRIDGE, Libra Gold Co.
Light White, A. Szabo Co., Inc.
Mastercast #3; 3C; #3H; Micro Mini Gold; Mini Gold; Midi Gold 50; Williams Gold Refining Co., Inc.
Midabrite, Pentron Corp.
MOWREY 120; S-3; SPECIAL INLAYS: TT, W.E. Mowrey Co.
NARK KIM IMPERIAL, Wilkinson Co.
Neycast III, J.M. Ney Co.
NEY-ORO B-2, J.M. Ney Co.
Ney-Oro B-20; CB, J.M. Ney Co.
NOBLE 3, Noble Metals & Alloys Co., Inc.
Nova; Paladin 3, Sterndent Corp.
Noble Lab Special; 3; 24; 39; 62, Noble Metals & Alloys Co., Inc.
Paliney CB; J.M. Ney Co.
Par-Cast Casting Gold, Type IV, I.L.G.S.
PENTRON III CASTING GOLD, Pentron Corp.
Pentron C&B; White, Pentron Corp.
PMW, Rx Jeneric Gold Co.
RX JENERIC C, Rx Jeneric Gold Co., Inc.
Rx LDG C&B; Midacast; Oryi Satin Cast, Rx Jeneric Gold Co.
SPECIAL INLAY CASTING GOLD, I.L.G.S.
SPEYER NO. 18; NO. 21, Speyer Smelting & Refining Co.
STERNGOLD 2; STERNGOLD B; STERN-GOLD BRIDGETTE INLAY; STERNGOLD 5, Sterndent Corp.
Sterngold 20; Sunrize, Sterndent Corp.
Szabo W, Heraeus Dental Gold Corp.
Tawny Cast, Heraeus Dental Gold Corp.
TICONIUM TG3, Ticonium Co.
Wilkinson Sierra M, Wilkinson Co.
WILKINSON SPECIAL, Wilkinson Co.
WILKINSON 9M, Wilkinson Co.
Wilkinson WD, Wilkinson Co.

WILLIAMS HARMONY LINE HARD; "KLONDIKER," Williams Gold Refining Co., Inc.
WLW, Williams Gold Refining Co., Inc.
XL, Williams Gold Refining Co., Inc.

TYPE IV, EXTRA HARD
VICKERS HARDNESS NUMBER
QUENCHED, MINIMUM 150;
HARDENED, MINIMUM 220

ADERER NO. 3 BRIDGE GOLD: PROCAST GOLD, J. Aderer, Inc.
BAKER INLAY EXTRA HARD, Baker Dental Dept. of Engelhard Industries, Engelhard Minerals & Chemicals Corp.
BRIDGE PARTIAL IV D, Direct Dental Sales & Supplies, Inc.
CODESCO PREMIUM TYPE IV, Codesco, Inc.
DEGULOR M, Degussa, Inc.
Dental Gold, Type C, #7; 8%, #24;#63, Heraeus Dental Gold Corp.
Econoplus, Rx Jeneric Gold Co., Inc.
HOWMEDICA A-18, Howmedica, Inc.
JELENKO NO. 7; J-13, J.F. Jelenko & Co., Pennwalt Corp.
LEFF HARD, Leff Dental Golds
LIBRA IV EXTRA HARD, Libra Gold Co.
Mastercast #4G, Ceramco, Inc.
MOWREY NO. 8; PAR-CAST, W.E. Mowrey Co.
NEY-ORO G-3, J.M. Ney Co.
NEY-ORO #5; 6, J. M. Ney Co.
NOBLE 4; 18; 19, Noble Metals & Alloys Co., Inc.
Noble 6%, 7; 8%; 14%, Noble Metals & Alloys Co., Inc.
Paladin 4, Sterndent Corp.
Paloy, Williams Gold Refining Co., Inc.
PAR-CAST CASTING GOLD, I.L.G.S.
PENTRON IV CASTING GOLD, Pentron Corp.
P-Hard, Pentron 44; 60, Pentron Corp.
RX JENERIC IV, Rx Jeneric Gold Co., Inc.
ORW; RxD; RxIV; Rx 41; Rx LDG 44; Rx LDG IV; Rx NYSp; Rx SEG; Special White, Rx Jeneric Gold Co., Inc.
STERNGOLD 3; STERNGOLD SUPERCAST, Sterndent Corp.
Sterngold APX; 40; 66; 90; 100; P, Sterndent Corp.
Szabo Spec.; Szabo-C-Spec., Heraeus Dental Gold Corp.
Szabo Premium, Heraeus Dental Gold Corp.
Szabo LG3; 666, Heraeus Dental Gold Corp.

TICONIUM TG4, Ticonium Co.

Tiffany, Sterndent Corp.

Tripli, Sterndent Corp.

Vantage, Sterndent Corp.

Wilkinson 4K; Sierra H; Imperial; Special; W60; 3K, Wilkinson Co.

Williams 49er, Williams Gold Refining Co., Inc.

Williams #6, All Purpose, Williams Gold Refining Co., Inc.

WILLIAMS HARMONY LINE EXTRA HARD, Williams Gold Refining Co., Inc.

Williams XL-S; XXX; Williams Gold Refining Co., Inc.

ALLOYS FOR PORCELAIN BONDING

Precious Metal Systems

Development of improved porcelain-alloy systems has enhanced both the usefulness and the status of the porcelain-fused-to-metal restoration. With skillful handling, these systems yield esthetically pleasing restorations that can withstand the stresses of mastication.

COMPOSITION AND PROPERTIES: Rational selection and clinical application of veneerable precious metal casting alloys require a fundamental appreciation of the inherent differences that exist among high-gold, low-gold and palladium-silver based alloys.

"High gold" is a term applicable to high-fusing crown-and-bridge alloys, the gold content of which exceeds 85 percent by weight. These alloys contain sufficient palladium (about 6 percent) and platinum (about 4 percent) to ensure that their fusion temperature range is higher than the fusion temperatures of dental porcelains. The high golds contain relatively small quantities of silver, iron, indium and tin.[19] High gold alloys exhibit a subdued yellow hue. Strength and hardness values of the cast materials are within the range of hardened Type IV golds and chromium-containing partial denture casting alloys.[19] Porcelain to metal bond strength is adequate.[20-24]

Hardening of some high-gold alloys occurs during the porcelain firing procedure.[19,25-27]

The aging mechanism appears to involve the transformation of an iron-platinum intermetallic compound (FePt) that forms during solidification or at temperatures just below the solidus to $FePt_3$ at temperatures below 982°C. It is likely that indium and tin influence to some extent the effects of the $FePt_3$ precipitate. The principal functions of indium and tin, however, are probably other than hardening or strengthening. Among such functions are perhaps grain refinement, control of the coefficient of thermal expansion and improvement of the porcelain-to-metal bond.

Light-colored precious metal crown-and-bridge alloys have been available for several years.[28,29] High fusion temperature ranges, low ductility and questionable tarnish resistance have discouraged the routine use of these materials in fixed prosthodontic procedures. Recently, however, seemingly new "white golds" or "low golds" have attracted increased attention as potential substitutes for the more costly yellow alloys.[30] Several white golds intended primarily for use in the ceramic-metal technique have appeared on the market.

The gold content of low gold systems varies from a minimum of about 20 percent by weight to a maximum of 60 percent by weight. The content of most available products is approximately 50 percent. Sufficient palladium is used in the production of alloys to raise the total noble metal content to at least 80 percent. The majority of low gold alloys contain silver which contributes to their whiteness. Minor quantities of base metals such as indium, tin, nickel and gallium play a significant role in the development of hardness and strength.[31,32] Strength characteristics of the low gold alloys are comparable to those of hardened Type III casting golds. These materials, however, are harder and less ductile than conventional crown-and-bridge alloys.[31,32] Porcelain-to-metal bond strength is adequate.[23,24]

The use of veneerable alloys containing substantial amounts of palladium (22 to 50 percent by weight) and silver (35 to 65 percent by weight) has increased in recent years. The palladium-silver based crown-and-bridge alloys contain very little or no gold.[30,32,33] Although the nobility of palladium is lower than that of platinum, the preference for palladium as a major component of these alloys is due probably to the lower melting point, lower cost per unit weight, and lower density of palladium.

The palladium-silver alloys used for fabrication of porcelain-fused-to-metal restorations contain minor amounts of low melting base metals such as zinc, indium or tin. These components increase the fluidity of the molten alloy and thereby improve its castability. Indium and tin also form intermetallic compounds with both palladium and silver. Age hardening of certain alloys appears to be related to the formation of these compounds.

From manufacturer's data and from limited independent laboratory investigations, it seems that the strength characteristics of the palladium-silver based materials are comparable to those of hardened Type III casting golds.[32-34] These alloys, however, are significantly harder and less ductile than Type III golds. The degree of bonding of porcelains to the alloys appears to be adequate.[23,24]

USES: Alloys bonded to porcelains are useful for casting veneerable substructures for the fabrication of individual full coverage restorations, and for manufacturing fixed partial dentures and pontics.

Porcelain-alloy systems are used also to fabricate veneerless components of fixed prosthetic devices.

DIRECTIONS FOR USE: The successful fabrication of fixed prostheses from the palladium-silver alloys requires strict adherence to meticulous laboratory technique. The alloys, in the molten state, readily occlude and interact with atmospheric gases. The entrapment of gases may result in the production of porous castings. The casting of multiple components, therefore, requires the use of a well designed sprue arrangement that provides adequate reservoirs and vents. The use of borax (reducing) flux is generally recommended to prevent excessive oxidation of the alloys during the fusion. However, to avoid possible contamination of the alloys, a

---

PRECIOUS METAL ALLOYS FOR PORCELAIN BONDING

Do:

1. Use phosphate-bonded investment molds for the casting of precious high-fusing alloys.
2. Employ electric induction equipment or a properly adjusted city gas-oxygen blow pipe for melting.
3. Immerse high-gold castings in HF for a minimum of 3 hours to remove tenacious investment debris.
4. Sandblast white alloys for removal of investment debris.
5. Rough grind all surfaces to which porcelain is to be applied with clean, hard stones.
6. Follow manufacturers' instructions for degassing and application of bonding agent and porcelain.

Don't:

1. Use contaminated crucibles or lined crucibles for melting alloy.
2. Use casting flux.
3. Use abrasive devices with high carbon content for preparation of surfaces to which porcelain is to be applied.

---

flux should not be used when the castings are to be veneered with porcelain. The alloys are attacked vigorously by mineral acids. Therefore, the removal of investment debris and cleaning of the cast pieces must be accomplished by liquid-honing or sandblasting.

In the use of palladium-silver alloys, certain specific points must be considered. Alloys with less than 50 percent palladium may tarnish in the oral environment, although their mechanical properties may be completely adequate to meet the requirement of long term function.

When porcelain is fired to alloys containing silver in excess of 8 to 10 percent, a yellowish green discoloration of the porcelain may occur during the firing operation. This difficulty may be precluded by application of a suitable colloidal gold coating agent to the metal substructure.

Since sufficient data based on long-term observations of fixed prostheses fabricated from palladium-silver based alloys are not available, the clinical efficacy of these materials cannot be ascertained. It appears, therefore, that caution and conservation should be exercised in their present use.

LIMITATIONS OF USE: High hardness and low ductility contraindicate the use of high fusing precious alloys for the fabrication of restorations other than those of the full coverage type.

Base Metal Systems

COMPOSITION: Since the late 1960's, more than twenty relatively inexpensive base metal alloys have been marketed for use in the porcelain-fused-to-metal technique. A number of features of these materials reflect obvious as well as subtle departures from the compositions of base metal partial denture alloys.[35,36] Nickel (about 60 to 80 percent by weight) and chromium (about 12 to 20 percent by weight) are the major constituents of most available products. At least one alloy is based on an iron (about 55 percent by weight)–chromium (about 27 percent by weight) system.

Modification of the nickel-chromium system by addition of varying amounts of minor alloying elements such as carbon, molybdenum, aluminum, manganese, tungsten, niobium, tantalum, boron, silicon and beryllium has made possible the availability of a broad selection of castable alloys, the structural features and properties of which are significantly diverse. Therefore, each base metal restorative alloy must be considered as a unique entity. Conclusions based on experience with one material cannot be used to predict the behavior of another.

The base metal crown-and-bridge alloys are platinum colored, lightweight and possess little or no scrap value. Available base metal alloys offer broad ranges of hardness and strength[37] Most base metal alloys, however, are harder, stronger and stiffer than precious metal crown-and-bridge alloys. Generally, the Vickers hardness of the base metal alloy is about twice that of precious metal-porcelain alloys. Ultimate tensile strength and yield have ranges of 552 to 1,024 MN/m² (32,000 to 110,000 psi), respectively. Modulus of elasticity values are close to 207×10^3 MN/m² (30 million psi). Elongation of most materials is relatively low (2 to 10 percent). At temperatures employed in porcelain veneering, the sag resistance of the base metals is greater than that of high-fusing precious alloys.[38]

High modulus of elasticity (rigidity) values and high yield strength (resistance to permanent deformation) suggest the potential usefulness of the base metal alloys for the casting of thin copings and retainers, as well as for the fabrication of long-span fixed partial dentures. These properties, however, when coupled with low ductility and high hardness, impede finishing and adaptation of margins. High hardness also complicates the adjustment of proximal areas and occlusal equilibration.

USES: Primarily used for the casting of veneerable substructures for the fabrication of individual full coverage restorations, base metal systems are used also to manufacture fixed partial dentures and pontics.

Porcelain-alloy systems using base metals in the alloy are also serviceable in the fabrication of veneerless components of fixed prosthetic devices.

DIRECTIONS FOR USE: The application of porcelain to the base metal crown-and-bridge alloys is a sensitive technique. Success of the procedure depends on meticulous surface preparation of the substrate castings. Evaluation of the apparent bond strength of various base-metal porcelain combinations has shown that some values are significantly lower than the bond strength of precious alloy-porcelain systems.[23,37,39] Excessive oxides which accrue at the surface of

---

BASE METAL ALLOYS FOR PORCELAIN BONDING

Do:

1. Recognize that sprueing, burnout temperature and casting techniques for base metal alloys differ markedly from those used with gold alloys.
2. Give critical attention to prescribed techniques.
3. Exercise rigid standards of laboratory and personal hygiene in the handling of nickel and beryllium containing alloys.

Don't:

1. Assume that techniques relevant to the management of one base metal alloy are applicable to others.

---

some base metal alloys during porcelain firing appear to preclude adequate porcelain-to-metal bonding.[39,40]

Some base metal crown-and-bridge alloys have higher *in vitro* corrosion rates than dental casting golds.[41] The clinical significance of this finding is not known. Additionally, sufficient research relevant to determination of the long term compatibility of fixed base metal prostheses with tissues of the human host is lacking.

Alloys that contain beryllium may be hazardous to laboratory workers.[37] (See Section I, "Safety in the Dental Office.")

LIMITATIONS OF USE: High hardness and low ductility contraindicate use of base metal crown-and-bridge alloys for fabrication of restorations other than those of the full coverage type.

The most perplexing problems associated with the use of available base metal crown-and-bridge alloys are difficulties encountered in the casting of these materials using procedures, investments and equipment designed for the centrifugal casting of gold alloys. Thin sections of

base metal castings often are incomplete. Fine detail of margins is prone to obliteration by rounding. Extracoronally retained castings made for preparations with relatively parallel walls (approximately 5° taper) often fail to seat completely.[42] Critical attention to individual technique differences is required to reduce the frequency of occurrence of these problems.[37]

AVAILABLE PRODUCTS

ACA CASTING ALLOY, Howmedica, Inc.
Auramic 2; 145; 210, Sterngold Div., Sterndent Corp.
Bak-On White; Yellow, Ceramco, Inc.
BIOBOND CROWN AND BRIDGE ALLOY, Dentsply International, Inc.
CAMEO, J.F. Jelenko and Co., Div. of Pennwalt Corp.
CERAMALLOY CROWN AND BRIDGE ALLOY, Johnson and Johnson Dental Products Co.
CERAMALLOY II, CROWN AND BRIDGE ALLOY, Johnson and Johnson Dental Products Co.
Condord, Rx Jeneric Gold Co.
Galaxy, Sterngold Div., Sterndent Corp.
Gnatho Ceram, Rx Jeneric Gold Co.
Gold Color Technic Casting Alloy, J.M. Ney Co.
JELENKO "O" PORCELAIN FUSED-TO-METAL ALLOY. J.F. Jelenko Co., Div. of Pennwalt Corp.
Litecast Hard, Williams Gold Refining Co., Inc.
Majestic II, Sterngold Div., Sterndent Corp.
MF-Y, Sterngold Div., Sterndent Corp.
MICRO BOND NP² ALLOY, Howmedica, Inc.
Ney 76; SMG-2; SMG-3; SMG-W; SMG-Y; Neydium Gold Ceramic, J.M. Ney Co.
Neydium Non Precious, J.M. Ney Co.
Noble ECW; #4869; J; M; YEC, Noble Metals and Alloys Co., Inc.
Omega Non-Precious Alloy, Sterngold Div., Sterndent Corp.
Paladine 4, Sterngold Div., Sterndent Corp.
Pentex 62; 77, Rx Jeneric Gold Co.
Pentillium, Rx Jeneric Gold Co.
Pentron PNP, Rx Jeneric Gold Co.
Prevox, Williams Gold Refining Co., Inc.
Rexalloy, Rx Jeneric Gold Co.
Rexillium III, Rx Jeneric Gold Co.
Royal, Sterngold Div., Sterndent Corp.
Rx Ceramic-Bond; CG; G; Imperial Ceramic;

SFC; SpCG; SWCG; WCG; Y Cermic; Rx 90, Rx Jeneric Gold Co.

Solar, Sterngold Div., Sterndent Corp.

Sterngold 66, Sterngold Div., Sterndent Corp.

Tripli, Sterngold Div., Sterndent Corp.

UTK Ceramic Gold Alloy — White, Unitek Corp.

UTK Ceramic Gold Alloy — Yellow, Unitek Corp.

UTK Ceramic Gold Alloy — Yellow Plus, Unitek Corp.

UTK UNIBOND NON PRECIOUS CERAMIC ALLOY, Unitek Corp.

VERABOND, Aalba-Dent, Inc.

Viking, Sterngold Div., Sterndent Corp.

Vista, Sterngold Div., Sterndent Corp.

White Ceramic Gold, Rx Jeneric Gold Co.

White Technic Casting Alloy, J.M. Ney Co.

Wilkinson Ceramicast; Ceramic White Classic; Hard; HFG; Wilkoro; Will-Ceram P; Will-Ceram W; Will-Ceram W-1; W-3; Y; Y-1; Y-2, Wilkinson Co.

Will-Ceram Litecast, Williams Gold Refining Co., Inc.

Wiron-S, Williams Gold Refining Co., Inc.

Yellow Ceramic I, Rx Jeneric Gold Co.

Yellow Ceramic II; III; IV, Rx Jeneric Gold Co.

BASE METAL ALLOYS FOR REMOVABLE PROSTHETIC APPLIANCES

Bright, lustrous, hard and tarnish resistant cobalt-based casting alloys were introduced to dentistry in the early 1930's. Since 1949, the use of alloys of this type in removable prosthodontic procedures has exceeded that of gold alloys.

COMPOSITION AND PROPERTIES: Most base metal partial denture alloys do not contain precious or noble metals. The alloys, must, by the composition requirement of American Dental Association Specification No. 14, contain a total of not less than 85 percent by weight of chromium, cobalt and nickel. Passivation of alloys meeting the requirement is sufficient to provide reasonable assurance of corrosion resistance. Cobalt (around 60 percent) and chromium (25 to 30 percent) are the major constituents of most available products. Molybdenum, carbon and tungsten are principal strengthening elements. The alloys may also contain minor additions of iron, manganese, tantalum, platinum, niobium, gallium, copper, iron, carbon and sil-

icon.[43,44]

One alloy acceptable for use in partial denture prostheses is formulated on a nickel (about 70 percent)–chromium (about 16 percent) system. This material contains relatively little cobalt. Important minor components of the nickel-chromium alloy include aluminum (about 2.5 percent) and beryllium (about 0.5 percent).

Some physical characteristics of the base metal alloys differ markedly from those of partial denture golds.[45-49] Comparatively, base metal alloys exhibit higher melting temperatures, greater casting shrinkage and lower density.

Base metal partial denture alloys are about 30 percent harder than Type IV golds. Typical Rockwell (R-30N) hardness values range between 50 and 60. Appliances cast from alloys exhibiting such hardness must be finished and polished with special laboratory equipment.

Rigidity of cast base metal partial denture alloys is approximately twice that of dental golds. Therefore, under a given load within its elastic limit, a structure cast from a base metal alloy will be deflected only half as much as a like structure made from gold alloy. Modulus of elasticity values of cobalt-chromium and nickel-chromium partial denture alloys approach 207×10^3 MN/m^2 (30 million psi).

USES: Alloys of base metals are the principal materials from which removable partial denture frameworks are fabricated. They are used to a lesser extent for construction of full denture bases.

Alloys of base metals, to a limited extent, are used in the fabrication of tooth-borne surgical and periodontal splints.

DIRECTIONS FOR USE: Base metal alloys tend to be brittle rather than ductile. Factors such as melting procedure, casting temperature and mold conditions affect microstructure, which, in turn, influences elongation.[50,51] Available base metal partial denture alloys exhibit "as-cast" elongation values of 2 to 10 percent.

The mechanical properties of cobalt-chromium partial denture alloys can be neither improved nor controlled by heat treatment. Properties of some nickel-chromium based materials, however, can be altered by high temperature treatment. For heat treatable materials, a softening treatment (15 minutes at 982°C followed by water quenching) may be used to improve workability. Subsequent rehardening (15 minutes at 704°C followed by water quenching) increases toughness of cast appliances.[52] Chromium-containing alloys are attacked by chlorine. Household bleaches should not be used to cleanse removable appliances made from base metal alloys.

LIMITATIONS OF USE: Allergic responses to the constituents of base metal alloys are observed occasionally. However, most adverse tissue reactions attributed to the wearing of a base metal prosthesis are manifestations of improper design or poor fit.

EVALUATION PROGRAM: The American Dental Association elucidates the requirements for base metal alloys in its Specification No. 14 for Dental Chromium-Cobalt Casting Alloy.

BASE METAL ALLOYS FOR REMOVABLE PROSTHETIC APPLIANCES

Do:

1. Recognize that casting and finishing procedures for base metal alloys are more complex than those for gold.
2. Adhere completely to manufacturer's instructions.
3. Use laboratory equipment designed specifically for the casting of high-heat alloys.
4. Use high speed lathes in metal finishing.

Don't:

1. Impair the luster of a base metal prosthesis by application of heavy pressure during polishing.
2. Cleanse chromium appliances in household bleaches.

AVAILABLE PRODUCTS

TYPE I, HIGH FUSING

ALLOY X-12, Federal Prosthetics, Inc.
DENTICON BERTRAM ALLOY, Denticon Dental Labs
DENTORIUM, Dentorium Products Co., Inc.
JD ALLOY: LG ALLOY, J. F. Jelenko & Co., Pennwalt Corp.
NEOLOY "N" PARTIAL ALLOY-REGULAR, Neoloy Products, Inc.
NIRANIUM, Niranium Corp.
NOBILIUM ALLOY, Nobilium Products, Inc.
PLATINORE, Allen Dynamics, Inc.
REGALLOY, Ransom & Randolph Co., Div. of Dentsply International, Inc.
STALITE CHROMIUM-COBALT ALLOY "S" INGOTS, Buffalo Dental Mfg. Co., Inc.
TICONIUM PREMIUM 100, Ticonium Co.
VITALLIUM, Howmedica, Inc., Dental Div.
VITALLIUM², Howmedica, Inc., Dental Div.
WIRONIUM, Williams Gold Refining Co., Inc.

WROUGHT WIRE

Precious Metal Wrought Wire

Gold wires have been used in the fabrication of prosthetic devices for more than 25 centuries. The continued usefulness of wrought structures in dental practice is derived mainly from their ability to transmit, store and resist forces.

COMPOSITION AND PROPERTIES: Precious alloys used in the manufacture of wire are complex materials containing gold, platinum, copper, palladium, silver, zinc and occasionally nickel. The specification for wrought gold wire alloys prescribes two grades of wire. One grade has a high precious metal content and is a white-colored wire, designated as Type II. The ranges in composition of Types I and II alloys are given in Table II.

Type I wire that complies with the specification requirement for composition contains no less than 75 percent gold and metals of the platinum group. The gold colored wire (Type II) must contain no less than 65 percent gold and metals of the platinum group.

Table II
Range of Percentage Composition of Wrought Gold Wire Alloys

Type of alloy	Component						
	Gold	Silver	Copper	Palladium	Platinum	Zinc	Nickel
I	53.6-63.2	8.5-12.4	10.2-15.2	0.0- 8.2	6.8-17.6	0.0-0.6	0.0-1.9
II	60.0-67.1	8.4-21.4	10.2-19.6	0.0-10.3	0.0- 6.5	0.0-1.7	0.0-6.2

Gold alloy wires obtain their properties from their composition and wrought structure. Pertinent physical properties of Type II wire are significantly lower than those of Type I. Nonetheless, the less expensive gold colored wire is used more frequently than the white gold wire.

USES: Wrought gold wires are used in the construction of orthodontic appliances and clasps for removable partial dentures. In addition, they may be used for retention pins for cast restorations.

DIRECTIONS FOR USE: Most gold wires, as supplied by the manufacturer, are annealed and normally do not require further annealing during fabrication. If, during processing, severe bending is necessary, then additional annealing may be required. The manufacturer's recommended annealing temperature should be followed. Care should be taken not to overheat the wire as overheating may destroy the wrought structure, thereby significantly reducing the properties of the wire.

Many wrought gold wires can be age hardened. The manufacturer's recommendation of temperature and time should be followed to obtain the best combination of high hardness, strength and ductility that can be developed in the alloy.

LIMITATIONS OF USE: Variations in the design of wrought wire clasps are limited. Generally, the circumferential-type clasp is the only design used. Because of its high resiliency, a wrought wire clasp may deliver insufficient bracing action.

EVALUATION PROGRAM: To be certified by the American Dental Association wrought wires of precious metals must conform to Specification No. 7 for Dental Wrought Gold Wire Alloy.

PRECIOUS METAL WROUGHT WIRE

Do:
1. Follow manufacturers' instructions for annealing.
2. Reanneal after completion of each major bend.
3. Use solder that fuses at about 100°C below the fusion temperature of the alloy being soldered.

Don't:
1. Nick or dent the wire.
2. Make bends too large, too sharp or too rapidly.

Base Metal Wrought Wire

In recent years, less expensive wrought stainless steels, nickel-chromium and cobalt-chromium alloys have largely displaced the gold-based materials in orthodontics. Excellent tarnish and corrosion resistance exhibited by the base metal wires is imparted principally by chromium.

USES: Wrought wires of base alloys are used primarily for orthodontic arch wires and surgical arch wires. They are also of value as retention pins for amalgam restorations and cores. To a limited extent, base wrought wires are used for clasps for transitional removable partial dentures.

DIRECTIONS FOR USE: The properties of base metal wrought wires can be altered adversely in bending. When repeated alteration of shape is necessary, annealing heat treatments should be used to relieve the deleterious effects of cold work. Proper stress-relief treatments decrease the possibility of fracture on further bending. For optimum results, annealing should be accomplished as prescribed by the manufacturer.

In soldering, special care must be exercised to prevent overheating of stainless steel wires. Prolonged exposure to temperatures in excess of 700°C (1,292°F) induces softening and reduces corrosion resistance. Property changes which accompany the recrystallization of stainless steel cannot be reversed by hardening heat treatments. The recrystallization temperatures of the nickel-chromium and cobalt-chromium wires are higher than the fusion temperatures of gold and silver solders. Therefore, on soldering, significant change in the mechanical properties of nickel-chromium and cobalt-chromium wires is unlikely.

BASE METAL WROUGHT WIRE

Do:
1. Follow the manufacturer's instructions for annealing.
2. Reanneal after completion of each major bend.

Don't:
1. Nick or dent wires.
2. Make bends too large, too sharp or too rapidly.

AVAILABLE PRODUCTS

TYPE I, HIGH PRECIOUS METAL

ADERER NO. 20 CLASP; NO. 4, J. Aderer, Inc.
CROWN HYLASTIC, General Refineries, Inc.
DEEPEP-HARD, Howmedica, Inc., Dental Div.
Elastic #4, #12, J.M. Ney Co.
JELENKO SUPER WIRE, J.F. Jelenko Co., Div. of Pennwalt Corp.

14K Lock & Ligature Wire, J.M. Ney Co.
Neylastic H.F. Wire, J.M. Ney Co.
MOWREY 12% WIRE, W.E. Mowrey Co.
Wilkinson A Wire; C Wire, Wilkinson Co.
WILLIAMS NO. 2, Williams Gold Refining Co.
Zepher Loops & Wires, J.M. Ney Co.

TYPE II, LOW PRECIOUS METALS

ADERER NO. 16; NO. 18 CLASP, J. Aderer, Inc.
Gold Color Elastic Wire, J.M. Ney Co.
MOWREY NO. 1 WIRE, W.E. Mowrey Co.
P.G.P. Wire, J.M. Ney Co.
P&I Wire, J.M. Ney Co.
Stainless Steel Clasp Wire, Williams Gold Refining Co., Inc.
STERNGOLD G-43, Sterndent Corp.
WILLIAMS NO. 4; NO. 70, Williams Gold Refining Co., Inc.
Wironit Wire, Williams Gold Refining Co., Inc.
Wirotom Clasp Wire, Williams Gold Refining Co., Inc.

OTHER PRODUCTS

Buffalo 5 Clasp Wire, Williams Gold Refining Co., Inc.
Crown Hylastic White Gold Wire, General Refineries, Inc.
Denture Clasp Wire, J.M. Ney Co.
Gold Case Staples, Williams Gold Refining Co., Inc.
Iridio-Platinum Wire, Williams Gold Refining Co., Inc.
Paliney Nos. 6 & 7, J.M. Ney Co.
Paloy Clasp Wire, Williams Gold Refining Co., Inc.
Unitek Nitinol Activ — Arch Wire, Unitek Corp.
Unitek HI-T II Wire, Unitek Corp.
Unitek Permachrome Wire, Unitek Corp.
Unitek Permachrome Resilient Wire, Unitek Corp.
Unitek Permachrome Unisil Wire, Unitek Corp.
Will Clasp Wire, Williams Gold Refining Co., Inc.

PREFORMED CROWNS

For the most part, preformed metal crowns are used for the fabrication of interim restorations. When properly fitted or contoured, these devices restore prepared and damaged teeth to function and assist in the maintenance of the integrity of soft and hard supporting tissues.

AVAILABLE PRODUCTS

Aluminum Shells, Williams Gold Refining Co., Inc.

Coin Gold Plate, J.M. Ney Co.

Getz Aluminum Shell Crowns, Teledyne Dental Products

Gold Plate, Williams Gold Refining Co., Inc.

Gold Shells, Williams Gold Refining Co., Inc.

Ion Brand Iso-form Temporary Crowns, 3M Company

Ion Brand Ni-Chro Permanent Molar Crowns, 3M Company

Ion Brand Polycarbonate Crown Sets, 3M Company

Lactona Polycarbonate Crowns, Lactona Corp.

Lactona Tin Crowns, Lactona Corp.

Tem-Crowns, L.D. Caulk Co.

22k Dark Color Plate, J.M. Ney Co.

Unitek Preformed Stainless Steel Primary Crowns, Anteriors, Cuspids, Molars, Unitek Corp.

Unitek Preformed Stainless Steel Permanent Crowns, Bicuspids, Molars, Unitek Corp.

Unitek Preformed Gold Anodized Aluminum Temporary Crowns, Unitek Corp.

Unitek Preformed Primary Polycarbonate Temporary Crown, Unitek Corp.

Unitek Preformed Polycarbonate Temporary Crown, Unitek Corp.

LITERATURE REFERENCES

1. Baum, L. The use of powdered gold in restorative dentistry: a preliminary report. J. South. Calif. Dent. Assoc. 12:392 Dec. 1962.

2. Baum, L. Gold foil (filling golds) in dental practice. Dent. Clin. N. Am., p. 199, Mar. 1965.

3. Lund, M.R., and Baum, L. Powdered gold as a restorative material. J. Prosthet. Dent. 13:1151 Nov.-Dec. 1963.

4. Cartwright, C.D. Powdered gold for single-surface restoration. J. Mich. Dent. Assoc. 47:122 Apr. 1965.

5. Mahan, J., and Charbeneau, G.T. A study of certain mechanical properties and the density of condensed specimens made from various forms of pure gold. J. Am. Acad. Gold Foil Oper. 8:6 Apr. 1965.

6. Richter, W.A., and Cantwell, K.R. A study of cohesive gold. J. Prosthet. Dent. 15:722 July-Aug. 1965.

7. Hollenback, G.M.; Lyons, N.E.; and Shell, J.S. A study of some of the physical properties of cohesive gold. J. Calif. Dent. Assoc. 42:9 Feb. 1966.

8. Shell, J.S., and Hollenback, G.M. Tensile strength and elongation of pure gold. J. South. Calif. Dent. Assoc. 34:219 Apr. 1966.

9. Burse, A.B., et al. Comparison of the in vitro and in vivo tarnish of three gold alloys. J. Biomed. Mater. Res. 6:267 May 1972.

10. Skinner, E.E. Effect of nucleation of gold alloys. IADR Program and Abstracts of Papers, Abstract 188, p. 85, 1966.

11. Nielsen, J.P., and Tuccillo, J.J. Grain size in cast gold alloys. J. Dent. Res. 45:964 May-June 1966.

12. Leinfelder, K.F.; O'Brien, W.J.; and Taylor, D.F. Hardening of dental gold-copper alloys. J. Dent. Res. 51:900 July-Aug. 1972.

13. Lane, J.G. The casting shrinkage as applied to inlays of gold and other dental uses. Dent. Digest 15:498 July 1909.

14. Shell, J.S. Gold castings–with special reference to cast gold inlays. JADA 10:187 Mar. 1923.

15. Coleman, R.L. Physical properties of dental materials (III). Progress report on research on the dental casting process. Dent. Cosmos 68:743 Aug. 1926.

16. Scheu, C.H. Precision casting utilizing the hygroscopic action of plaster in investment in making expanded molds. JADA 20:1205 July 1933.

17. Souder, W., and Paffenbarger, G.C. Physical properties of dental materials. Washington, D.C., Superintendent of Documents, 1942, p. 73.

18. Hollenback, G.M., and Skinner, E.W. Shrinkage during casting of gold and gold alloys. JADA 33:1931 Nov. 1946.

19. Shell, J.S., and Nielsen, J.P. Study of the bond between gold alloys and porcelain. J. Dent. Res. 41:1424 Nov.-Dec. 1962.

20. Lavine, M., and Custer, F. Variables affecting porcelain fused to gold bond. IADR Program and Abstracts of Papers, Abstract 140, 1963.

21. Civjan, S., et al. Determination of apparent bond strength of alloy-porcelain combinations. J. Dent. Res. 53(Special Issue):240, Abstract 742, Feb. 1974.

22. de Simon, L.B., et. al. Effect of laboratory procedures on alloy-porcelain bond strength. J. Dent. Res. 54(A):160, Abstract 459, Feb. 1975.

23. Leinfelder, K.F., et. al. Hardening of high-fusing gold alloys. J. Dent. Res. 45:392 Mar.-Apr. 1966.

24. Fairhurst, C.W., and Leinfelder, K.F. Heat treating porcelain-enameled restorations. J.

Prosthet. Dent. 16:554 May-June 1966.

25. Smith, L.L., et. al. Iron platinum hardening in casting golds for use with porcelain. J. Dent. Res. 49:283 Mar.-Apr. 1970.

26. Taylor, N.O. Precious metal alloy composition. U.S. Patent No. 1,965,012. Patented July 3, 1934.

27. Taylor, N.O. Precious metal alloy composition. U.S. Patent No. 1,987,452. Patented Jan. 8, 1935.

28. Huget, E.F., and Civjan, S. Status report on palladium-silver-based crown and bridge alloys. Prepared for the Council on Dental Materials and Devices. JADA 89:383 Aug. 1974.

29. Civjan, S., et. al. Further studies on gold alloys used in fabrication of porcelain-fused-to-metal restorations. JADA 90:659 Mar. 1975.

30. Huget, E.F.; Dvivedi, N.N.; and Cosner, H.E., Jr. Characterization of gold-palladium-silver and palladium-silver for ceramic-metal restorations. J. Prosthet. Dent. 36:58 July 1976.

31. Huget, E.F.; Dvivedi, N.N.; and Cosner, H.E., Jr. Characterization of Au-Pd-Ag and Pd-Ag alloys. J. Dent. Res. 54(A):161, Abstract 463, Feb. 1975.

32. Huget, E.F.; Dvivedi, N.N.; and Cosner, H.E., Jr. Characterization of "economy" crown and bridge alloys. J. Dent. Res. 55(B):B236, Abstract 697, Feb. 1976.

33. Huget E.F.; Dvivedi, N.N.; and Cosner, H.E., Jr. Properties of two nickel-chromium crown-and-bridge alloys for porcelain veneering. JADA 94:87 Jan. 1977.

34. Huget, E.F.; Civjan, S.; and Dvivedi, N.N. Characterization of two newly developed Ni-Cr alloys. J. Dent. Res. 53(Special Issue):238, Abstract 733, Feb. 1974.

35. Huget, E.F.; Vilca, J.M.; and Wall, R.M. Characterization of two base-metal crown-and-bridge alloys. J. Dent. Res. 56(B):B212, Abstract 642, June 1977.

36. Moffa, J.P., et al. An evaluation of non-precious alloys for use with porcelain veneers, Part 1. Physical properties. J. Prosthet. Dent. 30:424 Oct. 1973.

37. Huget E.F., and de Simon, L.B. Apparent bond strength of base metal-porcelain combinations. Transactions of the 3rd annual meeting, society for biomaterials and the 9th annual international biomaterials symposium, Vol. I. Paper No. 3, Apr. 1977.

38. Sced, I.R., and McLean, J.W. The strength of metal-ceramic bonds with base metals containing chromium. A preliminary report. Br. Dent. J. 132:232 Mar. 1972.

39. Sakar, N.K., and Greener, E.H. In vitro corrosion resistance of new dental alloys. Biomater. Med. Devices Artif. Organs 121:29, 1973.

40. Paffenbarger, G.C.; Caul, H.L.; and Dickson, G. Base metal alloys for oral restorations. JADA 30:852 June 1943.

41. Osborne, J. Improvement in cobalt-chromium alloys. Rev. Belg. Med. Dent. 21:303 July-Sept. 1966.

42. Moffa, J.P., and Jenkins, W.A. Status report on base-metal crown and bridge alloys. Prepared for the Council on Dental Materials and Devices. JADA 89:652 Sept. 1974.

43. Earnshaw, R. Fatigue tests on a dental cobalt-chromium alloy. Br. Dent. J. 110:341 May 1961.

44. Bates, J.F. Studies related to the fracture of partial dentures: flexural fatigue of a cobalt-chromium alloy. Br. Dent. J. 118:532 June 1965.

45. Harcourt, H.J.; Riddihough, M.; and Osborne, J. The properties of nickel-chromium casting alloys containing boron and silicon. Br. Dent. J. 129:419 Nov. 1970.

46. Evitmore, E., and Aleksiera, J. Some physical properties of the chrome-cobalt molybdenum and nickel-chromium alloys. Stomatologija (Sofia) 48:18, 1966.

47. Carter, T.J., and Kidd, J.N. The precision casting of cobalt-chromium alloy. Part 2. The influence of casting variables on microstructure properties. Br. Dent. J. 118:431 May 1965.

48. Asgar, K., and Peyton, F.A. Effect of casting conditions on some mechanical properties of cobalt-base alloys. J. Dent. Res. 40:73 Jan.-Feb. 1961.

49. Civjan, S., et al. Properties of two newly developed base metal dental casting alloys. IADR Program and Abstracts of Papers, Abstract 311, 1971.

50. Civjan, S., et al. Property optimization of dental casting alloys. J. Dent. Res. 53(Special Issue):237, Abstract 731, Feb. 1974.

51. Civjan, S., et al. Effects of heat treatment on mechanical properties of two nickel-chromium based alloys. J. Dent. Res. 51:1537 Nov.-Dec. 1972.

52. Phillips, R.W. Skinner's science of dental materials, ed. 7. Philadelphia, W.B. Saunders Co., 1973, p. 390.

CERAMICS

Porcelain teeth were conceived by Alexis Duchateau in an attempt to eliminate the staining, odors, and tastes due to ivory denture materials.[1] He worked with the Sevres China Factory and later with DeChemant. Dr. C. H. Land introduced what is considered to be the first successful porcelain jacket crown through the use of a platinum matrix which he patented in 1887. Around 1960, the current class of porcelain fused to metal materials was introduced and has become widely accepted.

COMPOSITION:[2-4] To define porcelains it is first necessary to define glass, since it is the major constituent of most dental porcelains. A glass is a non-crystalline solid with no long range molecular order. Inorganic glasses are produced from the melting of high fusing crystalline materials that form at their melting point a very viscous liquid. On cooling, the high viscosity which reduces molecular mobility makes recrystallization difficult. Thus, these materials, on cooling below their melting point, become more and more viscous until they are very hard, brittle solids without any sharp transition at any temperature from liquid to solid.

Dental porcelains are usually two or more phase systems. Typically, the matrix is glass with crystalline (unmelted) material dispersed throughout. The most important glass forming material is silica, usually in the quartz form. This is modified by additives to produce desired melting and physical properties. The crystalline material is often soluble in the molten glass at melting temperature. The degree of solution and the mechanical properties may vary with the time and temperature of the firing processes.

Dental porcelains range from 100 percent glass in the case of some porcelains for fusing to gold to about 50 percent glass in some high strength aluminous porcelains.

The early dental porcelains were derived from the conventional triaxial white ware formulations comprising clay, quartz, and feldspar. A wide variety of compositions are now available. There are also a wide variety of uses and fusing temperatures.

The glass phase usually comprises about 65 percent silica (SiO_2) with a significant portion of alumina (Al_2O_3), potassium oxide and sodium oxide (K_2O and Na_2O) as the balance. Minor ingredients include, among others, calcium oxide (CaO), lithium oxide (Li_2O), and boric oxide (B_2O_3). The porcelains are opacified by adding crystalline oxides of high index of refraction such as titanium dioxide (TiO_2), zirconium dioxide (ZrO_2) and colored oxides of cobalt, iron or chromium. For some uses such as the manufacture of porcelain teeth, ground powdered minerals are used in the molding of the article and then fired to the vitreous state as a finished tooth. For most laboratory uses such as for inlays, jacket crowns or porcelain bonded to metal, the raw materials are mixed together and fired to a high temperature to produce a melt that is subsequently ground to a fine powder for use in a dental laboratory.

Dental porcelains are classified by their fusion temperature as shown in Table I.

Table I.
Classification of Dental Porcelains

Class	Fusion Temperature
High fusing	1288-1371°C (2350-2500°F)
Medium fusing	1093-1260°C (2000-2300°F)
Low fusing	871-1066°C (1600-1950°F)

Pigments used in porcelains do not necessarily match the color adsorption curves of the pigments of natural teeth. Thus there may be metamerism (failure to match in all lights).

PROPERTIES AND PRECAUTIONS:[1,4] Porcelain materials have yields (elongations) of less than 0.10 percent and because of flaws on the surface and in the interior that are invariably present, they are much weaker in tension than in compression. Thus, any residual stresses should be minimized or kept slightly on a compressive side. When several layers are used or when porcelain is bonded to metal, the matching of the coefficients of expansion is extremely important.

A ceramic (or ceramic fused to gold) restoration must be rigid enough to withstand forces applied to it without appreciable strain or there will be fracture of the porcelain. In the case of multi-unit bridges, torsion must be restricted or eliminated by design to avoid failure.

Dental porcelains have been found to be biologically inert for oral use.

Of great significance and importance are the esthetic properties of the material, including the colorability and translucency. Porcelain materials that have been used in dentistry for many years can be readily colored and are now available in high translucency formulations. The composition of the enamel-simulating and the dentin-simulating materials are restricted in part by their translucency. The use of minerals with a large difference of index of refraction must be minimized. Consequently, techniques to strengthen dental porcelains by adding reinforcement crystalline materials of different indices of refraction or baking porcelain onto metal has compromised the esthetics. In the incisal third of a natural tooth there is about 70 percent light transmission. There is also a considerable degree of light transmission in the interproximal zones.[1,5]

Methods of Strengthening Dental Porcelains:[2,6] Methods used to increase the strength of glasses include the following:

a) Development of a finely dispersed crystalline phase through appropriate nucleating and heat treating techniques. To date this is largely experimental.

b) Introduction of a crystalline phase by mixing materials such as fine grain alumina with the glass powder and then fusing. If the bond of the two phases is good and the coefficients of expansion are closely matched, a strong crystalline phase will significantly increase the strength of the porcelain. This technique has been used in the aluminous porcelains. Unfortunately, the more alumina that is added, the less the translucency of the material, so that a compromise between strength and translucency must be made.

c) A glaze that is added with a slightly lower coefficient of expansion will produce a surface under compressive stress.

d) The technique of altering the surface through ion exchange also can produce a surface under a compressive stress.

Fabrication Processes: For dental laboratory procedures powders are applied to a die usually employing an aqueous phase with some additives that will improve the wetting ability. The material is condensed by vibration, blotting with paper, or by use of a spatula.

For artificial tooth manufacture, gums, starches, or other thickening agents are added to provide a temporary binder to facilitate the handling of a molded biscuit tooth prior to firing.

Teeth are molded in metal molds. Thus a "biscuit" tooth that is oversized is formed from the mold. On firing this may shrink between 15 and 20 percent linearly as the grains coalesce in much the same fashion as in the firing of crown and bridge restorations.

Fusion or Firing Techniques:[4,7,8] In the firing operation it is necessary to remove water at a rate sufficiently slow to prevent damage due to build-up of steam pressure.

Firing of porcelain restorations at normal atmospheric pressure to produce a form that is anatomically correct will result in about 5 percent internal porosity. If the porcelain is fired under a vacuum of about 50 mm of mercury up to about the peak temperature and then atmospheric air pressure is allowed to enter the furnace, the porosity will be less than 1 percent. This same pressure differential ratio and porosity reduction can be developed by employing atmospheric pressure during the initial firing stages and then introducing superatmospheric pressure at about the peak temperature with continuation through the cooling stages.

The final firing step should produce a sufficient glaze in the surface of the restoration. This may be accomplished by self glazing of the porcelains used or by the addition of a thin layer of a lower fusing glaze to the surface.

The shrinkage on firing is of the order of 30 to 50 percent by volume. For the manufacture of denture teeth, oversized molds are used to compensate for this. In the construction of crowns it is necessary to overbuild and to add additional porcelain in subsequent bakes. The fusion of porcelains is caused by the surface tension between particles that are in contact; the rate of fusion depends on the viscosity which in turn is temperature dependent. Thus, the degree of gloss is affected not only by the temperature but by the time exposed to that temperature. The rate of heating, the dwell and the rate of cooling are all critical.

Care must be exercised not to overheat because if the viscosity is sufficiently reduced or the firing time sufficiently long, the article will slump and lose shape.

PORCELAIN TEETH[9]

Porcelain artificial teeth are available in a wide range of molds and shades to provide a suitable selection for the individual patient. The posterior teeth are also available in a number of cusp designs. Some of the anterior lines include "characterization" such as stains, decalcified areas, and fillings.

Posterior teeth are retained on the organic denture bases by an undercut hole. This is molded into the tooth and escape vents are usually drilled to allow the denture base material to displace air.

Anterior teeth, because of their size, cannot use the same type of retention. Therefore, they depend on gold clad nickel pins that are soldered into baked-in anchorages. Thus, when the tooth is molded, platinum alloy anchorages are molded into the tooth and fired with it. Subsequently, the gold pin is soldered with a silver alloy solder. The pins have heads which provide a mechanical anchorage in the denture base material.

Esthetically, porcelain artificial teeth are highly satisfactory. They are free from staining, and abrasion is virtually no problem. The two most often defects are (1) the brittleness or tendency to fracture, either across the pins in the anterior teeth or cusp sections in the posterior teeth, and (2) the click that comes through premature striking of the teeth.

The co-use of flat plane porcelain posterior teeth in one arch opposing flat plane plastic teeth in the other has been proposed as a means of minimizing the "click" of all porcelain teeth and reducing the fracture when opposing porcelain teeth are used. The abrasion resistance of the combination is also reported to be better than that of opposing plastic teeth because of the reduced coefficient of friction between the porcelain and plastic teeth when contrasted to the all plastic combination.

DIRECTIONS FOR USE: Porcelain denture teeth when ground for adjustments should be finished to an approximation of the fired glaze by using a rubber wheel and then polishing with the appropriate polishing media. This will minimize retention of plaque and, more importantly, minimize abrasion and damage to opposing occlusal surfaces.

Deflasking of a processed denture should be done with care to avoid fracture of the porcelain teeth. Essentially this requires the use of a deflasking press and the avoidance of any wedging action in opening the mold. Further, the use of a "topping" in the original flasking will allow the top layer investment to be removed readily and show precisely the incisal and occlusal surfaces of the teeth.

AVAILABLE PRODUCTS

Check-Bite Kits Positive Centric Teeth, Charles Development Co.
Imperial Facing, H.D. Justi Co., Div. of Williams Gold Refining Co., Inc.
Kenson Porcelain Anterior Teeth, Kenson Mfg. Co.
Kenson Porcelain Posterior Teeth, Kenson Mfg. Co.
Myerson's Aesthetic Multi-fired Anterior Teeth, Myerson Tooth Corp.
Myerson and Sears Multi-fired Posterior Teeth, Myerson Tooth Corp.
Myerson's Modern Blend Multi-fired Anterior Teeth, Myerson Tooth Corp.
Myerson's Porcelain Special Multi-fired Anterior Teeth, Myerson Tooth Corp.
Myerson's Synchronized Posterior Teeth, Myerson Tooth Corp.
Naturadent Porcelain Denture Teeth, Charles B. Schwed Co., Inc.

Steele's Facings, Columbus Dental Co.
Trubyte Bioblend; Bioform; New Hue, Vacuum-fired; New Hue; Solila-Vac Anteriors, Dentsply International
Trubyte New Hue 33°; New Hue 20°; Fournet Posteriors, Dentsply International
Trubyte 33° Vacuum-fired; Pilkington-Turner 30°; 20° Vacuum-fired; Functional Vacuum Fired; Rational Vacuum-fired; Solila Vac Posteriors, Dentsply International
Trubyte Vacuum-fired Long Pointed Pin Facings, Dentsply International
Vita Lumin Vacuum Porcelain Teeth, Unitek Corp.
Vita Lumin Acryl-V Acrylic Teeth, Unitek Corp.
Vita Lumin Acryl-V Markant Teeth, Unitek Corp.

JACKET CROWNS [5,10-14]

The use of alumina and aluminous porcelain have expanded the capability of dental porcelains. Aluminous porcelain is significantly stronger than regular dental porcelain and thereby improves the chances for success of a porcelain jacket. The prefered alumina pieces provide very high strength reinforcement to local areas of weakness.

Both alumina and high alumina content aluminous porcelains are opaque and must be used in conjunction with compatible conventional dental porcelains of closely matched coefficients of expansion. For esthetic reasons, aluminous porcelain of high alumina content is used lingually and for the core of a jacket. The prefered alumina pieces also are used lingually or at interproximal junctures.

Through the use of alumina and aluminous porcelain, esthetically pleasing jackets and bridges of a few teeth can be made without metal.

McLean and Hughes have reported on two approaches toward improving the strength of a dental porcelain restoration.[6]

1. The first of these is through the use of a reinforcing piece of prefired alumina. In this case, a tube or disc of alumina which can be as much as ten times as strong as dental porcelain, is inserted in the restoration during the fabrication phase and

significantly reinforces the material. For instance, in an anterior jacket, the usual weak point is in the lingual portion. If a disc of alumina is placed in the lingual section, it will help prevent fracture.

2. The second approach involves mixing into the dental porcelain about 40 to 50 percent of fine granulated alumina. Compared to strengths for conventional porcelain of about 10,000 psi, aluminous porcelain can be made in the 20,000 to 25,000 psi range. The prefired alumina referred to above can approach 100,000 psi in strength.

Aluminous porcelain has less pyroplastic flow than regular dental porcelain, hence, it is not distorted as much by overfiring. In its normal use, it is the first layer fired. Thus, this ability to withstand repeated firings is important.

Because of the difference of coefficient of expansion between gold alloys and alumina, aluminous porcelain is not used in conjunction with gold alloys.

A technique has been reported wherein aluminous porcelain is bonded to pure platinum foil through the application of a tin plate to the platinum foil of 0.2 to 2 microns. In the firing operation the tin oxidizes and a bond to the porcelain is developed. The purpose of this is to minimize the microcracks at the metal-porcelain interface and thus strengthen the interior surfaces of a porcelain jacket. This technique then allows a significant reduction of the metal thickness required when porcelain is fused to gold and thereby increases the thickness of porcelain, allowing the use of a more translucent core material than the opaque that is required for gold and nonprecious bake-on alloy copings.

Discs fired of aluminous porcelain bonded to platinum foil that have been electroplated with the tin as described above, show a strength improvement of about 80 percent in contrast to an aluminous porcelain disc without the metal foil.

DIRECTIONS FOR USE:[15] The technique developed for construction of the aluminous porcelain crown bonded to a tin plated foil includes the following steps:

1. Two layers of platinum foil are adapted to a die. The inner foil provides a matrix space for cementing and is removed after the fusing of the porcelain. The outer foil is to be bonded to the crown.

2. The outer foil is tin plated to produce a thickness of tin of about 2 microns.

3. Aluminous porcelains or porcelains of similar coefficients of expansion (about $8.0 \times 10^{-6}/°C$) are then baked onto the tin plated outer foil in the normal fashion.

AVAILABLE PRODUCTS

Air Fired Incisal, Ceramco, Inc.
B Vacuum Porcelain, Ceramco, Inc.
Ceramco Glaze, Ceramco, Inc.
Ceramco Low Temperature Glaze, Ceramco, Inc.
Ceramco Stain System Stain Wet; Stain Set; Sta-Wet, Ceramco, Inc.
G Vacuum Porcelain, Ceramco, Inc.
Liquidisk, Williams Gold Refining Co., Inc.
Neydium Porcelain, J.M. Ney Co.
N.H. Vacuum Porcelain, Ceramco, Inc.
Palladium Foil, J.M. Ney Co.
Platinum Foil, Williams Gold Refining Co., Inc.
Prox-O-Pake Porcelain, Ceramco, Inc.
1600 Porcelain, Ceramco, Inc.
Steele's Aluminous Porcelain, Columbus Dental Co.
Tissue Tint Porcelain, Ceramco, Inc.
Vita Vitadur-N Aluminous Porcelain, Unitek Corp.
Will-Ceram Porcelain, Williams Gold Refining Co., Inc.

PORCELAIN INLAYS[16-20]

Porcelain inlays, introduced in 1862, are in many ways an excellent restorative filling material. Techniques include use of the platinum foil matrix for fabrication and refractory models. With these techniques it has been found that the success of the inlay depends to a great extent on the cementing medium. The traditional silicate cements and zinc oxyphosphate both show a cement line and lack of complete seal when tested with thermal cycling. A porcelain inlay silane treated and cemented in place with composite resin was reported as having improved esthetic appearance and good resistance to leakage during thermal cycling.

In all porcelain inlay techniques the procedure is considerably more involved than the use of composite resins and this has sharply limited their use.

PORCELAIN FUSED-TO-METAL[3,21-27]

Requirements for the bond between porcelain and metal include a matched or nearly matched coefficient of expansion. The porcelain should not change significantly in repeated bakes, and the porcelain should fuse at a low enough tension temperature such that the metal does not sag.

Explanations of the porcelain to metal bond include the proposition that there is a chemical reaction and that a primary chemical bond develops at the interface. There is also the surface energy theory which postulates that the wetting of the surface can produce a strong bond via Van der Waal's bonds. Finally, a mechanical type of bond has been proposed involving the penetration of the glass into the crevices on the metallic surface.

The presence of base metal elements in both porcelain and metal that can diffuse to the surface and react, aid in the formation of a bond. The factors that should be considered in the bonding of porcelain to metal include preoxidation procedures, firing time and temperature, initial concentrations of active diffusing elements in both the porcelain and metal, the oxidation-reduction behavior between the metal and the ceramic, the rate of solution and the saturation point of the metal oxide in the ceramic and furnace atmosphere.

Bonding dental porcelain to nickel chrome alloys is technique sensitive. For instance, too high a vacuum or a reducing atmosphere results in an undesirable reaction between the alloy and porcelain. Further, it was shown that when chromic oxide is dissolved by the porcelain, the thermal expansion coefficient of the porcelain interface layer is reduced. Nickel oxide behaves similarly but at a slower rate. It was proposed that this reduction of the coefficient of expansion of the bonding layer of the porcelain would introduce stresses that would weaken the bond.

DIRECTIONS FOR USE:[5,26,28-32] It has been repeatedly suggested by many authors and by instructions of manufacturers that all surfaces should be rounded to avoid sharp contours in the metal design. Thus in the preparation of the tooth for receiving the metal coping, this factor should be kept in mind. It has been recommended for anterior teeth to remove about 2 mm in the incisal area and if full coverage is to be used in the posterior teeth, to remove about 1½ mm in the occlusal area. The porcelain layer should not exceed 1½ to 2 mm for the best compromise of strength and esthetics. In soldering the porcelain after firing, it is important not to have the flux come in contact with the porcelain.

Important in the judgment of color are the light source characteristics, the angle of incidence of the light to the tooth, and the movement of the light. Color matching should be done with short interval views of no more than 5 seconds to avoid fatigue. Usually a combination of shade matching in north light, incandescent light and normal fluorescent lighting is considered to approach natural daylight. The matching of natural teeth requires more than a simple determination of the shade (that is, the definition of the three dimensions of color— hue, value, and chroma). The definition must also include the blending of the enamel and dentin, in other words, the relative overlay that is desired for the enamel-simulating material. It also must include a prescription defining the varied effects present in the natural tooth such as gingival staining, check lines, and decalcified areas, among others.

Important in the prescription for the restoration is the form and surface texture of the natural tooth. Form is important not only because it is one of the most visible characteristics of the natural tooth but also because the form and surface characteristics significantly affect the reflection of incident light.

The illusion of depth in bridge work utilizing porcelain fused to metal can be produced by darkening the shade interproximally.

It has been recommended that for optimizing the esthetics of restorations made with porcelain fused to metal sufficient depth be provided in the interproximal zones. This would suggest the use of a shoulder preparation or modified shoulder preparation.

Corrections in color can be made by applying a surface stain to a porcelain restoration. It should be borne in mind that surface stains darken a tooth or make it greyer. Thus when in doubt, a shade should be selected to be slightly light and slightly less grey than the goal.

In order to minimize shrinkage, porosity, and voids, it is necessary to condense the ceramic powder while molding it to the form of the restoration. This is accomplished by vibration, the use of capillary forces, and spatulation or combinations of these.

Manufacturers' time-temperature schedules and furnace atmosphere conditions should be followed carefully. These will affect not only the degree of fusion and the maintenance of shape but also the bond between the porcelain and the metal, primarily because of variations in the degree of oxidation.

LIMITATIONS OF USE:[2,3,5,21,33-43] The bonding of porcelain to the metal copings is technique sensitive, particularly in the case of the base metal alloys. This requires careful technique in the casting, the treatment of the casting, and the baking techniques.

In the case of jacket crowns, normal masticating loads tending to seat the jacket will set up circumferential tensile stresses. The material must have adequate strength and cross section to withstand these.

Because of the nature of the brittle failure of porcelain caused by static fatigue, restorations should be free of undercuts and bridge work should seat without any torsional stresses. As there is a significant stress concentration at the porcelain-metal junction, it is desirable to avoid having contact points at this junction. If porcelain occluding surfaces are used in posterior restorations, there may be increased wear on opposing surfaces.

With repeated baking it is possible to change the crystalline content of a porcelain that will alter its opacity and thermal expansion. Manufacturers' instructions usually designed to minimize the high temperature exposure should be followed, including the prescribed rate of heating and cooling.

CERAMICS[3,9,21,24,29,31,32,38-44]

Do:

1. Follow the manufacturer's firing instructions for time, temperature and prescribed rate of heating and cooling.
2. Follow carefully casting metal preparation and baking techniques.
3. Allow sufficient time after building up the porcelain for a jacket or a crown to dry prior to firing to avoid damage to the shape through steam pressure.
4. Reduce teeth sufficiently to provide the space for the metal substructure and for the bulk of porcelain required to achieve the desired shade match without overcontouring the crowns.

5. Adjust occlusion by selective grinding before tooth preparation to eliminate interferences that could apply undue stress during excursive movements.

6. Remove tooth structure uniformly from the coronal surfaces of abutment teeth such that they will be contoured as miniatures of the original natural teeth. Porcelain can then be applied in uniform layers to minimize stress development during firing cycles.

7. Reduce tooth structure to provide the required clearance for metal substructures strong enough to resist deformation under mastication forces.

8. Design the restoration so that it is free of undercuts and in the case of bridge work so that it will seat without torsional stresses.

9. Design metal framework so that it minimizes tension forces on the porcelain.

10. Avoid having contact points at the porcelain-metal junction.

11. Use gold occluding surfaces if wear on opposing surfaces is considered a problem.

12. Avoid fatigue in color matching by use of a series of short interval views of no more than 5 seconds.

13. Bear in mind that stain corrections will darken a tooth or make it greyer. Thus any error in shade selection should be in the direction of being slightly light and slightly less grey.

14. Use, if possible, in shade determination, a combination of three determinations in north day light, incandescent and fluorescent lighting. Major reflective surfaces such as ceilings and walls should be neutral or a light grey.

15. Encourage patients to wear only natural shade cosmetics to appointments. Mask or remove any unnatural shade cosmetics if they are worn, as they might interfere with shade selection.

16. Make several shade determinations before tooth preparation. If the desired shade falls between two shade tabs, choose the lighter shade.

17. Include in the prescription such characteristics of patient as sex, age, and hair, eye, and skin colors.

18. Send diagnostic casts as visual aids to indicate the location of any characterizing features, such as cracks, stains, or simulated restorations.

19. Provide drawings to show the desired body and incisal shade distributions and the location of characterizing features not indicated on study casts.

Don't:

1. Permit excessive oxidation to occur through overfiring and in the preparation of the metal.

2. Use nickel-containing alloys if a patient has nickel allergies or sensitivities.

3. Contaminate the metal surface, particularly by oil from fingers, prior to firing the porcelain.

4. Overheat porcelain in grinding. The use of a heatless stone or lubricant can avoid this.

5. Design abutment restorations with sharp angles at the porcelain-to-metal junction.

6. Allow soldering fluxes to come in contact with the porcelain during soldering procedures.

7. Attempt shade selections under poor lighting conditions such as may exist on overcast days or when eyes are fatigued.

EVALUATION PROGRAM: The American Dental Association Specification No. 52 applies to all dental porcelains, including artificial teeth, jacket crown porcelains, and bake-on porcelains. Specifically, this limits the use of uranium as a fluorescing agent to 300 ppm. Two other specifications are being developed through the International Standards Organization. One of these is for porcelain artificial teeth, and the other for porcelains for use in jackets and inlays. These specifications have not been internationally accepted to date.

LITERATURE REFERENCES

1. Sproull, R. C. The history of porcelain. In Yamada, H. N. (ed.) Dental porcelain: The state of the art—1977. Los Angeles, University of Southern California School of Dentistry, p. 17, 1977.

2. Binns, D. B. The physical and chemical properties of porcelain. In Yamada, H. N. (ed.) Dental porcelain: The state of the art—1977. Los Angeles, University of Southern California School of Dentistry, p. 25, 1977.

3. Lacy, A. M. The chemical nature of dental porcelain. In Yamada, H. N. (ed.) Dental porcelain: The state of the art—1977. Los Angeles, University of Southern California School of Dentistry, p. 47, 1977.

4. O'Brien, W. J. Dental porcelains. In Dental materials review. Ann Arbor, University of Michigan, p. 123, 1977.

5. McLean, J. W. Introduction: The state of the art and its problems. In Yamada, H. N. (ed.) Dental porcelain: The state of the art—1977. Los Angeles, University of Southern California School of Dentistry, p. 11, 1977.

6. McLean, J. W., and Hughes, T. H. The reinforcement of dental porcelain with ceramic oxides. Br. Dent. J. 119:251 Sept.1965.

7. Vines, R. F., and Semmelman, J. O. Densification of dental porcelains. J. Dent. Res. 36:950 Dec.1957.

8. Meyer, J. M.; O'Brien, W. J.; and Yu, R. Sintering behavior of porcelain enamels. J. Dent. Res. 55:696 July-Aug. 1976.

9. Myerson, R. L. Use of porcelain and plastic teeth in opposing complete dentures. J. Prosthet. Dent.7:625 Sept.1957.

10. McLean, J. W. High-alumina ceramics for bridge pontic construction. Br. Dent. J. 123:571 Dec. 1967.

11. McLean, J. W., and Sced, I. R. The bonded alumina crown. I. The bonding of platinum to aluminous dental porcelain using tin-oxide coatings. Austr. Dent. J. 21:119, 1976.

12. McLean, J. W.; Kedge, M. I.; and Hubbard, J. R. The bonded alumina crown. 2. Construction using the tin-foil technique. Austr. Dent. J. 21: 262, 1976.

13. Sced, I. R.; McLean, J. W.; and Hotz, P. The strengthening of aluminous porcelain with bonded platinum foils. J. Dent. Res. 56:1067 Sept. 1977.

14. McLean, J. W., and Sced, I. R. The bonded alumina crown. I. The bonding of platinum to aluminous dental porcelain using tin oxide coatings. Austr. Dent. J. 21:119 Apr. 1976

15. McLean, J. W.; Kedge, M. I.; and Hubbard, J. R. The bonded alumina crown. 2. Construction using the tin-foil technique. Austr. Dent. J. 21:262 June 1976.

16. Myerson, R. L., and Dogan, I. L. The role of the porcelain inlay in restorative dentistry. J. Biomed. Mat. Res. Symp. No. 2 (Part 2), p. 405, 1972.

17. McGehee, W. H. O.; True, H. A.; and Inskipp, E. F. A textbook of operative dentistry. New York, McGraw-Hill, p. 498, 1956.

18. Charbeneau, G. T. An evaluation of porcelain inlay investment materials and a reverse platinum matrix technic. JADA 75:142 July 1967.

19. Smith, B. B. Porcelain inlays for the general practitioner. Dent. Clin. N. Am., p. 191, Mar. 1967.

20. Christensen, G. J., et al. Accuracy of fit of direct-firing porcelain inlays. J. Prosthet. Dent. 22:46 July 1969.

21. McLean, J. W. Physical and chemical characteristics of alloys used for ceramic bonding. In Yamada, H. N. (ed.) Dental porcelain: The state of the art—1977. Los Angeles, University of Southern California School of Dentistry, p. 79, 1977.

22. Shell, J. S., and Nielson, J. P. Study of the bond between gold alloys and porcelain. J. Dent. Res. 41:1424 Nov.-Dec. 1962.

23. O'Brien, W. J., and Ryge, G. Contact angles of drops of enamels on metals. J. Prosthet. Dent. 15:1094 Nov.-Dec. 1965.

24. McLean, J. W., and Sced, I. R. Bonding of dental porcelain to metal, II. The base metal alloy porcelain bond. Trans. J. Br. Ceram. Soc. 72:235 July 1973.

25. Kelley, M.; Asgar, K.; and O'Brien, W. J. Tensile strength determination of the interface between porcelain fused to gold. J. Biomed. Mat. Res. 3:403 Sept.1969.

26. Anusavice, K. J.; Horner, J. A.; and Fairhurst, C. W. Adherence controlling elements in ceramic-metal systems. I. Precious alloys. J. Dent. Res. 56:1045 Sept. 1977.

27. Anusavice, K. J.; Ringle, R. D.; and Fairhurst, C. W. Adherence controlling elements in ceramic-metal systems. II. Non-precious alloys. J. Dent. Res. 56:1053 Sept. 1977.

28. Berger, R. P. The art of dental ceramic sculpturing. In Yamada, H. N. (ed.) Dental porcelain: The state of the art—1977. Los Angeles, University of Southern California School of Dentistry, p. 229, 1977.

29. Braze, G. W. Achieving esthetic effects through internal characterization. In Yamada, H. N. (ed.) Dental porcelain: The state of the art—1977. Los Angeles, University of Southern California School of Dentistry, p. 237, 1977.

30. Eissman, J. Visual perception and tooth contour. In Yamada, H. N. (ed.) Dental porcelain: The state of the art —1977. Los Angeles, University of Southern California School of Dentistry, p. 297, 1977.

31. Pincus, C. L. Color and esthetics. In Yamada, H. N. (ed.) Dental porcelain: The state of the art—1977. Los Angeles, University of Southern California School of Dentistry, p. 303, 1977.

32. Preston, J. D. Color and esthetics. In Yamada, H. N. (ed.) Dental porcelain: The state of the art—1977. Los Angeles, University of Southern California School of Dentistry, p. 307, 1977.

33. Lehman, M. L., and Hampson, E. L. Study of strain patterns in jacket crowns on anterior teeth resulting from different tooth preparations. Br. Dent. J. 113:337 Nov. 1962.

34. El-Ebrashi, M. K.; Craig, R. G.; Peyton, F. A. Experimental stress analysis of dental restorations, Part III. The concept of the geometry of proximal margins. J. Prosthet. Dent. 22:333 Sept. 1969.

35. Culpepper, W. D. A comparative study of shade-matching procedures. J. Prosthet. Dent. 24:166 Aug. 1970.

36. Mariu, M. J. Japan. Stomatological Soc. 35:412, 1963.

37. Sproull, R. C. Color matching in dentistry. II. Practical applications of the organization of color. J. Prosthet. Dent. 29:566 May 1973.

38. Barreto, M. T. Porcelain-fused-to-metal framework design. In Yamada, H. N. (ed.) Dental porcelain: The state of the art—1977. Los Angeles, University of Southern California School of Dentistry, p. 181, 1977.

39. Nally, J. N.; Farah, J. W.; and Craig, R. G. Experimental stress analysis of dental restorations. Part IX. Two-dimensional photoelastic stress analysis of porcelain-bonded-to-gold crowns. J. Prosthet. Dent. 25:307, 1971.

40. Craig, R. G.; El-Ebrashi, M. K.; and Peyton, F. A. Stress distribution in porcelain-fused-to-gold crowns and preparations constructed with photoelastic plastics. J. Dent. Res. 50:1278, 1971.

41. Hobo, S., and Shillingburg, H. T. Porcelain-fused-to-metal: Tooth preparation and coping design. J. Prosthet. Dent. 31:28, 1973.

42. Craig, R.G.; El-Ebrashi, M. K.; and Farah, J. W. Stress distribution in photoelastic models of transverse sections of porcelain-fused-to-gold crowns and preparations. J. Dent. Res. 52:1060 Oct. 1973.

43. Hobo, S., and Shillingburg, H. T. Porcelain-fused-to-metal: Framework design. In Yamada, H. N. (ed.) Dental porcelain: The state of the art—1977. Los Angeles, University of Southern California School of Dentistry, p. 195, 1977.

44. Cascone, P. J. The theory of bonding for porcelain-to-metal systems. In Yamada, H. N. (ed.) Dental porcelain: The state of the art—1977. Los Angeles, University of Southern California School of Dentistry, p. 109, 1977.

CEMENTS

Historically, cement has been used in dentistry for nearly a century. There has been a new interest in cements over the last few years and a number of new formulations have been entering the market. Much effort and research has been directed toward cements but they are, in general, far from ideal. Dental cements usually consist of a powder and liquid which, when mixed, form a plastic mass that subsequently sets or hardens. All cements shrink on setting, all have relatively poor mechanical properties, and some are irritants to the pulp. Notwithstanding their defects, cements have been used for decades as bases and luting agents and will continue to be important in the dentist's armamentarium.

ZINC OXIDE-EUGENOL CEMENT

COMPOSITION AND PROPERTIES: Zinc oxide-eugenol (ZOE) cement, with a pH of 7 to 8, is recognized as the least irritating of the dental cements, and the most palliative to the pulp. Although the eugenol itself may act as an obtundent, it is also possible that the sedative effect on the pulp may be related to the ability of ZOE initially to seal the cavity preparation. The ingress of saliva and bacterial organisms, which further irritates the pulp at a critical time of cavity preparation, is reduced, and postoperative sensitivity is thus abated.

Attempts to improve zinc oxide-eugenol cements include adding hydrogenated rosin[1] which improves the working and handling characteristics of the cement as well as the compressive strength. In addition, the rosin reduces the solubility of the cement.[2] The addition of plastics such as poly(methyl methacrylate)[3] and polystyrene[4] increases the strength. The best agents to increase the strength are orthoethoxybenzoic acid (EBA)[5] and alumina.[6]

USES: ZOE and reinforced ZOE products are available for use as bases, temporary restorations, root canal fillings, surgical dressings and luting agents.

DIRECTIONS FOR USE: Since the dental market provides such a variety of cements, it is important to follow carefully the manufacturer's instructions. It is most important to choose the cement that is specifically designed for the use intended.

In recent years, the increasing use of fixed prostheses for reconstruction of mutilated dentitions has increased the number of restorations on sound teeth with large areas of exposed dentin. The problems of cementing temporary restorations and temporarily cementing finished prostheses have directed attention more closely to the physical qualities of the zinc oxide-eugenol cements which are relatively bland to the pulp. The retention of restorations for the required time without undue difficulties of removal when necessary is related to the compressive strength of the cement. Suitable compressive strength for various clinical situations have been defined and the selection of an appropriate cement is less empirical as a result.[7-9] Fortified experimental zinc oxide-eugenol cements have been prepared with one week compressive strengths up to 103.4 MN/m^2 (15,000 psi). Current clinical evaluation of one experimental cement with a compressive strength between 55.1 MN/m^2 (8,000 psi) and 63.4 MN/m^2 (9,000 psi) showed it suitable for the final cementation of fixed prostheses.[10]

These cements eliminate most of the post-cementation problems experienced with zinc phosphate cements such as pulp irritation or pulp death. A status report on the zinc oxide-eugenol cements was published by the Council on Dental Materials, Instruments and Equipment.[11]

LIMITATIONS OF USE: Many of the improved ZOE materials have been designed for a specific use. It is important to select a product while recognizing its limitations. Film thickness is generally a limitation for use as a luting agent.

Because of their disintegration in water, zinc oxide-eugenol cements require additional clinical testing before they are recommended for routine use as a permanent cementing medium.

EVALUATION PROGRAM: The American Dental Association's specification program includes No. 30 for zinc oxide-eugenol type restorative materials. There are acceptance programs for zinc oxide-eugenol cements and zinc oxide-eugenol EBA cements.

ZINC OXIDE AND EUGENOL CEMENT

Do:
1. Choose carefully the type of cement for each use.
2. Use an alumina-EBA for permanent cementation.
3. Use a "softer" cement for temporary cementation.
4. Follow the manufacturer's instructions.

Don't:
1. Use an unreinforced ZOE for a base.
2. Try to use one type for all purposes.
3. Intermix powders and liquids from different products.
4. Try to mix too small a portion.

AVAILABLE PRODUCTS

CAULK ZOE B & T, L.D. Caulk Co., Div. of Dentsply International, Inc.

CAULK ZOE 2200, L.D. Caulk Co., Div. of Dentsply International, Inc.

CAVITEC, Kerr Mfg. Co., Div. of Sybron Corp.

Dentin, Moyco Industries, Inc.

Eugenol, Pulpdent Corp. of America

FYNAL, L.D. Caulk Co., Div. of Dentsply International, Inc.

Healthco Eugenol, Healthco, Inc.

IRM, L.D. Caulk Co., Div. of Dentsply International, Inc.

Opotow After-Prep Cement, Teledyne Dental Products

Opotow Alumina EBA Cement, Teledyne Dental Products

Opotow EBA Cement, Teledyne Dental Products

Opotow Temporary Cement, Teledyne Dental Products

Pulprotex, L.D. Caulk Co., Div. of Dentsply International, Inc.

Scutabond, Premier Dental Products Co.

Temp-Bond, Kerr Mfg. Co., Div. of Sybron Corp.

ZABECEM, L.D. Caulk Co., Div. of Dentsply International, Inc.

Zinc Oxide, Pulpdent Corp. of America

ZINC OXIDE-ROSIN-EUGENOL CEMENT WITH MENTROL AND THYMOL IODIDE, Moyco Industries, Inc.

ZOE Powder, Moyco Industries, Inc.

ZOE Cement No. 2 with Fiber, S.S. White Dental Products International, Div. of Pennwalt Corp.

ZOE TEMPORARY CEMENT, L.D. Caulk Co., Div. of Dentsply International, Inc.

ZOGENOL, Stratford-Cookson Co.

ZINC PHOSPHATE CEMENTS

COMPOSITION AND PROPERTIES: Zinc phosphate cement powders consist of calcined zinc oxide and magnesium oxide in the approximate ratio of 9 to 1. Zinc phosphate cement liquids are phosphoric acid solutions buffered by alumina salts and in some instances by both alumina and zinc salts or metals; the water content is 33 ± 5 percent.[12]

The compounds formed by reaction of the powder and liquid are noncrystalline phosphates of zinc, magnesium and aluminum.[13] The exact mechanism of setting is not known, but these phosphates form only part of the set cement. The rest is unreacted cores of larger powder particles. Thus, set cement consists of powder particles cemented together with phosphates. The proportion of powder particles and phosphate matrix varies with the amount of powder incorporated into a given amount of liquid. The set cement having the minimum amount of matrix has the best values for physical properties and is most suitable for use in the mouth.

USES: Luting agent is the primary use for zinc phosphate cement. It is still widely used as a base and temporary restoration even though it can be irritating to the unprotected pulp.

DIRECTIONS FOR USE: Zinc phosphate cement should be mixed on a cool slab for approximately 2 minutes. The increments of powder should be small. If mixing is carried out on a cool slab over a wide area, reaction between powder and liquid proceeds at a slow pace and considerably more powder can be incorporated for a given consistency. Setting zinc phosphate cements liberate heat, hence the rationale for slow mixing on a cool slab.

Consistency of mix, which is determined by the amount of powder incorporated into a given amount of liquid, governs values for pertinent physical properties. Generally stated, the more powder incorporated in the mix, the better the physical properties and the less irritation to the pulp. A heavier mix should be used for a base rather than for a luting agent. Pulp protection should be employed before using this cement in either instance.

By using the maximum amount of powder in a given quantity of liquid to produce a workable consistency, one produces, generally, a cement with ample working time and with comparatively high strength, low shrinkage on hardening and low solubility.

The compressive strength of cement may be correlated with its durability in withstanding occlusal forces, although no determination has yet been made of the minimum compressive strength required for final cementation of a cast restoration. Under specific situations of cavity preparation and occlusal loading, the cement bond may fail under tensile forces. Therefore, the tensile or shear strengths may be more appropriate properties to evaluate.

Proper seating of castings requires that the film of cement between the casting and tooth should be as thin as possible. The film thickness is governed by the particle size of the powder, the viscosity of the cement and the type of appliance being cemented. To obtain the thinnest possible cement film between tooth and restoration, it is important to bring about the greatest flow in the seating stage of cementation. A uniform but thin film thickness of the luting cement will result in the closest adaptation of the margins of a cast restoration. This can be accomplished through the use of heavy and sustained forces during seating of the casting, by venting the occlusal or lingual surface to relieve pressure during seating, by electrolytically or chemically stripping the internal surface of the casting, and by utilizing a "die relief" technique in which the enlargement of the die is accomplished by the addition of a spacing material.[14]

LIMITATIONS OF USE: The main limitation to use of zinc phosphate cement is the potential irritation of the pulp by the acid of the unset cement. Teeth that have not previously been restored and exhibit large areas of fresh cut dentin are most susceptible. Conversely, teeth with large restorations and/or bases have more resistance to the penetration of acid. Proper mixing to raise the powder/liquid ratio will reduce the damage potential as will the use of certain forms of cavity varnish.

EVALUATION PROGRAM: American Dental Association Specification No. 8 for zinc phosphate cement lists two types of cement based on particle size. Type I, a fine grain cement, has a permissible maximum film thickness of 25μm (0.001 in.). This permits a thin film for seating of precision castings. Type II, a medium grain cement has a maximum film thickness of 40μm (0.0016 in.). This type is suitable for uses other than luting.

AVAILABLE PRODUCTS

TYPE I, FINE GRAIN

FLECK'S EXTRAORDINARY, Mizzy, Inc.
MODERN TENACIN, L. D. Caulk Co., Div. of Dentsply International, Inc.
SMITH'S ZINC, Teledyne Getz-Opotow
ULTRABOND ZINC PHOSPHATE CEMENT, Doric Corp.
S. S. WHITE ZINC IMPROVED, S. S. White, Div. of Pennwalt Corp.

TYPE II, MEDIUM GRAIN

AMES Z-M, Teledyne Dental Products Co.
Ames Temporary Cement, Teledyne Dental Products Co.
Unitek Blend-Eye Zinc Oxyphosphate, Unitek Corp.

ZINC PHOSPHATE CEMENT

Do:

1. Take time to mix properly and to the proper consistency for the use indicated.
2. Protect fresh cut dentin from acid attack.
3. Insure that preparations are clean and dry, but not desiccated.
4. Use some form of cement escape, especially in long crowns (vents, grooves, stripping or die spacing).

Don't:

1. Place cement on preparations before placing on castings.
2. Use as deep bases without liner or varnish.
3. Try to mix too small a volume.
4. Forget to use a glass slab and a wide area to mix.
5. Allow moisture to contact the cement until set.

ZINC SILICO-PHOSPHATE CEMENTS

COMPOSITION AND PROPERTIES: The silico-phosphate cements are combinations of silicate cement and zinc phosphate cement. These cements are manipulated quickly like silicate cements. Their characteristics, such as working time and film thickness, are somewhat inferior to zinc phosphate cements, but in general they exhibit greater strength and less solubility than the zinc phosphate type. Since this cement is acidic, pulp protection must be provided.

USES: They are primarily used as a temporary filling material and for cementation of porcelain crowns, orthodontic bands, and cast restorations.

DIRECTIONS FOR USE: As with any cement, the manufacturer's directions should be followed. Most suggest incorporating large amounts of powder into the liquid at one time and spatulating with long strokes. The mix should be completed in one minute or less, since overmixing interferes with the setting reaction of the cement. Powder and liquid should be measured for any of the consistencies for luting or for other uses.

These cements are more translucent than other luting agents and can be selected according to shade. The shade of the cement can alter the shade of certain porcelain restorations. This makes them the material of choice by some dentists for the cementation of fused feldspathic porcelain restorations where the film thickness

may be of less importance, and maintaining the correct shade is of the utmost concern.

A satisfactory cement should develop a relatively high compressive strength rather quickly. The 24 hour minimum value for compressive strength required in the American Dental Association Specification Program is 137.3 MN/m² (19,800 psi). This is about twice that required for zinc phosphate cements.

LIMITATIONS OF USE: The film thickness of the zinc silico-phosphate cements makes them unsuitable for cementation of precision castings, although a film thickness of 25 μm can be obtained in the laboratory. The pH of this cement is low, so pulp protection must be used.

EVALUATION PROGRAM: American Dental Association Specification No. 21 classifies the zinc silico-phosphate cements into three types according to usage: Type I to be used as a cementing medium, Type II as a temporary posterior filling material and Type III for dual purposes including the uses of the previous two types.

ZINC SILICO-PHOSPHATE CEMENTS

Do:
1. Incorporate some form of pulp protection.
2. Mix properly to manufacturer's instructions.
3. Use for band cementation and porcelain jacket crowns.

Don't:
1. Use for general cementation until the resultant film thickness has been checked. (25 μ range).
2. Place cement on preparations before placing on castings.
3. Use as deep bases without liner or varnish.
4. Try to mix too small a volume.
5. Forget to use a glass slab and a wide area to mix.
6. Allow moisture to contact the cement until set.

AVAILABLE PRODUCTS

TYPE I, CEMENTING MEDIA

Bondalcaps Red, H. D. Justi Co., Div. of Williams Gold Refining Co., Inc.
FLUORO-THIN, S. S. White, Div. Pennwalt Corp.
LUCENT, L. D. Caulk Co., Div. of Dentsply International, Inc.
New Germicidal Kryptex, S. S. White Dental Products International, Div. Pennwalt Corp.
Petralit, Premier Dental Products Co.

TYPE II, TEMPORARY POSTERIOR FILLING MATERIAL

DORCATE, L. D. Caulk Co., Div. of Dentsply International, Inc.

POLYMER CEMENTS

There are three types of cements considered as polymer cements: poly(methyl methacrylate) resin, BIS-GMA resin and cyanoacrylate.

Uses: The methyl methacrylate type has been marketed as a luting agent. The BIS-GMA resin cements are also adapted for luting agents. Suggested uses for the cyanoacrylates are pin retention, wound suturing, pulp capping and pit and fissure sealants.

Directions for Use: There is some degree of variance among the polymer cement products, so that following the specific manufacturer's instructions is essential.

Resin cements based primarily on poly (methyl methacrylate) with mineral fillers, have been available since 1952.

A newer resin cement[15] based on the BIS-GMA formulation for composite restorative materials is also available for use in combination with a solution of 50 percent citric acid. Cavity cleansing with the acid solution is suggested by the manufacturer to create a clean surface into which a degree of "tag" retention can develop. This appears to open the dentinal tubules and results in pulpal irritation.

Despite improved retention, neither material has found wide clinical acceptance, except in the temporary seating of a loose-fitting casting until it can be reconstructed.

Cyanoacrylates have been researched as a possible addition to the luting agents presently being used in dentistry. Among the properties that attract attention is their ability to polymerize at room temperature without the addition of a catalyst. The cyanoacrylates most studied are methyl 2, ethyl 2, and isobutyl.

Limitations of Use: Drawbacks associated with the use of resin cements include: high film thickness values, high water absorption values, short working time, difficulty in the removal of excess material at the gingival margins, and pulpal irritation.

The cyanoacrylate polymers undergo degradation in the biologic system and may form cyanoacetate and possibly formaldehyde, both of which may give rise to local irritation.[16,17]

The Council has published a Status Report on the cyanoacrylates which states that on the basis of current knowledge, they cannot be recommended for routine use in dentistry.

Evaluation Program: There is currently no specification for these cements.

POLYCARBOXYLATE (POLYACRYLATE) CEMENTS

Composition and Properties: Investigations at the University of Manchester in England led to the development of the polycarboxylate or polyacrylate cements in the late 1960's.[18] The new cement is a powder containing a modified zinc oxide and a liquid composed of an aqueous solution of polyacrylic acid of sufficient molecular weight. Most products have a molecular weight of 25,000 to 50,000. Variation in the molecular weight of the polyacrylic acid influences the viscosity of the mix and determines handling characteristics.[19] The setting reaction is thought to take place between the zinc ions and the carboxyl groups on the polyacrylic acid chain, resulting in a crosslinked matrix holding unreacted powder particles together. Any bonding which develops as the material polymerizes is thought to be the result of a chelation reaction involving the calcium ions of tooth structure and the available carboxyl groups.[20]

Uses: This cement is a luting agent and is also useful as a non-irritating base. It is especially recommended for cementation of stainless steel crowns. Its use for direct bonding of orthodontic brackets has been reported.

Directions for Use: It is important to measure both powder and liquid. They must be mixed very rapidly (within 30 seconds) because the setting gelation starts quickly. The usable viscosity for a polycarboxylate cement is of a thicker consistency than that obtained with a primary mix of zinc phosphate or zinc oxide-eugenol-EBA cement. This "thixotropic" property can be misleading, however, because a powder to liquid ratio of approximately 1.5 to 1.0 will produce an apparently viscous mix, but one that will flow readily under the sustained pressures used to seat a metal casting.[21]

Pulpal reaction to the polycarboxylate cements has been relatively bland and has been an important asset in their use.[18,22,23] Only a minimal reaction appears to be evident during the first seven days, but it is reversible and after that time the reaction is similar to a zinc oxide-eugenol control.[24] The polycarboxylate cements can be used effectively as a cement base under amalgam or composite resins where they will be bland to pulpal tissue and also will not interfere with resin polymerization.

Castings should be sandblasted or stripped electrolytically in preparation for cementation in order to increase the bonding potential of the cement to the metal.

Physical properties for the polycarboxylate cements are in much the same range as those for other types.[22,25,26] The compressive strength values are somewhat less than those for zinc phosphate cement, but clinical studies on the retention of castings have shown little difference among the major types of cement.[21,27] Optimum retention is still best obtained by creating it within the cavity preparation and not relying on the cement.

POLYCARBOXYLATE CEMENTS

Do:

1. Premeasure both powder and liquid.
2. Incorporate all powder into the liquid and mix within 30 seconds.
3. Use the cement quickly.
4. Use airbrasive on the intalgio of the casting to ensure a clean surface for cementing.

Don't:

1. Desiccate teeth; blow dry or wipe dry.
2. Use after a eugenol containing temporary cement without cleansing teeth carefully.
3. Expect the same mixing viscosity as a zinc phosphate cement.

LIMITATIONS OF USE: The available working time is more limited than with other cements[25] and may suggest a contraindication for its use with multiple castings in long span fixed restorations.

EVALUATION PROGRAM: There is no specification for the polycarboxylate cements at this time, but they are being considered under an Acceptance Program.

AVAILABLE PRODUCTS

Bondalcaps Blue, H. D. Justi Co., Div. of Williams Gold Refining Co., Inc.

CARBOXYLON POLYCARBOXYLATE CEMENT, 3M Company

CHEMIT CARBOXYLATE CEMENT, Harry J. Bosworth Co.

DURELON, Premier Dental Products

Intra-Oral Solvenex I-O, Den-Mat Inc.

Oxicaps, H. D. Justi Co., Div. of Williams Gold Refining Co., Inc.

PCA CEMENT, S. S. White, Div. of Pennwalt Corp.

POLYBOND CARBOXYLATE CEMENT, Doric Corp.

SHOFU POLYCARBOXYLATE CEMENT, Shofu Dental Corp.

TYLOK POLYCARBOXYLATE CEMENT, L.D. Caulk Co., Div. of Dentsply International, Inc.

GLASS IONOMER CEMENTS

COMPOSITION AND PROPERTIES: A new translucent cement for dentistry was first reported in the literature in 1972.[28] This cement is based on the hardening reaction between aluminosilicate glass powders and aqueous solutions of polymers of acrylic acid. The material is given the generic name of glass ionomer cement; it is also called ASPA from aluminosilicate polyacrylate. Current research is being done to show that the siliceous hydrogel which develops at the surface of the glass particles in the set cement provides an effective bond between filler and matrix with improved resistance to abrasion and thermal cycling. Glass ionomer cement has compressive strength comparable to that of silicate cement and has a higher tensile strength.

USES: It is being developed for a variety of dental applications such as restoration of erosion/abrasion lesions and inconspicuous lesions on anterior teeth, fissure sealing and filling, and as a luting agent.

DIRECTIONS FOR USE: Proper measuring and dispensing of the powder and liquid is more critical with this cement than any other. Large increments are added until the "putty-like" consistency is reached. Mixing must be completed in one minute. Matrices and protective coatings must be used. Moisture contamination must be avoided. Attention to detail is very important in handling this material.

It is suggested by the manufacturer that the ionic bonds formed at the tooth/restorative interface negate the need for mechanical retention. During the intermediate setting stage it can be carved like amalgam.

This cement has good strength properties, resistance to abrasion, low solubility and resistance to staining.

LIMITATIONS OF USE: This material is too opaque for use where esthetics is a primary concern. Cervical erosion should be greater than 1 mm in depth to be considered for this material. A return visit for finishing is required.

The currently available form has too high a film thickness for a luting agent, but a luting agent formulation is being clinically evaluated.

EVALUATION PROGRAM: There is currently no American Dental Association specification for glass ionomer cements but they are being considered under an Acceptance Program.

AVAILABLE PRODUCTS

ASPA, L.D. Caulk Co., Div. of Dentsply International, Inc.
Fuji, G-C International

SILICATE CEMENTS

COMPOSITION AND PROPERTIES: Powders used for silicate cements are pulverized complex glasses consisting essentially of alumino-silicates containing magnesium, fluorine, calcium, sodium and phosphorus.[29] All modern silicate cement powders are stable and contain large quantities of fluorides, as much as 15 percent by weight. The high fluoride content is associated with the apparent anti-cariogenic properties of silicate cement.

Liquids of currently used silicate cements, like those employed for zinc phosphate cements, are aqueous solutions of phosphoric acid buffered by aluminum or zinc salts, or both.[29] Their water content runs about 40 ± 5 percent, which is higher on the average than the liquids used with zinc phosphate cements. The liquids have a pH of approximately 2, and can create severe inflammatory reactions in pulpal tissue when a fresh mix is placed directly against exposed dentin.

USES: The silicate cements are primarily used as a restorative material in the anterior teeth, where esthetics and color match are of primary importance.

DIRECTIONS FOR USE: Optimum properties and durability can be obtained with silicate restorations by adhering to the prescribed techniques for mixing, insertion and finishing. Silicate cements set by the formation of a noncrystalline gel which should not be disturbed after its initiation. Silicate cements should be mixed quickly (no longer than thirty seconds) on a cool slab or mechanically with proportioned powder and liquid in a closed container.

The permanence and esthetic qualities of silicate cement restorations are closely related to the powder-liquid ratio. Consistencies which are either too thin or too thick will not produce durable or esthetic restorations.

The compressive strength of a dental filling material gives an indication of its resistance to masticatory forces. The minimum value in the current specification is 166.9 MN/m^2 (24,200 psi).

One of the principal reasons for using silicate cement in anterior restorations is its lifelike appearance, at least when first inserted. The pleasing esthetic qualities depend upon the optical properties of the cement closely matching those of the tooth. Translucency (reciprocal of opacity) and shading are the most critical qualities in obtaining a good visual match between filling and tooth. Translucency increases with time; the greatest change occurs within 24 hours in most cements. The shade guide is the practical method for selection of the appropriate shade of cement in each individual application. It represents the final shade of the restoration after it has been in place several weeks.

LIMITATIONS OF USE: A major weakness of silicate cements is their tendency to dissolve and disintegrate in the mouth especially when placed in areas of the mouth where oral hygiene is difficult to maintain and plaque tends to accumulate. The solubility of current silicate cements is about 0.8 percent when one hour old specimens are immersed for 24 hours in distilled water. The present maximum value permitted in the specification is 1.0 percent. Most of the soluble material is a mixture of sodium salts of dihydrogen phosphate and complex fluorides, silica, and very small amounts of alumina, zinc and calcium.[30] Desiccation that would occur with mouth breathers is extremely detrimental to silicate cement restorations. Effective isolation with a rubber dam can prevent early contamination with moisture, and the lubrication of existing restorations to prevent desiccation will help to maintain translucency of shade and dimensional stability.[31] Final finishing or unnecessary manipulation should be postponed for 24 hours after insertion to allow the gel matrix to set more completely. Pulp protection should always be used under silicate restorations.

The use of silicate cement as an anterior restorative material for esthetic purposes has greatly diminished in recent years. Composite restorative resins have proven to be more satisfactory for use in this capacity, since they compensate for some of the detrimental properties of the silicate cement and are more stable in the oral environment.

EVALUATION PROGRAM: American Dental Association Specification No. 9 delineates the requirements for the silicate cements.

SILICATE CEMENTS

Do:
1. Use a base or liner to protect pulp.
2. Mix properly according to manufacturer's instructions.
3. Use a matrix strip.
4. Cover the restoration with varnish for protection.

Don't:
1. Polish for at least 24 hours.
2. Use coarse abrasives or high speeds.
3. Allow silicates to dry out (coat finished ones while working on others).

AVAILABLE PRODUCTS

ACHATITE: ACHATITE BIOCHROMATIC, W.H. Byron, Inc.

Caulk Grip Cement, L.D. Caulk Co., Div. of Dentsply International, Inc.

Caulk Celluloid Strips, L.D. Caulk Co., Div. of Dentsply International, Inc.

Caulk Silicote Protective Coating, L.D. Caulk Co., Div. of Dentsply International, Inc.

CAULK SYNTREX F, L.D. Caulk Co., Div. of Dentsply International, Inc.

EBAC, The Lorvic Corp.

Fleck's Cement, Mizzy, Inc.

Justi Resin Cement, H.D. Justi Co., Div. of Williams Gold Refining Co., Inc.

MQ CEMENT, S.S. White, Div. of Pennwalt Corp.

Opotow Dental Paraben, Teledyne Dental Products

Opotow Trial Cement, Teledyne Dental Products

SILICAP, H.D. Justi Co., Div. of Williams Gold Refining Co., Inc.

Solvenex Concentrate, Den-Mat, Inc.

ZRE Liquid, Moyco Industries, Inc.

CAVITY LINERS

Cavity liners are used to provide a barrier for the protection of pulpal tissue from chemical irritation. These liners are relatively fluid and can be applied to dentinal surfaces as thin layers. Liners are not to be confused with varnishes which are described in the following section.

USES: Cavity liners become a barrier to irritation from cements and composites and help reduce the sensitivity of fresh cut dentin.[32] Liners are either a zinc oxide and eugenol formula or a calcium hydroxide type. The latter is especially useful under composites. Neither is strong enough to be used in bulk as a base. Some can be used as pulp capping agents. There is some overlapping of usage between liners and varnishes but substitution of one for another is not necessarily appropriate.

DIRECTIONS FOR USE: Since there are many liners packaged in different forms, it is mandatory to follow instructions and to know that the product will perform the use intended. Lining agents are applied as relatively thin layers and are painted or flowed over the cut dentin surface. It is sometimes necessary to add a cement base over the lining agent.

LIMITATIONS OF USE: Cavity liners usually lack both the strength and thickness to be used without an overlying base in deep cavities.[33] Liners should not be left on cavity margins since they are soluble in saliva and will allow increased marginal leakage.

AVAILABLE PRODUCTS

Caulk Cavity Primer, L.D. Caulk Co.
Cavity Lining, Moyco Industries, Inc.
Dycal Calcium Hydroxide Compositions, L.D. Caulk Co.
Handi-Liner (kit), Mizzy, Inc.
Hydrox, Kerr Mfg. Co., Div. of Sybron Dental Products
Hydroxyline, George Taub Products, Inc.
Kerr MPC, Kerr Mfg. Co., Div. of Sybron Dental Products

Opotow Dental Silicone, Teledyne Dental Products
Opotow Intermediate Filling Material, Teledyne Dental Products
Poly-Liner Kit, Mizzy, Inc.
Procal, 3M Company
Pulpdent Cavity Liner, Pulpdent Corp. of America
Vitec, Kerr Mfg. Co., Div. of Sybron Dental Products

CAVITY VARNISHES

Cavity varnishes are solutions of one or more resins in an organic solvent. They are utilized primarily for protection of pulpal tissue.

USES: Varnishes provide an adequate marginal seal during the early contraction of the newly placed amalgam restoration. They reduce postoperative sensitivity by decreasing the microleakage around the restoration.[33] Several layers of varnish will significantly reduce the penetration of acid from cement into the dentinal tubules.

DIRECTIONS FOR USE: Cavity varnishes are usually applied with cotton pellets or other appropriate instruments. They should be applied in two or three layers. When used prior to amalgam placement, it is not necessary to keep varnishes off the margins; when used to protect a deep cavity from a cement base, the varnish should be applied before the base is placed. Bases containing calcium hydroxide or zinc oxide-eugenol should be applied directly to the dentin and subsequently covered by varnish.[33]

LIMITATIONS OF USE: Varnishes provide inadequate insulation against the thermal conduction of metal restorations. Varnishes are contraindicated for use under resins including composites, because the solvent of the varnish may soften the resin and the residual monomer of the resin may dissolve the varnish film. In addition, the varnish may also prevent the wetting of the cavity surface by the resin.[33]

Table I.

Classification of Dental Cements

Class	Cement Type		Composition			Uses	
			Powder	Liquid	Set Cement	Primary	Secondary
I	Zinc oxide-eugenol		Zinc oxide (uncalcined) rosin polymer	Eugenol with mineral and/or vegetable oils as diluents	Unreacted zinc oxide and eugenol plus zinc eugenolate	Temporary	
	Zinc oxide-eugenol-EBA		Zinc oxide (uncalcined) quartz or alumina, rosin	Eugenol EBA (orthoeth-oxybenzoic acid)if-300	(Not known)	Cement base, temporary filling	Luting agent
II	Zinc phosphate	Regular	Calcined Zinc oxide and magnesium oxide. Sometimes copper, silver or salts	Orthophos-phoric acid plus aluminum phosphate and/or zinc phosphate	Unreacted powder in a noncrystalline phosphate matrix	Luting agent, cement	Temporary
III	Zinc silico-phosphate		Mechanical mixture of Class II regular & Class VII	Class VII	Probably combination of Class II regular & Class VII	Luting agent	Semi-permanent filling
IV	Polymers	BIS GMA resin	Acrylic polymers, mineral fillers	Acrylic monomers	Acrylic polymers & inert mineral fillers	Luting agent	
		Methyl methacry-late resin	Polymer	Monomer	Polymer	Luting agent	
		Cyano-acrylate	None	Methyl 2 cyano-acrylate	Polymerized fiber	Luting agent for pins	Pulp cap, fissure sealant

V	Polycarboxy-late	Zinc oxide & magnesium oxide	Polycarboxy-lic acid	Unreacted zinc oxide polycarboxy-late	Luting agent	
VI	Glass Ionomer	Alumino-silicate glass	Polyacrylic, tartaric, & itaconic acid	Siliceous hydrogel	Semi-permanent filling & fissure sealant	Luting agent
VII	Silicate	Complex glass alumino-silicates containing magnesium fluorine, calcium, sodium & phosphorus	Class II regular with less acid & more water	Unreacted glass particles sheathed by silicate gel & colloidal phosphates	Semi-permanent filling	

AVAILABLE PRODUCTS

Cavity Lining-Varnish, S.S. White Dental Products International, Div. of Pennwalt Corp.
Copalite Cavity Varnish, Teledyne Dental Products
Plus Protector, H.D. Justi Co., Div. of Williams Gold Refining Co.
Varnal, Cetylite Industrial Inc.

LITERATURE REFERENCES

1. Wallace, D.A., And Hansen, H.L. Zinc oxide-eugenol cements. JADA 26:1536 Sept. 1939.
2. Phillips, R.W.; Swartz, M.L.; and Norman, R.D. Materials for the practicing dentist. St. Louis, The C.V. Mosby Co., 1969.
3. Weiss, M.H. Improved zinc oxide-eugenol cement. Ill. Dent. J. 27:261 Apr. 1958.
4. Messing, J.J. Polystyrene-fortified zinc oxide-eugenol cement. Br. Dent. J. 110:95 Feb. 1961.
5. Copeland, H.I., Jr., et al. Setting reaction of zinc oxide and eugenol. J. Research NBS 55:133 Sept. 1955.
6. Brauer, G.M.; McLaughlin, R.; and Huget, E. Aluminum oxide as a reinforcing agent for zinc oxide-eugenol o-cthoxybenzoic acid. J. Dent. Res. 47:622 July-Aug. 1968.
7. Coleman, J.M., and Kirk, E.E. An assessment of modified zinc oxide-eugenol cement. Br. Dent. J. 118:482 June 1965.
8. Anderson, J.R., and Myers, G.E. Physical properties of some zinc oxide-eugenol cements. J. Dent. Res. 45:379 Mar.-Apr. 1966.
9. Gilson, T.D., and Myers, G.E. Clinical studies of dental cements. IV. A preliminary study of a zinc oxide-eugenol cement for final cementation. J. Dent. Res. 49:75 Jan.-Feb. 1970.
10. Phillips, R.W., et al. Retentive properties of dental cements. J. Prosthet. Dent. 14:760 July-Aug. 1964.
11. Wilson, A.D., and Batchelor, R.F. Zinc oxide-eugenol cements: II. Study erosion and disintegration. J. Dent. Res. 49:593 May-June 1970.
12. Paffenbarger. G.C.; Sweeney, W.T.; and Isaacs, A. A preliminary report on the zinc phosphate cements. JADA 20:1960 Nov. 1933.
13. Servais, G.E., and Cartz, L. Structure of zinc phosphate cements. J. Dent. Res. 50:613 May-June 1971.
14. Going, R.E., and Mitchem, J.C. Cements for permanent luting: a summarizing review. JADA 91:107 July 1975.
15. Lee, H., and Swartz, M.L. Evaluation of a composite resin crown and bridge luting agent. J.Dent. Res. 51:756 May-June 1972.

16. Dennison, J.D., and Powers, J.M. A review of dental cements used for the permanent retention of restorations. Part 1. Composition and manipulation. Mich. Dent. Assoc. J. 56:116 Apr. 1974.

17. Brannstrom, M., and Nyborg, H. Bacterial growth and pulpal changes under inlays cemented with zinc phosphate cement and Epoxylite CBA 9080. J. Prosthet. Dent. 31:556 May 1974.

18. Smith, D.C. A new dental cement. Br. Dent. J. 124:381 Nov. 1968.

19. Powers, J.M.; Johnson, Z.G.; and Craig, R.G. Physical and mechanical properties of zinc polyacrylate dental cements. JADA 88:380 Feb. 1974.

20. Beech, D.R. Improvement in the adhesion of polyacrylate cements to human dentine. Br. Dent. J. 135:442 Nov. 1973.

21. McLean, J.W. Polycarboxylate cements, five years' experience in general practice. Br. Dent. J. 132:9 Jan. 1972.

22. Jendresen, M.D., and Trowbridge, H.O. Biologic and physical properties of a zinc polycarboxylate cement. J. Prosthet. Dent. 28:264 Sept. 1972.

23. Truelove, E.L.; Mitchell, D.F.; and Phillips, R.W. Biological evaluation of a carboxylate cement. J. Dent. Res. 50:166 Jan.-Feb. 1971.

24. Plant, C.G. The effect of polycarboxylate cement on the dental pulp. Br. Dent. J. 129:424 Nov. 1970.

25. Powers, J.M., and Dennison, J.D. A review of dental cements used for the permanent retention of restorations. Part 2. Properties and criteria for selection. Mich. Dent. Assoc. J. 56:218 July-Aug. 1974.

26. Phillips, R.W.; Swartz, M.L.; and Rhodes, B. An evaluation of a carboxylate adhesive cement. JADA 81:1353 Dec. 1970.

27. Silvey, R.G., and Myers, G.E. Preliminary report of a three year study of three luting cements. J. Dent. Res. 53 (Special Issue): 191, Abstract 548, Feb. 1974.

28. Wilson, A.D., and Kent, B.E. A new translucent cement for dentistry. Br. Dent. J. 132:133 Feb. 1972.

29. Paffenbarger, G.C.; Schoonover, I.C.; and Souder, W. Dental silicate cements: physical and chemical properties and a specification, JADA 25:32 Jan. 1938.

30. Wilson, A.D., and Batchelor, R.F. Dental silicate cements: I. The chemistry of erosion. J. Dent. Res. 46:1075 Sept.-Oct. 1967.

31. Smith, D.C. Protection of silicate restorations from contamination by moisture. Br. Dent. J. 122:382 May 1967.

32. Seltzer, S., and Bender, I.B. The dental pulp. Philadelphia, J.B. Lippincott Co., 1965.

33. Going, R.E. Status report on cavity liners, varnishes, primers and cleansers. JADA 85:654 Sept. 1972.

DENTURE BASE RESINS

A denture base is the portion of a complete or removable partial denture which rests on the oral mucosa and retains the artificial teeth. The most common resin used for the fabrication of denture bases is poly(methyl methacrylate), an acrylic resin. This resin is colorless in its pure state and can be pigmented and characterized easily, which makes it possible for the dental profession to produce virtually undetectable complete dentures.[1]

Historically, vulcanized rubber, discovered in 1839 by Charles Goodyear, had early widespread use as a denture base. Until the introduction of methyl methacrylate to dentistry, many other materials were tried, including cellulose nitrate (celluloid), phenolformaldehyde (bakelite), and mixtures of polymerized vinyl chloride and vinyl acetate, but rubber remained the only satisfactory denture base material.

Vernonite was the first of the acrylic resin compounds formulated for dentistry to be introduced in the United States and was perhaps the first application of the monomer-polymer principle anywhere. It was developed by Harold M. Vernon and Lester B. Vernon with the collaboration of members of the research and development staffs of Rohn & Haas Company. Initial clinical testing of the new synthetic resin was begun by the Department of Clinical Prosthesis at the School of Dentistry, University of Pittsburgh, in late 1936 under the supervision of Dr. Walter H. Wright.

The acrylic resins represented such significant improvements in the construction of denture bases that by 1946 it was estimated that more than 95 percent of all dentures were constructed of methyl methacrylate polymer or copolymers for use with porcelain teeth.[2]

While the properties of acrylic denture base resins are not ideal in every respect, it is the combination of virtues rather than one single desirable property that accounts for their popularity and universal use. Acrylic resins have excellent esthetic properties, adequate strength, low water sorption and low solubility. In addition, they are free from toxicity, can be easily repaired, have the ability to reproduce accurately and retain indefinitely the details and dimensions of a pattern, and can be used with a simple molding and processing technique for the construction of denture bases.

ACRYLIC DENTURE BASE RESINS

COMPOSITION: Acrylic denture base resins are available in two forms.

(1) *Gel or plastic cake:* With the gel or plastic cake, the monomer and polymer have been premixed and packaged as soft, rubbery one-unit cakes ready for immediate use. While the gels possess several advantages over the powder-liquid form such as accuracy of proportioning and thoroughness of mixing,[3] they are not as popular and their use has been diminishing throughout the years. Perhaps this is due in part to their limited shelf life, even when stored under refrigeration.

(2) *Powder-liquid:* The powder-liquid type is more common. The liquid (monomer) is mixed with the powder (polymer); the monomer plasticizes the polymer to a dough-like consistency, which is packed into the mold prior to polymerization of the monomer. The resulting denture base is composed of solid, homogeneous resin.

The liquid is composed of the methyl methacrylate monomer; a cross-linking agent, such as ethylene or butylene glycol dimethacrylate, which improves craze resistance, solvent resistance, heat resistance, and the hardness of the final polymer; an accelerator which is added to the cold-curing or autopolymerizing monomer; and an inhibitor, such as hydroquinone or the monomethyl ether of hydroquinone, which protects against premature polymerization. A minimum amount of inhibitor is used consistent with stability and safety, as an excess of inhibitor may interfere with efficient conversion of monomer to polymer. Certain inhibitors may affect the color of the final product. Some manufacturers add plasticizers, such as dibutyl phthalate to produce a softer final polymer or to increase the solubility of the polymer in the monomer.

The plasticizer is usually added to the monomer, but it can also be added to the polymer by ball milling.

The powder is composed primarily of methyl methacrylate polymer beads that may have been modified with small amounts of ethyl acrylate to produce a somewhat softer final product. Benzoyl peroxide, an initiator, is added to the polymer in small amounts. Usually sufficient benzoyl peroxide is present as a residual catalyst from the initial polymerization reaction to preclude its addition. Inorganic pigments are used by the majority of denture base manufacturers for coloration. The dry finely ground pigments are mechanically blended with the polymer particles for a specific amount of time. Some denture base polymers are internally colored, with the pigment added to the reactor kettle during production of the polymer. Characterizing fibers are present in some powders. Acrylic fibers have been found to be more serviceable than rayon fibers.[1]

PROPERTIES: *Thermal Expansion*—Acrylic denture base resins have high coefficients of thermal expansion. Whenever they are heat processed in rigid gypsum molds having low thermal expansion characteristics, internal stress is induced in the final denture. Stress formation can be held to a minimum by following procedures recommended by the manufacturer for powder-liquid ratio, mixing, packing, curing, and cooling during processing of the denture.

Wettability—The wettability of poly(methyl methacrylate) can be increased by the surface deposition of a silicon tetrachloride coating.[4,5] Silica coated acrylic dentures are said to be easier to clean and more retentive than non-coated dentures. Extensive data giving the length of time the coating will last are not available. Conditions of use, such as cleaning procedures, play an important role. The coating has been reported to last a very limited time, which would question the extra expense of this procedure for most patients.[6]

A special denture base material (Hydrocryl) is marketed on the basis of its inherent hydrophilic nature. However, long term water sorption, dimensional stability, and the ability of the material to resist staining and possible absorption of odor-producing substances have not been determined. In a recent investigation, Hydrocryl was found to offer no significant advantage over methyl methacrylate as to wettability when used as a denture base material.[6]

As wettability of a denture base can be markedly improved by sandblasting, periodic sandblasting of the basal surface, regardless of the denture base resin used, is advantageous. Denture bases should not be processed against a separating medium which would give them a smooth, highly polished tissue surface.[6]

Toxicity—The use of plastics in various phases of medical practice has revealed that the components and degradation products of various resins stimulate adverse tissue reactions.[7] However, evidence suggesting that acrylic denture bases induce inflammatory and neoplastic changes of the oral tissues does not exist. Implantation of polymeric methyl methacrylate into mice was not found to provoke tumor growth.[8]

Radiopacity—In recognition of the difficulties encountered in the detection of fragments of dentures that have been swallowed or inhaled accidentally, there have been continuing efforts to formulate radiopaque denture materials. Among the materials researchers have attempted to incorporate into acrylic resin to render it radiopaque are silver alloy, lead acetate, finely ground gold, gold leaf, magnesium oxide, bismuth subcarbonate, barium sulfate, poly(barium acrylate), and barium fluoride. Radiopaque materials developed in the past have been deficient with respect to accepted standards for strength and/or color stability. A recent report, however, describes a radiopaque material which satisfies current American Dental Association specifications for denture base polymers, although the material is noted to be more difficult to finish and polish than materials now in use.[9] Investigations in this area should be continued.

Characterization of Denture Bases for People of Color—Pigmentation of the oral tissues is a frequent clinical observation in many people of all races and nationalities.[10] It is evident in the gingiva, mucous membranes, hard and soft palate, tongue, and tissues of the floor of the mouth.

Dental manufacturers have responded with special shades for patients with heavily pigmented oral tissues, as the use of conventional pink denture base resins for these patients can be distracting and conspicuous, especially for those who have a high lip line when smiling.

Researchers have also described various techniques for the characterization of denture bases for people of color.[11-14] These techniques provide esthetic denture bases for patients who have pigmented gingivae.

Heat-cured vs. Cold-cured Acrylic Denture Base Resins: Most acrylic dentures are fabricated from heat-cured denture base materials. However, cold-curing (autopolymerizing, self-curing, chemically activated) acrylic denture base materials also produce durable and stable dentures[15,16] and are readily available to the profession.

The principal difference between heat-curing and cold-curing acrylic denture base resins is the method of activation of the benzoyl peroxide catalyst, which initiates polymerization of the monomer. With heat-cured resins, polymerization is started by free radicals from the benzoyl peroxide, which is activated by heat. In cold-curing, a tertiary amine chemical accelerator, usually N,N-dimethyl-p-toluidine, is added to the monomer so polymerization can be completed at room temperature.

The color of cold-curing resins is not as stable as that of the heat-curing type because of subsequent oxidation of the tertiary amine accelerator, which forms a colored end product. In an attempt to improve the color stability of cold-curing resins, many dental manufacturers have resorted to the use of ultraviolet absorbers, either incorporated into polymers by dry blending, or added to the monomer.

Analysis of spectral-transmittance curves of heat and cold-curing acrylic monomers of seven major dental manufacturers showed that while none utilized ultraviolet absorbers in their heat-curing monomers, all added an ultraviolet absorber to their cold-curing monomers.[17]

Polymerization of cold-curing resins is exothermic and like heat-curing resins results in a volumetric shrinkage. However, they do not reach the peak temperatures observed with the heat-curing types.

DIRECTIONS FOR USE: Cold-curing denture base resins may be processed by the same compression molding technique utilized for heat-curing resins or by pouring a fluid resin mixture into a hydrocolloid mold.

Compression Molding Technique: As the working time for cold-curing resins is undoubtedly shorter than that of heat-curing resins, an extended initiation period before polymerization begins is required to allow ample time for trial closures when compression molding is utilized. A simple method to prolong the initiation period is to cool the mixing jar and the monomer, which will maintain the mixed resin longer in the dough state and thereby increase the working time. Cold-curing resins must be workable for at least a five minute period to meet the requirements of American Dental Association Specification No. 12 for Denture Base Polymers.

Unfortunately the polymerization of cold-curing resins is never as complete as that of the heat-curing type. This results in a higher residual monomer content. Most of this monomer, which is extractable by water or saliva, disappears in a few hours when the denture is either immersed in water or worn by the patient.[18] There is probably no relationship between residual monomer and denture sore mouth. Allergy to acrylic resin denture base material is very rare.[19]

At best the transverse strength of cold-curing resins is approximately 80 percent that of heat-curing resins. It is likely that room temperature curing aids in eliminating many of the processing stresses introduced during heat-curing, with the resultant dentures possessing better fit and more dimensional stability. [20]

The Curing Cycle of Heat-cured Acrylic Resins: Because polymerization is an exothermic reaction and it is essential to heat the resin in the flask slowly to the critical range, the internal mass of resin reaches temperatures much higher than the temperature of the water bath.

In general, the critical range is between 65°C (149°F) and 80°C (176°F). At these temperatures the reaction is quite fast and most, but not all, of the polymerization is completed in about three to five minutes. A longer time in the water bath or a higher temperature is required to complete the cure.[21]

When a resin reaches the critical temperature, it begins to generate heat faster than it can be conducted away. The denture base resin as well as the stone or plaster surrounding it are poor conductors, so the heat of reaction tends to accumulate in the resin. The higher the temperature, the faster the polymerization takes place. When the polymerization temperature is reached, the denture base resin reaches higher temperatures than the temperature surrounding it and completes the polymerization on its own internally generated heat.

The maximum temperature obtained during polymerization is dependent upon the bulk of the denture and the rate of heating. In the case of a rapid curing cycle, the temperature inside the denture is much higher than that of the water bath. The internal temperature will rise much higher than the boiling point of methyl methacrylate monomer (100.3°C) and the monomer vapor produced can become trapped in the hard polymerized resin and cause porosity (bubbles) in the resultant denture base.

During a runaway polymerization, the lingual flanges of a lower denture are most prone to porosity. This is because they usually represent the largest bulk of resin and are nearest to the center of the flask. The closer to the center of the flask the bulk of the resin is placed, the greater the danger of porosity in that area because the exothermic heat cannot be conducted away easily.

The internal temperature of the resin can be controlled by a slow run-up time or by a lower curing temperature. With a slow heat-up, most of the polymerization takes place at a low safe temperature.

After extensive research on heat curing

cycles, the two time-temperature schedules shown in Table I have been accepted as most satisfactory.

Table I.

Temperature	Time
165°F (73.9°C)	9 hours
165°F (73.9°C) + 212°F (100°C)	1.5 hours 0.5 hour

Construction of Denture Bases from Pour Resins:[22] The use of pour type or fluid cold-curing resins in specially designed flasks with a colloidal investing medium for the construction of complete and partial denture bases has been increasing since their introduction to the profession a little more than a decade ago. Clinical and laboratory studies have indicated that satisfactory dentures can be produced by this method at a considerable savings in processing time.

The technique for the use of pour resins consists of waxing the denture in the usual manner to resemble the finished case and placing it in a specially designed flask, which is then filled with reversible hydrocolloid duplicating material. After the hydrocolloid has chilled and gelled, the cast and wax-up are removed. The case is sprued and vented to the highest portion of the mold. The wax is removed from the cast and the teeth, and the cleaned teeth are carefully replaced in the mold. After painting the cast with separating medium, it is reseated into the mold. The flask is reassembled to permit pouring the resin into the mold.

The flask is carefully transferred to a pressure pot and positioned so that the sprue and vent holes are upright and the flask is away from the air inlet. A pourable resin is mixed and poured into the mold. After standing for approximately four minutes, the case is allowed to cure under 20 pounds of air pressure for 30 minutes. The denture is then removed from the mold and finished in the usual manner.

It is imperative to handle the flask carefully and as little as possible after pouring the fluid resin. Careless handling can cause tooth movement and flash formation. Hence the resin should be poured after the flask has been positioned in the pressure pot; this will eliminate all movement and handling.

Advantages of Pour Resins: One of the advantages of the pour resin technique is the elimination of the increase in occlusal vertical dimension noted following processing in compression and injection molded dentures. This reduction is mainly due to the absence of a split flask and gypsum investing materials.

The reduction of the time required for processing is another advantage. The usual flasking and deflasking procedures are eliminated. Deflasking of the finished denture is easy, fast, and there is little danger of tooth breakage and framework distortion or scratching. Frameworks are recovered from the hydrocolloid mold with the same high luster that they had before the processing procedure.

Because of the clean recovery of the casts, the use of the splitcast technique is facilitated. Finishing time for the processed denture is reduced due to the clean separation of the denture from the hydrocolloid.

The same acrylic resin used to fabricate the prosthesis can be used for any subsequent repairs, rebases, or duplicate dentures.

Because of the confinement of the acrylic resin during curing and greater thermal contraction caused by higher processing temperatures, compression molding places greater stress on a denture than does the pour resin technique.

Limitations of Pour Resins: The pour technique for denture base processing is more complicated, delicate, and demanding than the compression molding procedure. More production problems can result. The time saved in processing, recovery, and finishing can be offset by the correction of processing errors.

The artificial teeth must be cleaned thoroughly in a strainer and not disturbed when replaced in the hydrocolloid mold. Tooth movement can occasionally occur due to vibration of the flask during reassembly or when transferring the flask to the pressure pot.

Voids or porosity in the resin can occur. This can be attributed to incorrect sprue positioning or to pouring resin that is too viscous into the mold. Some removable partial dentures require complicated spruing.

Pour resins do not bond well with cross-linked acrylic resin teeth. "Pop-outs" occasionally occur. Adequate retention can be obtained by grinding the ridge laps of the teeth.

A reduction in the occlusal vertical dimension occurs when dentures are processed with pour acrylic resins due to shrinkage of the resin during polymerization. Although this decrease is minimal, the combination of shrinkage in both upper and lower dentures and the loss from selective grinding of the teeth can result in some reduction of the vertical dimension.

Untoward color changes in the resin base have been recognized. Manufacturers have added ultraviolet absorbers and stabilizers to the existing products in an attempt to remedy the situation.

Dentures fabricated from pour resins cannot be individually characterized. Only stock denture base shades can be utilized in hydrocolloid molds.

In summary, satisfactory dentures can be produced from pour resins at a considerable savings of processing time. The problems of porosity, voids, and heavy anterior tooth contact resulting from shrinkage of the resin during curing present difficulties which must be understood and compensated. The use of alginate and a modified gypsum product as investing media, as well as centrifugation of the pour resin into the flask, offer no significant advantages over the originally introduced procedure. Further critical research will conceivably improve the pour resins and the corresponding processing techniques to the point that they can challenge heat-curing resins for the largest percentage of denture bases.

EPOXY DENTURE BASE RESINS

Although the thermosetting epoxy resins possess several properties which would be desirable for a denture base resin, they have seen limited use due to their handling problems, toxicity and porosity, among other disadvantages.

The polyamine accelerators needed for rapid hardening are toxic. They are also quite irritating and can cause patient sensitivity and allergic reactions. The high water sorption and solubility and poor dimensional stability of epoxy resins noted clinically result from incomplete curing of the material.[23]

When modified epoxy resins, supplied as a slurry-liquid combination, are used as denture base materials, the mixed resin is poured into the mold and cured at room or low temperatures. Epoxy resins are difficult to mold and must be handled with extreme care. Color stability presents a problem. Epoxy resins do not bond well to acrylic resin teeth.

The inferior physical properties of epoxy resins greatly outweigh the advantages of chemical stability, hardness, strength, and a low curing shrinkage.

POLYSTYRENE DENTURE BASE RESINS

A polystyrene resin (Jectron) was available commercially for fabricating denture bases by an injection molding technique, but has since been withdrawn from the market.

The resin was softened under heat to the molding temperature and forced into the mold in a preheated flask. It softened and flowed easily and produced clinically satisfactory dentures when the recommended technique was strictly followed. Advantages of polystyrene dentures are low water sorption and favorable fatigue resistance.

POLYCARBONATE DENTURE BASE RESINS

Infrequently, polycarbonates have been used as denture base resins. Their limited use may be due to the complicated injection molding technique required. The high softening temperature prior to injection of the resin into the mold is critical. If allowed to go too high, decomposition and discoloration of the resin results.

The outstanding feature of the polycarbonates is their very high impact strength. However, when compared to acrylic resins, they exhibit greater distortion on water sorption, higher flexibility, lower hardness, and poorer adhesion of resin teeth.[24] Due to the high curing temperatures involved, only porcelain teeth may be used safely with polycarbonate denture base resins.[23] However, crazing is often observed around the necks of porcelain teeth due to the different rates of thermal contraction.

Polycarbonates are polished by a solvent technique which requires dissolving a surface layer of the resin with ethylene dichloride or methylene chloride.[25]

NYLON

Nylon has been used experimentally as a denture base material and been found to be unsatisfactory due to its high molding shrinkage which leads to warpage, its high water sorption which results in swelling, softening, and a loss of surface finish, and its color instability.[26]

Nylon has also been used in the construction of removable partial dentures (connecting bars, saddles, rests, and clasps). Such removable partial dentures cannot maintain their shape and original positions in clinical situations. This lack of rigidity eventually leads to movement of the abutment teeth and in time serious periodontal complications may develop.[27]

ACRYLIC-VINYL COPOLYMER DENTURE BASE RESINS

The polyvinyl acrylics, mixtures of vinyl acetate-vinyl chloride copolymer and methyl methacrylate, are supplied in gel form and require special injection molding equipment for processing. Next to the acrylic resins, the polyvinyl acrylics are perhaps the most commonly used denture base material, but at best they are only a very distant second in popularity. Although they are also supplied in powder-liquid form (the vinyl copolymer is mixed with monomeric methyl methacrylate), a plastic cake is probably the sales leader among polyvinyl acrylics. The injection molding technique involves feeding compressed air into a cylinder which drives a piston that forces the resin into the mold.

The outstanding advantage of the polyvinyl acrylics is their superior toughness, which permits larger deformations to take place before fracture, but dentures made from these materials are not more stable in dimension than dentures fabricated from acrylic resins. Clinically, the polyvinyl acrylics produce satisfactory dentures which have withstood the test of time.

In summary, numerous investigations have concluded that the conventional acrylic resins, processed with the usual technique of compression molding, produce dentures that are just as stable in dimension and as satisfactory as dentures produced with special resins and elaborate processing equipment. The physical properties of injection molded dentures are not superior to those of acrylic resin dentures produced by the usual carefully controlled compression molding techniques. Cold-curing acrylic resins produce dentures that are as satisfactory as those made from heat-curing resins.[15,28-31]

EVALUATION PROGRAM: The scope, requirements and procedures for evaluating denture base polymers are presented in American Dental Association Specification No. 12. The specification includes acrylic, vinyl, and polystyrene polymers and copolymers, or mixtures of any of these three polymers. The denture base resins may be of the heat-curing or cold-curing types. The heat-curing types include powder-liquids, plastic cakes (gels), and prepolymerized blanks. Pink, clear, and fiber containing resins are included. Materials formulated for use with the pour technique have been admitted to coverage under the fourth revision of the specification. Accordingly, these materials are required to exhibit properties and characteristics comparable to those of the other materials previously included.

AVAILABLE PRODUCTS

TYPE I, HEAT CURING

ACRATON, FIBERED DARK, MEDIUM PINK, TYPE I, CLASS 1, Kerr Mfg. Co., Div. of Sybron Corp.

ACRA-TONE EASY FLOW ACRYLIC, Zahn Dental Co., Inc.

ACRYL-O-DENT FLESH TONE SERIES, Den-Tal-Ez Mfg. Co.

ACUPAC ACRYLIC (FIBERED) LIGHT, MEDIUM AND CHARACTERIZED MEDIUM, Howmedica, Inc., Dental Division

DENTIST'S RESPONSIBILITIES IN DENTURE BASE PROCESSING[32,33]

Do:

1. Provide to the dental laboratory technician a complete and explicit work authorization form (one form for each case) containing as much guidance as possible.
2. Visit your commercial dental laboratory occasionally and inform the technicians of any specific techniques and materials you prefer.
3. Specify a denture base resin that meets American Dental Association Specification No. 12 for Denture Base Polymers.
4. Specify the processing cycle.
5. Inspect the dentures carefully upon return from the laboratory for nodules of resin, thickness (especially palatal), correct depth and contour of frenal notches, and proper festooning and finishing.
6. Store the dentures in water until insertion to allow any small amounts of residual monomer to leach out and to permit some water sorption.
7. Place the dentures in a cold sterilization solution for 30 minutes prior to insertion.
8. Remount the dentures on an articulator from a new centric relation record and make the necessary occlusal corrections *before* allowing the patient to wear them home in order to compensate for changes in tooth position as a result of denture base processing.
9. Treat dental laboratory technicians with respect for their skills, knowledge, experience, and value to the dental team.

Don't:

1. Patronize a commercial dental laboratory that does not utilize a standardized procedure with adequate quality control, that does not follow instructions, or that substitutes materials.
2. Accept incomplete or unsatisfactory laboratory work. Return it to the laboratory with the deficiencies identified.

ASTRON 77, Astron Corp.

BIOLUX; SHADES 206, 207, 209, 220, 285, 483, 485, 506, 521, CLEAR, B. L. Dental Co., Inc.

CHARACTERIZED (VEINED) LUCITONE LIGHT; REDDISH PINK; LIGHT REDDISH PINK; BLUISH PINK; powder/liquid, L. D. Caulk Co., Div. of Dentsply International, Inc.

DENTURE CO-POLYMER PINK; powder/liquid, Teledyne Getz-Opotow

DURAFLOW PINK; CHARACTERIZED; LIGHT CHARACTERIZED; LIGHT VEINED; DARK VEINED; TRANSLUCENT VEINED; powder/liquid, Product Research Laboratories

Estron, Teledyne Dental Products

FEDERAL ACRYLIC, FORMULA 139, CLASS I, Federal Prosthetics, Inc.

Getz Co-Polymer, Teledyne Dental Products

HIRCOE LIGHT FIBERED; DARK FIBERED, Coe Laboratories, Inc.

Hydrocryl Denture Base Material, Solar Dental Co., Inc.

HYGIENE ACRYLIC PINK, Hygienic Dental Mfg. Co.

HY-PRO LUCITONE PINK; FIBERED PINK; FIBERED LIGHT; FIBERED DARK; powder/liquid, L. D. Caulk Co., Div. of Dentsply International, Inc.

IMPACT 76' FIBERED LIGHT, TRANS VEINED, TRANS PINK, TYPE I, CLASS 2, Kerr Mfg. Co., Div. of Sybron Corp.

K-33, K-33 Pur-Cryl, Modern Materials Mfg. Co.

LANG'S PREMIUM DENTURE ACRYLIC, Lang Dental Mfg. Co., Inc.

Lee Smlth Certified Acrylic, Teledyne Dental Products

LUCITONE CLEAR: PINK: 199 FIBERED LIGHT; powder/liquid, L. D. Caulk Co., Div. of Dentsply International Inc.

LUXENE PINK; PLASTIC CAKE, Howmedica, Inc., Dental Div.

LUXENE PINK, REGULAR, LIGHT, MOTTLED LIGHT, MOTTLED DARK, ESTHETIC-COLOR, MODIFIED C-TONE LIGHT, MODIFIED C-TONE DARK, CHARACTERIZED LIGHT, CHARACTERIZED DARK, NATURALUCENT, TRANSLUCENT, Howmedica, Inc. Dental Div.

MICROLON ACRYLIC PINK; LW PINK; powder/liquid, Hygienic Dental Mfg. Co.

MIRACRYL CLEAR; PINK; powder/liquid, Motloid Co.

NATURAL COE-LOR, Coe Laboratories, Inc.

ORA TONE REGULAR, International Dental Products, Inc.

Oryl Denture Base, Teledyne Dental Products

PALATEX PINK; powder/liquid, Moyco Industries, Inc.

PARAGON DENTURE ACRYLIC PINK; powder/liquid, Hygienic Dental Mfg. Co.

PERMA-CRYL CLEAR; LIGHT & DARK PINK; LIGHT & DARK FIBERED; powder/liquid, Coe Laboratories, Inc.

PERMATONE CLEAR; PINK; powder/liquid, Kerr Mfg. Co., Div. of Sybron Corp.

PLASTODENT DENTURE ACRYLIC, TYPE I, CLASS 1, CLEAR, PINK AND PINK VEINED, Plastodent, Inc.

PORIT DENTURE BASE RESIN, TRANSLUCENT PINK, CHARACTERIZED LIGHT VEINED, Product Research Laboratories

Premier Denture Resin, Healthco, Inc.

RX CO-POLYMER DENTURE RESIN CLEAR; FIBERED D PINK; FIBERED M PINK; LONG FIBERED M PINK; M PINK, Codesco, Inc.

SETATONE STANDARD DENTURE ACRYLIC, CROSSLINKED, TYPE I, CLASS 1, TRANSVEINED, LIGHT NATURAL, NATURAL, MEHARRY, PLAIN PINK, A1-19, CLEAR, Accurate Set, Inc.

TILON LIGHTONE; BRITONE; DUOTONE; V-TONE; GEL, Ticonium Co.

TRULEX DENTURE ACRYLIC, NATURAL AND CLEAR, Teledyne Dental Products

TRU-POUR FLUID DENTURE RESIN, Dentsply International, Inc.

T-3 Denture Base, H. D. Justi Co., Div. Williams Gold Refining Co., Inc.

UNITEK FIBERED ACRYLIC TYPE I LIGHT; MEDIUM; DARK; NON-FIBERED LABORATORY ACRYLIC LIGHT GRANULAR; LIGHT FINE; MEDIUM GRANULAR; MEDIUM FINE; SPECIAL MIX GRANULAR; CLEAR; powder/liquid, Unitek Corp.

VB VERNOCHROME PINK; GEL; powder/liquid, Vernon-Benshoff Co., Inc., Subsidiary of CMP Industries, Inc.

VB VERNONITE REALIST GEL; powder/liquid, Vernon-Benshoff Co., Inc., Subsidiary of CMP Industries, Inc.

VITALON 10/60; CLEAR; PINK; (FIBERED) LIGHT REDDISH PINK, TISSUETONE

MEDIUM, ETHNIC MILD, ETHNIC DARK, Howmedica, Inc., Dental Div.

TYPE II, COLD-CURING

Autocure, L. D. Caulk Co., Div. of Dentsply International, Inc.

Cold-Dent, Modern Materials Mfg. Co.

HYFLO DENTURE BASE POLYMER PINK, PINK #53, VEINED, SPECIAL VEINED, HEAVY VEINED, DARK VEINED, Hygienic Dental Mfg. Co.

HYGIENIC COLD-CURING CROSS LINKED DENTURE ACRYLIC, Hygienic Dental Mfg. Co.

PALATEX 51 PINK; powder/liquid, Moyco Industries, Inc.

Unitek Cold Cure Acrylics, Unitek Corp.

LITERATURE REFERENCES

1. Winkler, S., and Vernon, H. M. Coloring acrylic denture base resins. J. Prosthet. Dent. 40:4 July 1978.

2. Peyton, F. A. History of resins in dentistry. Dent. Clin. N. Am. 19:211 Apr. 1975.

3. Winkler, S. The advantages of gels in denture prosthesis. Cert. Dent. Tech. 1:8 Mar. 1964.

4. O'Brien, W. J., and Ryge, G. Wettability of poly-(methyl methacrylate) treated with silicon tetrachloride. J. Prosthet. Dent. 15:304 Mar.-Apr. 1965.

5. Boucher, L. J., et al. The effects of a microlayer of silica on the retention of mandibular complete dentures. J. Prosthet. Dent. 19:581 June 1968.

6. Winkler, S.; Ortman, H. R.; and Ryczek, M. T. Improving the retention of complete dentures. J. Prosthet. Dent. 34:11 July 1975.

7. Leonard, F., and Margetis, P. M. Polymers in dentistry and medicine. SPE Journal 24:60 Feb. 1968.

8. Spealman, C. R., et al. Monomeric methyl methacrylate. Ind. Med. 14:292 Apr. 1945.

9. Chandler, H. H.; Bowen, R.L.; and Paffenbarger, G. C. Physical properties of a radiopaque denture base material. J. Bio. Med. Mat. Res. 5:335 July 1971.

10. Dummett, C. O. Oral pigmentation. J. Periodont. 31:356 Oct. 1960.

11. Choudhary, S. C.; Craig, J. F.; and Suls, F.J. Characterizing the denture base for non-Caucasian patients. J. Prosthet. Dent. 33:73 Jan. 1975.

12. Gerhard, R., and Sawyer, N. Dentures to harmonize with heavily pigmented tissues. JADA 73:94 July 1966.

13. Quinlivan, J. T. Characterization of denture bases. Dent. Clin. N. Am. 19:321 Apr. 1975.

14. Winkler, S., et al. Characterization of denture bases for people of color. JADA 81:1349 Dec. 1970.

15. Woelfel, J. B.; Paffenbarger, G. C.; and Sweeney, W. T. Clinical evaluation of complete dentures made of 11 different types of denture base materials. JADA 70:1170 May 1965.

16. Mowery, W. E., et al. Dimensional stability of denture base resins. JADA 57:345 Sept. 1958.

17. Winkler, S.; Powell, J. P.; and Ortman, H. R. Ultraviolet absorbers in dental monomers. Dent. Dig. 77:460 Aug. 1971.

18. Smith, D. C., and Bains, M. E. D. Residual methyl methacrylate in the denture base and its relation to denture sore mouth. Br. Dent. J. 98:55 Jan. 1955.

19. Turrell, A. J. W. Allergy to denture base materials—fallacy or reality. Br. Dent. J. 120: 415 May 1966.

20. Phillips, R. W. Science of dental materials. ed. 7, Philadelphia, W. B. Saunders Company, 1973.

21. Sweeney, W. T. Acrylic resins in prosthetic dentistry. Dent. Clin. N. Am. 2:593 Nov. 1958.

22. Winkler, S. Construction of denture bases from pour resins. Dent. Clin. N. Am. 19:243 Apr. 1975.

23. Brauer, G. M. Dental applications of polymers: a review. JADA 72:1151 May 1966.

24. Stafford, G. D., and Smith, D. C. Polycarbonates. A preliminary report on the use of polycarbonates as a denture base material. Dent. Pract. 17:217 Feb. 1967.

25. Anderson, J. N. Applied dental materials. ed. 3, Oxford, Blackwell Scientific Publications, 1967.

26. Smith, D. C. Recent developments and prospects in dental polymers. J. Prosthet. Dent. 12: 1066 Nov.-Dec. 1962.

27. George, W. A. Notes and comments. Dent. Abs. 10:9 Jan. 1965.

28. Woelfel, J. B.; Paffenbarger, G. C.; and Sweeney, W. T. Some physical properties of organic denture base materials. JADA 67:489 Oct. 1963.

29. Woelfel, J. B.; Paffenbarger, G. C.; and Sweeney, W. T. Dimensional changes in complete dentures on drying, wetting and heating in water. JADA 65:495 Oct. 1962.

30. Paffenbarger, G. C.; Woelfel, J. B.; and Sweeney, W. T. Dimensional changes in dentures. Dent. Pract. 13:64 Oct. 1962.

31. Paffenbarger, G. C.; Woelfel, J. B.; and Sweeney, W. T. Resins and techniques used in constructing dentures. Dent. Clin. N. Am. 9:251 Mar. 1965.

32. Ward, J. E. Laboratory procedure authorizations and communicating with dental laboratory technicians. In Winkler, S. (ed.) Essentials of complete denture prosthodontics. Philadelphia, W. B. Saunders Company, Ch. 18, 1979.

33. Woelfel, J. B. Processing dentures. In Winkler, S. (ed.) Essentials of complete denture prosthodontics. Philadelphia, W. B. Saunders Company, Ch. 19, 1979.

PRECISION ATTACHMENTS

The development of attachments has been largely due to the inventive genius of restorative dentists around the world. Most attachments are identified by the designer's name and there is considerable variation among the attachments available in different countries. Many attempts have been made to classify the vast number of attachments.[1-10]

Matsuo[9] in 1970 developed a color-coded millimeter attachment gauge to measure the vertical distance available for the placement of an attachment. Mensor[7] refers to this gauge as the E.M. (after E. Matsuo) selector gauge and has since developed a most comprehensive attachment classification and compendium based on the E.M. Attachment Selector.[10]

In attempt to design a classification based on the function of the attachment and the indication for its use, the authors propose the classification system depicted in Table I.

USES: Precision attachments are used to provide retention and stabilization for removable partial and overlay dentures as well as for fixed restorations where there is difficulty in aligning abutment preparations and hence a problem in inserting a one-piece rigid casting.

COMPOSITION: A precision attachment consists of two precisely fitted parts: the matrix and the patrix. The matrix or female is soldered into a recess or cast directly within the abutment casting, so that it is within the normal contour of the abutment tooth. The patrix or male unit is joined to the removable partial denture and splints the partial to the abutment tooth when the patrix is seated firmly in the matrix.

EVALUATION PROGRAM: There is no Specification or Acceptance Program for precision attachments at the present time.

REST ATTACHMENTS

A slider attachment is a round dovetailed or rectangular section (patrix) sliding in an appropriate matrix. It is an interlocking device; its only retention derives from friction. It is usual to use a lingual retentive clasp arm on the partial denture framework to supplement retention.

Rest attachments are slide attachments that facilitate the transfer of the load. Cecconi[11] has shown that the closer the occlusal rest is to the gingival margin, the more effective the rest is in opposing movement of the tooth.

Plastic Patterns (Fig. 1): The Ney M.S. (minimal space) plastic pattern comprises a matrix with cylindrical slide and proximal flanges. The outside dimension of the matrix is 1.1 mm which makes it very suitable for use in anterior teeth. The Ney mini, contrary to its name, is a large tapered slider attachment for use in posterior teeth. Both of these intracoronal rests can be used for partial dentures or to break a fixed unit.

The Ney McKay Mortice is a mortice-shaped interlock whose use is restricted to "stress-broken" fixed restorations. The Stern Connector

Patterns and Howmedica P.D. attachments are designed for use with removable partial dentures and are incorporated in crowns on the abutment teeth.

Ceramic Cores: The Strauss system comprises ceramic cores plus complementary plastic patterns. One side of the core is a tapered slider attachment and the other is a cylindrical matrix. The ceramic cores are dissolved out of the gold castings with hydrofluoric acid.

Metal Mandrels (Fig. 2): The Ticon P.R.P. mandrels are for forming deep-seated, sharply tapered rests. The mandrels are inserted into the wax pattern. When cast, the mandrels are removed leaving a sharply defined rest in the gold crown.

The Scherer mandrel, used in a similar fashion, comes with a spring-lock.[12,13] The Stern-gold T-shaped slide has a base metal former for establishing the matrix.

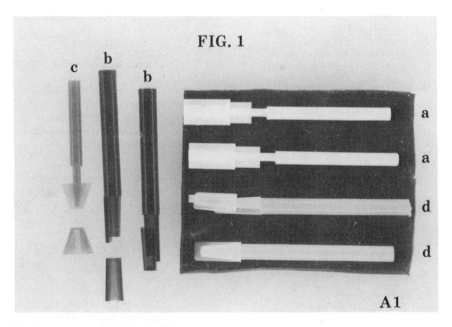

Fig. 1 Plastic Patterns (A1.)* **a.** Ney M.S.; **b.** Ney Mini; **c.** Ney McKay Mortice; **d.** P.D. Attachments.

---

*Letter and number in parenthesis e.g. (A1.) after the title and in the left hand corner of the figure provides a cross reference to the classification of precision attachments in Table I.

Table I.

A. *Rest Attachments—Intracoronal Slider Attachments*

A1. Plastic Patterns (Fig. 1)
   a. Ney M.S.
   b. Ney Mini
   c. Ney McKay Mortice
   d. Sterngold Connector Patterns
   e. P.D. Attachments (Howmedica)

A2. Ceramic Cores
   a. Strauss

A3. Metal Mandrels or Formers (Fig. 2)
   a. P.R.P. Mandrels (Ticonium)
   b. Scherer
   c. Sterngold—T shaped slide

A4. Milled Rests

B. *Slider Attachments—Intracoronal*

B1. Frictional (Fig. 3)
   a. Steiger Milled C.S.P.
   b. CM 639 and 639B (Sterngold), (Beyeler)
   c. CM 617, 643 (Sterngold)
   d. Des Marets (Sterngold)
   e. Sterngold T-shaped
   f. Austenal External (Howmedica)

B2. Frictional and Adjustable (Fig. 4)
   a. CM 633A (McCollum) (Sterngold)
   b. Sterngold Type 7
   c. Sterngold G/A
   d. Ney—Chayes, No. 9
   e. Ney—Chayes, No. 9 split lingual

B3. Frictional with Retentive Device (Fig. 5)
   a. CM 669 (Crismani) (Sterngold)
   b. CM 606 (Schatzmann) (Sterngold)
   c. Sterngold G/L Micro
   d. Sterngold G/L Dovetail
   e. Ney-Lock
   f. Ney-Lock split lingual

C. *Stud Attachments—Overlay Denture Anchors*

C1. Intraradicular (Fig. 6)
   a. Zest Regular (Sterngold)
   b. Zest Mini (Sterngold)

C2. Supraradicular

   C2.1 Frictional and adjustable (Fig. 7)
   a. CM 604A [Dalla Bona] (Sterngold)

b. CM 615 [Gmür] (Sterngold)
c. Kurer Press Stud (Union Broach)

C2.2 Frictional with retentive device (Fig. 8)
a. CM 686 [Gerber] (Sterngold)
b. CM 695 [Huser] (Sterngold)
c. CM 746 [Rothermann] (Sterngold)

C2.3 Frictional, adjustable and providing for tissueward movement (Fig. 9)
a. CM 604 [Dalla Bona] (Sterngold) (Fig. 10)
b. CM 604P [Dalla Bona] (Sterngold)
c. CM 684A [Biaggi] (Sterngold)
d. Ceka 691 (Jelenko)
e. Sandri-2 Pressure Button (Bell)

C2.4 Frictional with retentive device and providing for tissueward movement (Fig. 11)
a. CM 747 [Rothermann] (Sterngold)
b. CM 696 [Gerber] (Sterngold)

D. *Bar Attachments—Bar Splint Anchors*

D1. Rigid bar unit—no tissueward movement or rotation
   a. Andrews anterior and posterior curved bar (ICD) (Fig. 12)
   b. CM 336A and 336 Dolder (Sterngold) (Fig. 13)
   c. Steiger-Boitel Attachment
   d. CM Milled Bar (Sterngold)
   e. Ceka Bar (Jelenko)
   f. Octolink Bridge System (Sterngold)

D2. Rigid bar unit—allows rotation but no tissueward movement (Fig. 14)
   a. Baker (gauges 11 and 14) (Englehard) (Fig. 15)
   b. Ackermann (Sterngold)
   c. CM 342 (Sterngold) (gauge 13 with retentive riders) (Fig. 16)
   d. Hader Bar and Rider System (Sterngold)

D3. Resilient bar joint—allows rotation and tissueward movement (Fig. 17)
   a. CM 334A and 334 [Dolder] (Sterngold)
   b. Baker Bar (gauge 11) used with Dolder CM 334 (Ticonium)
   c. CM 342 (Sterngold) round bar with riders

E. *Distal Extension Attachments—Extracoronal* (Fig. 18)

E1. Frictional, adjustable and with rigid vertical stop
   a. Stabilex [Spang] (Sterngold)
   b. Conex (Sterngold)
   c. CM 612 [Roach] (Sterngold)

E2. Hinge or rotational movement (Fig. 19)
   a. CM 750A [Steiger Ro/lock] (Sterngold)
   b. D-E Hinge [Vitallium] (Howmedica)
   c. Ti-Hinge [TD-60] (Ticonium)
   d. CM 671 [Strini] (Sterngold)
   e. CM 697A and 697 [Gerber] (Sterngold)
   f. CM 716A and 716 [Gerber] (Sterngold)
   g. Ceka 691 (Jelenko)

E3. Frictional with retentive device and providing for tissueward and hinge movement (Fig. 20)
   a. CM 750 [Steiger Ax-Ro joint] (Sterngold)
   b. CM 613 [Roach] (Sterngold)
   c. Ceka 691 (Jelenko)
   d. Octolink 81 (Sterngold)
   e. CM 789 [Crismani] (Sterngold)
   f. CM 689 [Crismani] (Sterngold)
   g. CM 667B [Dalbo] (Sterngold)
   h. Dalbo-M [ultra-M] (Sterngold)
   i. ASC-52 (Bell)

F. *Cross Arch Attachments*

F1. Rigid, retentive and adjustable—only

vertical movement (Fig. 21)
   a. CM 653A and 653 (Sterngold)
   b. CM 717 [Snaprox] (Sterngold)
   c. Ney-Chayes,No. 9 (Ney) split-lingual
   d. Ney-Loc (Ney) split-lingual

F2. Rotational
   a. CM 750A [Steiger Ro lock] (Sterngold)
   b. CM 750 [Steiger Ax-Ro joint] (Sterngold)
   c. CM 665 [Huser] (Sterngold)

F3. Rotational, retentive and adjustable (Fig. 22)
   a. Push Lock [Spang] (Sterngold)
   b. Push Lock [Spang] (Sterngold)
   c. CM 613 [Roach] (Sterngold)

G. *Auxiliary Attachments*

G1. Screwblock anchors (Fig.23)
   a. CM 658A and 658 [Schubiger] (Sterngold)
   b. CM 659A and 659 [Schubiger] (Sterngold)
   c. CM 709A, 709 and 709C [Hruska] (Sterngold)

G2. Retentive anchors (Fig. 24)
   a. CM 783 [Ipsoclip] (Sterngold)
   b. CM 784 [Ipsoclip] (Sterngold)

G3. Hinged labial retentive units
   a. Swing-Lock (Idea Development Co.) (Fig. 25)
   b. Nobil-Latch (American Gold-Nobilium) (Fig. 26)

INTRACORONAL SLIDER ATTACHMENTS

Frictional (Fig. 3): Intracoronal frictional slider attachments with the exception of the Steiger C.S.P. (channel, shoulder, pin) attachment which is milled into a gold crown, are all carefully machined, prefabricated commercial attachments.[1] They are most commonly used as accurate interlocking slides where the only retention is due to the frictional resistance opposing the separation of the two components.

The Steiger C.S.P. attachment is made by milling a lingual shoulder on a three-quarter or full crown. The shoulder terminates mesially and distally, with a channel in the proximal areas. Additional retention is obtained by drilling pin holes. The patrix is then waxed to restore normal contour and then it is cast, fitted, soldered to a removable partial framework and finished.

The CM 639 Beyeler comprises an intracoronal matrix with a dovetailed slide. The matching patrix has an extension for soldering to the partial denture framework or to a fixed pontic. The CM 643 and CM 617 interlock slides are very similar to the Beyeler attachment, except that the slot in the matrix is round. The smaller

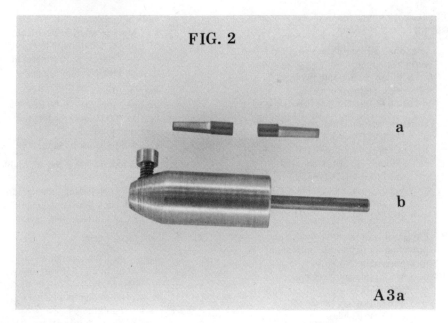

Fig. 2   Metal Mandrels (A3.) **a.** P.R.P. Mandrel; **b.** Surveyor attachment for mandrel.

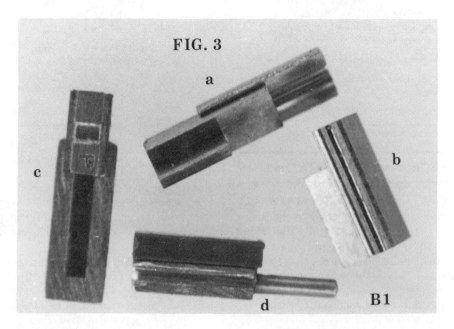

Fig. 3   Slider Attachments—Frictional (B1.) **a.** CM 639 Beyeler; **b.** CM 643 Interlock; **c.** Sterngold—T shaped slide; **d.** Austenal E.F.

CM 643 is used in anterior teeth, while the CM 617 is for posterior teeth.

The matrix of the Des Marets intracoronal slide attachment does not have a gingival floor; however, one side of the patrix is tapered towards the gingival margin to prevent the patrix from sliding too far down the matrix. The T-shaped Sterngold rest is a standard slider attachment and comes in a variety of alloys.

The Austenal External Frictional attachment is a regular T-shaped slider attachment.

These attachments, being factory made, fit more accurately than custom-made rest attachments and, therefore, are more positive in locking together sections of a fixed restoration or a removable appliance to an abutment tooth. They should not be used in distal extension cases.

Frictional and Adjustable (Fig. 4): Although the intracoronal attachments in this group depend on friction for retention, the patrix of each attachment can be adjusted to overcome the loss of friction with wear. As the retentive capacity of these attachments can be maintained, it is not necessary to use retentive arms on the cast framework. All of the attachments listed in this class are designed to provide support and retention for tooth supported partial dentures.

The CM 633A was developed by McCollum. It is an H-shaped slide, the patrix of which has a slot running the full length. The Sterngold Type 7, H-shaped slide has a longitudinal expansion slot on either side of the patrix. The patrix must be soldered to the partial denture framework. The Sterngold G/A (gingival adjustment) is H-shaped, has a retentive adjustment slot in the patrix, and is designed to be soldered to the cast framework.

The Ney-Chayes No. 9, regular and split-lingual, are H-shaped slide attachments in which the patrix can be adjusted to maintain retention. The split-lingual attachment is designed with a wide proximal plate to reduce rotation and is useful as a cross-arch stabilizer.

Frictional with Retentive Device (Fig. 5): Positive retention is supplied by a retentive device which is usually a spring-loaded ball-catch or a spring-leaf in the form of a gingival latch.

The retentive device of the CM 699 Crismani is a spring clip in the base of the dovetail patrix which engages the sides of the opening of the matrix. A screw on the face of the patrix allows for each replacement of the clip.

The Schatzmann CM 606 dovetailed slide includes a spring-loaded ball in the contacting surface of the dovetail in the patrix. The ball engages a corresponding dimple in the wall of the matrix.

Sterngold G/L (gingival latch) H-shaped slider attachments have a gingival spring-leaf latch that clicks over a ridge near the gingival floor of the matrix. The Sterngold Micro G/L is perhaps the smallest frictional with retentive device attachment available.

The Ney-Loc attachments have, in addition to a gingival spring-leaf, a ridge on the wall of the matrix close to the floor of the attachment over which a ridge on the spring-leaf of the patrix grips. This mechanism provides positive retention to resist vertical dislodgement. The Ney-Loc and #9 matrices are available in a platinum-iridium alloy which may be used in combination with porcelain bonded to metal crowns.

STUD ATTACHMENTS—OVERLAY DENTURE ANCHORS

Intraradicular Anchors (Fig. 6): An intraradicular anchor is one in which the matrix is positioned within the root itself.[14] The best known is the Zest anchor which is available in two sizes: the regular Zest and Mini Zest. The Zest system of intraradicular anchors is based on the use of a prefabricated nonmagnet stainless steel matrix which is cemented within the root and a nylon patrix which is held in the acrylic base of the denture. To allow for variation in root size the matrix is available in two sizes, regular and mini, the patrix for each being interchangeable.

The other components of the Zest system comprise a sizing bar (regular and mini) for cutting the cavity in the root for the matrix and a

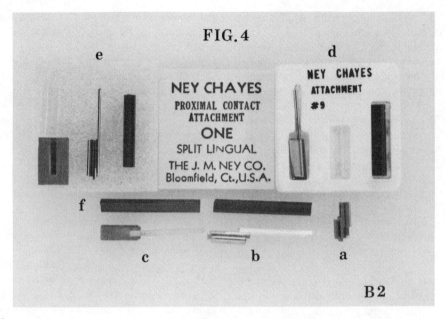

Fig. 4 Slider Attachments—Frictional & Adjustable (B2.) **a.** CM 633A McCollum; **b.** Sterngold G/A; **c.** Sterngold Type 7; **d.** Ney Chayes No. 9; **e.** Ney Chayes No. 9 Split Lingual; **f.** Carbon soldering patrix.

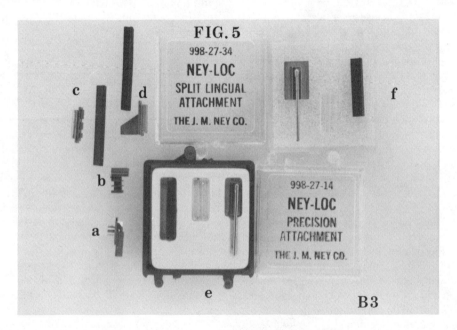

Fig. 5 Slider Attachments—Frictional with Retentive Device (B3.) **a.** CM 669 Crismani; **b.** CM 606 Schatzmann; **c.** Sterngold G/L Micro; **d.** Sterngold G/L Dovetail; **e.** Ney-Loc; **f.** Ney-Loc Split lingual.

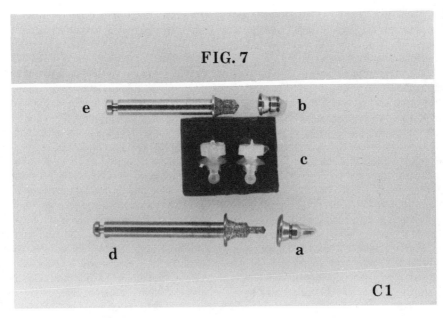

FIG. 7

Fig. 6   Stud Attachments—Intraradicular (C1.) **a.** Zest Regular Matrix; **b.** Zest Mini Matrix; **c.** Zest Regular and Mini Patrices; **d.** Zest Regular sizing bur; **e.** Zest Mini sizing bur.

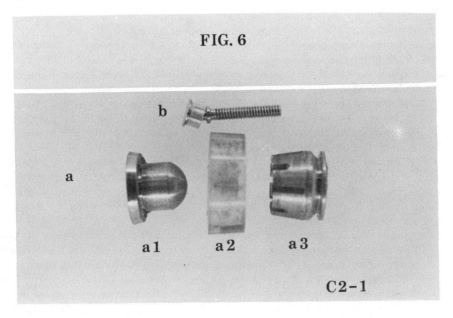

FIG. 6

Fig. 7   Stud Attachments—Supraradicular (C2.) C2.1 Frictional and Adjustable **a.** CM 604A Dalla Bona (3x mag.) eight lamellae; **a1.** patrix; **a2.** P.V.C. Ring; **a3.** Matrix; **b.** Kurer Press Stud.

transfer patrix that is used in making the impression and positioning the processing jig in the cast which, in turn, locates the permanent nylon patrix in the denture base.

Zest attachments are almost exclusively used for overlay dentures. They are easy to use, relatively inexpensive and provide dramatic retention for the complete overlay denture. As exposed dentin is left surrounding the matrix on the root face, it is imperative that the dentin be treated regularly with fluoride and that the patient maintain strict oral hygiene and a plaque control program.

Supraradicular Anchors: A supraradicular anchor comprises a prefabricated patrix and matrix with the patrix being soldered to a gold rootcap which is held in place on the root face by a post in the root canal. In the case of the Kurer Press Stud, the patrix ball-attachment screws onto a stainless steel threaded post. In all cases, the matrix fits directly over the patrix and is processed into the acrylic base of the denture.

Frictional and Adjustable Anchors (Fig 7): The CM 604A Dalla Bona and CM 615 Gmur are frictional fitting, cylindrical snap-grips that grasp a cylindrical patrix. In each case they can be adjusted to maintain the frictional contact. Because the patrices have parallel sides, there is resistance to lateral movement and rotation and therefore they are not suited for overlay dentures but are suitable as tooth or root supporting abutment attachments. The Kurer stainless steel press stud is more like a universal joint and serves as a good anchor for overlay dentures.

Frictional with Retentive Device (Fig. 8): These three attachments, CM 686 Gerber, CM 695 Huser and CM 746 Rothermann, are designed to facilitate tooth support for a removable partial denture. They may be used as an abutment, intermediate pier or root anchor on which the partial denture rests.[15] Each has a specific retentive device which, in the case of the Gerber and Huser, is easily and inexpensively replaced whereas the arms of the CM 746 can be tightened or loosened.

(3) *Frictional, Adjustable and Providing for Tissueward Movement* (Fig. 9): The five anchors in this group are specifically designed to pro-

vide retention for overlay dentures.[16] In each case the patrix is a ball attached to a flat base which is soldered to a gold root-cap which, in turn, is cemented in the anchor root. The cylindrical matrix grasps the patrix thereby creating a near universal joint. With the exception of Ceka 691 the lamellae or fingers of the matrices can be adjusted to increase or decrease the amount of retention. In the case of the Ceka, the patrix is both adjustable and replaceable.

They are designed to allow 0.4 mm of tissueward movement (CM 604P-0.8 mm) and because they are virtually universal joints they provide retention of the overlay denture without torquing the anchor roots.[17]

The Dalla Bona CM 604 (Fig. 10) is perhaps the best known and most versatile of this group.[18] It is essentially a universal joint that allows movement in all directions but resists dislodgement. A spacer washer is used during processing to provide 0.4 mm tissueward movement. The cylindrical matrix is enclosed in a polyvinyl chloride (P.V.C.) sheath to form a resilient layer between the lamellae and the surrounding acrylic. This resilient P.V.C. layer permits the lamellae to open and close over the spherical patrix.

CM 604P is very similar to CM 604 except that the matrix is taller and wider to allow the inclusion of a recoil-spring in the matrix. It is doubtful if such a spring is necessary and it has the disadvantage of increasing the height of the attachment by 1.20 mm over the CM 604. Even the height of the shorter CM 604 can be a problem.

The Biaggi CM 648A is similar to CM 604 but has an adjustable split-ball patrix with a threaded split-ring insert inside the cylindrical matrix.

The Ceka 691[19] comprises a patrix in the form of a cone, with rounded top, which is split longitudinally in two directions at right angles to each other. The patrix is threaded at the base for screwing into a base-ring which is incorporated in the root-face casting. The cylindrical matrix is held in the acrylic of the overlay denture, and during processing is kept above the base-ring by a 0.4 mm spacer washer. The attachment is available in three different alloys of

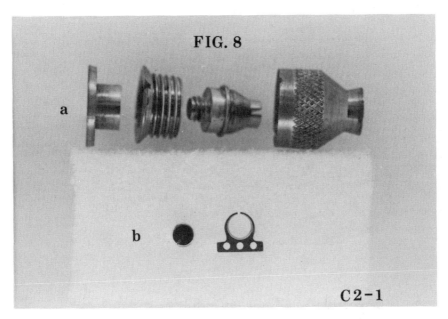

Fig. 8 Stud Attachments—Supraradicular (C2.) C2.2 Frictional with Retentive Device **a.** CM 686 Gerber (3x mag.); **b.** CM 746 Rothermann.

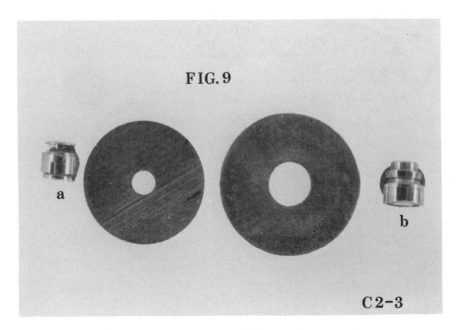

Fig. 9 Stud Attachments—Supraradicular (C2.) C2.3 Frictional, Adjustable & Providing for Tissueward Movement **a.** CM 604 Dalla Bona with spacer **b.** Ceka 691 with spacer.

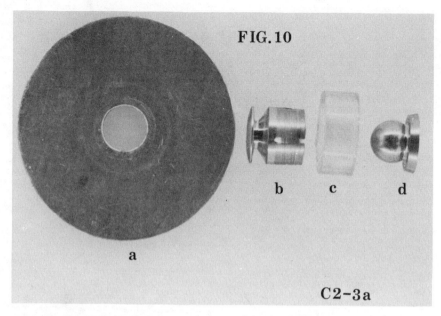

Fig. 10   CM 604 Dalla Bona (3x mag.) **a.** spacer; **b.** matrix with four lamellae; **c.** P.V.C. ring; **d.** spherical patrix.

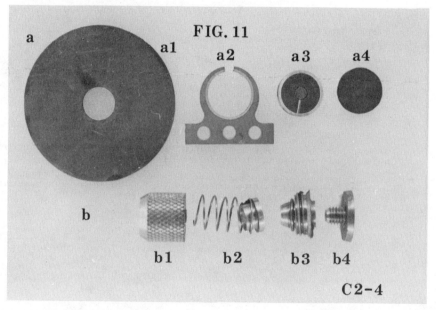

Fig. 11   Stud Attachments—Supraradicular (C2.) C2.4 Frictional with Retentive Device and Providing for Tissueward Movement **a.** CM 747 Rothermann; **a1.** root-face spacer; **a2.** matrix; **a3.** grooved patrix with solder core; **a4.** occlusal spacer (3x mag.); **b.** CM 696 Gerber; **b1.** matrix housing; **b2.** coiled spring and snap-grip; **b3.** patrix grip; **b4.** patrix base (3x mag.).

varying melting points. The patrix is subject to wear[20] but is easily replaced in the base ring on the anchor root.

The Sandri-2 pressure button is the smallest stud attachment available, being only 2.5 mm high.[21] The patrix comprises a threaded gold soldering base which is incorporated into the root-face casting. A stainless steel ball with a female thread screws down into the base to complete the patrix. The stainless steel matrix consists of a threaded housing which carries the adjustable split-ring retentive cylinder. The matrix is closed at the top by a frictional fitting cap. The outside threads of the matrix lock it into the acrylic of the overlay denture. Provisions may be made for tissueward movement by using 0.4 mm spacer washers during processing of the acrylic.

(4) *Frictional with Retentive Device and Providing for Tissueward Movement* (Fig. 11): The CM 747 Rothermann attachment, which comprises two spring arms embracing a grooved patrix, is perhaps the best attachment to use when there is minimal vertical space available. The patrix is only 1.7 mm high and after allowing for the two 0.6 mm spacers above and below the attachment, as well as providing for adequate acrylic coverage in the overlay denture, only a total of 5.0 mm vertical space is required. The snap-grip of the attachment is both adjustable and serviceable. The CM 696 Gerber is a more complicated attachment which, in addition to a snap-grip with split-ring retention, has a coil-spring that returns the matrix and of course the overlay denture to the resting position after each tissueward movement. Unfortunately, the CM 696 is 5.2 mm high, which limits its usefulness.

BAR ATTACHMENTS— BAR SPLIT ANCHORS

Rigid Bar Unit—No Tissueward Movement or Rotation: The seven bars in this class are designed to splint together the remaining teeth, usually in groups, and to make provision for the tooth-support of the removable prosthesis. The shape of the bars prevents both tissueward movement and rotation of the prosthesis around the bar. It is for this reason that the bar unit is described as "rigid."

The Andrews[22] bar is specifically designed to allow for the esthetic restoration of lost bone and tissue, especially in anterior saddles. Otherwise it is very difficult to make a satisfactory fixed esthetic restoration. However, with the bar completing the arch and with the removable section restoring the lost labial alveolus, a favorable esthetic result can be obtained.

The anterior Andrews bar and sleeve is precurved and is available in four different ring curvatures: A, B, C, and D. (Fig. 12). The selection of the ring curvature is made using a clear plastic template, "Guide for Selecting Bar Curvature," supplied by the distributors.[22]

In addition, the bars (patrices) and sleeves (matrices) are available in three different vertical heights: Regular, Thin-line and Low-set. Whenever possible the regular height is used as it provides maximum resistance to rotation and hence greater stability. In cases where the muco-occlusal height is limited, the Thin-line is indicated. In those cases where there is a space problem, the Low-set bar is used as it is only half the height of the Regular bar but twice as thick to achieve the required strength. The distributors now advise that the single bar has also proved effective in posterior restorations[23] but suggest that the bar with maximum curvature and size that can be accommodated in the space be used. However, many would advocate that the partial denture should be extended to the opposite side of the arch to ensure stability rather than risk rotation to the restoration around the bar.

The CM Dolder bar, which comes in two sizes, is a "U" shaped bar with a channel-section matrix (Fig. 13). The bar or patrix is soldered between splinted abutments and the matrix is held in the acrylic anchorage of the saddle. A combination of bar units and a removable partial denture provides a very satisfactory economical alternative to a complete arch porcelain bonded-to-metal splint.

The Steiger-Boitel[1] and the CM milled bar

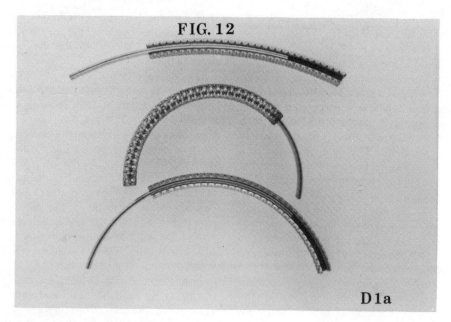

Fig. 12   Bar Attachments, Rigid Bar Unit—No Tissueward Movement or Rotation (D1.a) Andrews bar, patrix inside matrix, three different curvatures.

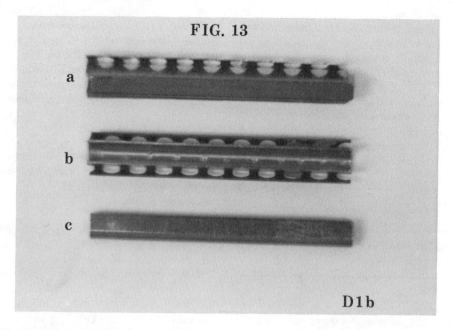

Fig. 13   Rigid Bar Unit (D1.b) CM 336 Dolder **a.** patrix in matrix; **b.** matrix showing acrylic anchorage; **c.** patrix.

require extensive precision work in the laboratory, along with a close working relationship between the doctor and technician. Both the Ceka bar[19] and the Octolink Bridge System[8] make use of plastic patterns for casting the bars. The gold matrices are incorporated in the plastic bar patterns. After warming, bending and adjusting the bar-pattern, the bar is cast in an appropriate gold alloy directly around the gold matrices. In both cases the patrices are expandable press-studs which, when secured in the acrylic of the partial denture saddle, provide positive retention.

Rigid Bar Unit—Allows Rotation but no Tissueward Movement (Fig. 14): These bars are used when it is desired to excuse the abutments from resisting rotary movement about the bar and also in those cases where it is thought that at some future occasion it may be necessary to extract posterior abutments and to convert the case into a distal-extention partial denture. The Baker (Fig. 15), Achermann and CM 342 (Fig. 16) bars are round with small matching female retentive riders. The bars can be annealed to allow bending to follow tissue contour either around the arch or along the crest of the ridge. After the bars have been bent and soldered to the crowns on the splintered abutments they should be heat treated, before cementation, to restore optimal properties to the metal.

The Hader bar system includes a plastic pattern for the bar with a flange to contact the ridge crest. The bar plus flange is heated in hot water and bent or ground to the desired shape. It is then cast in an appropriate gold alloy, soldered to the abutment crowns, heat treated and cemented in place.

During processing of the acrylic saddle, teflon spacers are used to create the recesses for the half-round nylon matrices which are pushed into place when the teflon spacers are removed from the processed acrylic.

Resilient Bar Joint—Allows Rotation and Tissueward Movement (Fig. 17): The Dolder CM 334 bar, being oval in cross section, permits limited rotation without traumatizing the abutment.[24] Both the Baker and CM 342 bars are round and hence allow rotation. CM 334 and

CM 342 are supplied with throw-away brass spacers which are used during processing to hold the matrices (CM 334—channel section, CM 342 metal riders) above the bar. When it is required to use the Baker bar to provide retention without involving bar support, it is necessary to use small sections of the Dolder CM 334 spacer and matrix as the Baker bar is only supplied with small tight fitting retentive clips.

DISTAL EXTENSION ATTACHMENTS—EXTRACORONAL

Frictional, Adjustable and with Vertical Stop (Fig. 18): The Stabilex and Conex attachments are designed to carry distal-extension saddles as cantilevered units off splinted abutment teeth. The Stabilex matrix extends some 6.0 mm distal to the abutment tooth and receives two adjustable split-pins which comprise the retentive mechanism of the patrix which unit is, in turn, incorporated in the acrylic of the saddle. The Conex attachment is similar but smaller, having only one retentive pin.

The CM 612 Roach is one of the oldest attachments and was designed by Roach to allow the free-end saddle to move tissueward parallel to the basal seat.[2] Usually the tube matrix of the attachment is soldered to the distal surface of the abutment restoration and the adjustable ball patrix with flange is imbedded in the proximal surface of the acrylic saddle.

Hinge or Rotational Movement (Fig. 19): These attachments are designed to allow rotational or hinge movement between the distal-extension saddle and the abutment tooth. CM 750A Steiger Ro/lock comprises a rectangular bar (patrix) mounted in a rectangular tube section (matrix) held together by a screw. The bar can be ground on each side of either end to permit limited rotation and the screw hole in the matrix may be cut as a vertical slot to allow tissueward movement. Commonly the attachment is a resilient unit between the saddle connector and the partial denture retentive unit, usually a C.S.P. attachment, embracing the

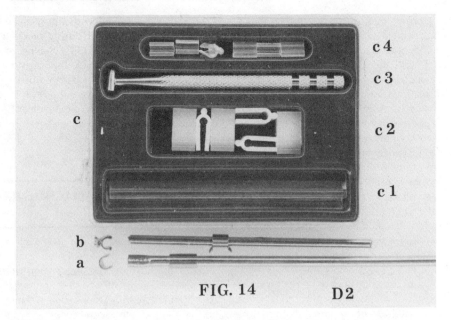

Fig. 14   Rigid Bar Unit—Allows Rotation but no Tissueward Movement (D2.) **a.** Baker bar with two retentive clips; **b.** CM 342 with two retentive riders; **c.** Hader bar system; **c1.** plastic pattern for bar; **c2.** teflon spacers; **c3.** tool for inserting matrix; **c4.** nylon matrices.

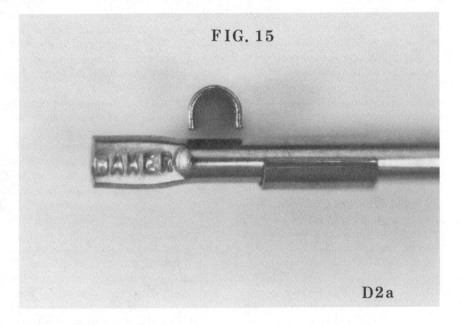

Fig. 15   Baker Bar gauge 11 with two retentive clips.

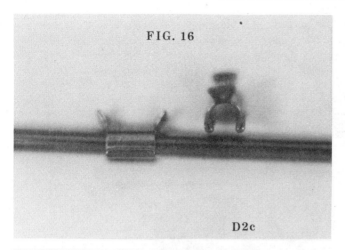

FIG. 16

D2c

Fig. 16 CM 342 gauge 13 with two retentive riders.

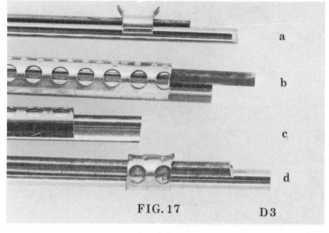

a

b

c

d

FIG. 17   D3

Fig. 17 Resilient Bar Joint, Allows Rotation and Tissueward Movement (D3.) **a.** CM 342 with rider and spacer allowing 0.75mm tissueward movement; **b.** CM 344 Dolder, oval patrix with matrix and 1.05mm spacer; **c.** CM 344A Dolder, oval patrix with matrix and 0.75mm spacer; **d.** Baker bar gauge 11 with section of Dolder CM 344 clip and spacer.

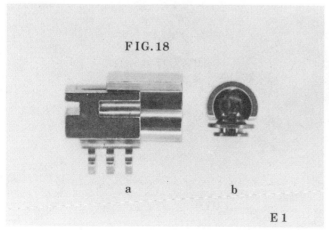

FIG. 18

a   b

E 1

Fig. 18 Distal Extension Attachment—Frictional, Adjustable and with Rigid Vertical Stop (E1.) **a.** Conex, matrix sliding on patrix; **b.** CM 612 Roach, patrix inside tube matrix.

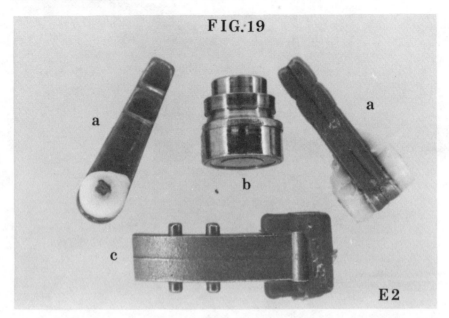

Fig. 19   Distal Extension Attachment—Hinge or Rotational Movement (E2.) **a.** TI-Hinge; **b.** Ceka 691; **c.** D-E Hinge.

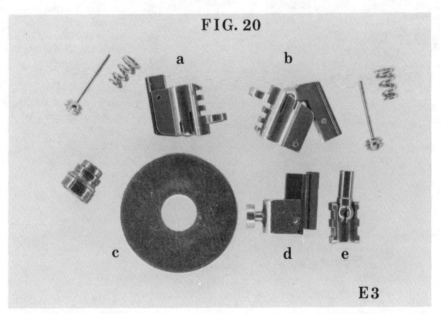

Fig. 20   Distal Extension Attachment with Frictional Retentive Device & Providing for Tissueward Movement and Hinge Movement (E3.) **a.** CM 667B Dalbo, matrix on patrix, recoil spring and locking pin; **b.** CM 667B, matrix hinging on ball of patrix; **c.** Ceka 691 with spacer; **d.** CM 689 Crismani matrix hinging on patrix; **e.** CM 613 patrix sliding in matrix.

abutment teeth.

The D-E Vitallium hinge and TI-Ticonium hinge are positioned close to the distal end of the abutment teeth allowing the saddle to hinge about a horizontal axis. The DE and TI come in plastic pattern forms to be incorporated in Vitallium and Ticonium cast frameworks respectively.

The CM 671 Strini, CM 697 Gerber and CM 716 Gerber are gold prefabricated hinges that may be used to attach the free-end saddle to the cast framework embracing the abutment teeth. However, although hinge movement allows the posterior periphery of the saddle to move tissueward, the attachment at the abutment tooth is still rigid.

The adjustable press-stud patrix of the Ceka 691 is held in the acrylic of the saddle and upon insertion engages the projecting female ring at the gingival of the abutment tooth restoration. A simulated hinge action may be achieved by cutting the superior surface of the matrix thereby reducing the height progressively posteriorly.

Frictional with Retentive Device and Providing for Tissueward and Hinge Movement (Fig. 20): The attachments in this group, perhaps the largest, are designed with an adjustable retentive device and allow for both tissueward and hinge movement. CM 750 Steiger Ax-Ro joint is composed of a rectangular bar fitted into a rectangular hollow section held together by a central screw. A varying length slot in the hollow section provides for vertical movement and is rounded and tapered towards each end to permit rotation. Unlike most other attachments, it is positioned in the partial denture between the distal-extension saddle and the clasp unit which embraces the abutment teeth. The Roach CM 613 is a tube with an adjustable split ball that slides up and down. Unlike CM 612 there is no flange at the base of the ball so that the patrix moves freely in the tube without the risk of binding on the edge of the matrix. Ceka 691 and Octolink 81 are similar rotating anchors which can be adjusted to allow tissueward and hinge movement. The patrices can also be adjusted to maintain retention in spite of wear. One disadvantage of this type of attachment is

that the matrix is entirely extracoronal which may cause torquing of the abutment and also covers considerable gingival tissue.

The patrices have a poor reputation[20] for wear but are capable of quick and easy replacement. Crismani CM 789 and CM 689 each comprise an intracoronal dovetail-shaped matrix with a correspondingly shaped slider patrix (either rectangular CM 789 or tapered CM 689) which is fitted with a snap-grip to which is attached a hinge-like yoke for retention in the acrylic.

A return coil-spring is included in the matrix and the range of movement of the yoke may be adjusted to allow varying amounts of hinge movement. As a matter of considerable practical interest, the matrix for these two attachments is the same as for the CM 699 Crismani. Consequently, when the posterior abutment is lost in a tooth supported saddle, where CM 699 has been used on the anterior abutment, it is possible to convert the unit into a distal-extension saddle simply by replacing the CM 699 patrix by either CM 789 or CM 689 patrices.

Dalbo CM 667 and Dalbo MK[25] have a male rectangular slide which runs occluso-gingivally and projects from the distal of the abutment crown. At the gingival margin there is a further extension of the patrix away from the tooth on which a ball is supported. The matrix slides down the rectangular section thereby preventing side to side movement and finally its two lamellae grip the ball. Between the top of the ball and the inside of the roof of the cylindrical-like matrix is a resilient coil-spring which returns the attachment to the rest position after each tissueward movement. The attachment has a frictional and spring-controlled sliding movement toward the tissue, followed by hinge movement. It is an excellent attachment for use in restoring distal-extension saddles.

The ASC-52[26] is the smallest, simplest and cheapest attachment for use with free-end saddles. It comprises a vertical extracoronal tube matrix in which slides a ball, secured to a long metal rodlike projection, which fits into a spring-loaded housing. A projection of the housing extends over the top of the matrix thus keeping out debris but, more importantly, preventing the saddle from moving away from its mucosal support.

CROSS ARCH ATTACHMENTS

Rigid, Retentive and Adjustable with only Vertical Movement: These four attachments are designed to provide retention and stability on the opposite side of the arch to a unilateral tooth-supported saddle. They are very effective in preventing lateral rotation of the saddle, thereby ensuring cross-arch support.

The CM 653 is a cylindrical interlocking slide in which the patrix has adjustable leaves or "teeth" that can be opened to maintain frictional contact. The matrix is positioned within a crown or large inlay. Should it be possible to have only a short length of attachment, such as less than 3.0 mm, the frictional retention should be supplemented by using a clasp arm on the partial denture framework.

The Schatzmann, snaprox CM 717 is designed to fit in the interproximal space involving adjoining proximal restorations. It is a very neat and convenient attachment having a small, grip-hook on the buccal side so that the patient may more easily remove the partial denture. The split ring retentive device is replaceable thereby maintaining the very effective retention of the attachment.

The Ney split-lingual attachments (Ney-Chayes and Ney-Loc) are designed to be used on the lingual surface of the crown or within the pontic of a fixed restoration on the opposite side of the arch to the tooth-supported saddle. The attachments are the same as the regular Ney-Chayes No. 9 and the Ney-Loc except that the matrix has a wider "proximal" plate to provide greater resistance to side-to-side rotation and hence greater stability. (Fig. 21)

The Roach CM 613 (Fig. 22) is a small versatile cross-arch stabilizer for unilateral distal-extension base partial dentures. It is very effective when used in conjunction with the resilient Dalbo CM 667 attachments. Usually the matrix is mounted in a fixed pontic on the opposite side and the ball patrix is soldered to the minor connector from either a palatal or lingual bar.

AUXILIARY ATTACHMENTS

Screwblock Anchors (Fig 23): The Schubiger CM 658 and 659 screw-blocks are available in different sizes and provide a convenient method for inserting and cementing bar-splint anchors attached to root-caps with non-aligned post retention. They comprise a soldering base with threaded patrix post over which is placed a matrix sleeve or ferrule which has a shoulder on the inside near the top of the sleeve. The locking screw engages this shoulder and the male post by means of a female thread. The bases are soldered to root-caps and the bar is soldered between the ferrules; the bar assembly is then locked in place by a locking screw on each attachment.

The soldering bases are identical to the bases for the Gerber CM 686 and CM 696 attachments making it a simple matter to change from a bar anchor to a stud anchor for an overlay denture.

The tall screw-block CM 659 may also be used for attaching milled bars to posterior abutments thus facilitating the cementation when the abutments cannot be aligned.

The Hruska CM 709 series of tapered block-anchors with fixing screw on top are useful for securing cast or milled custom bars to cast root-caps in either the anterior or posterior arches.

Retentive Anchors (Fig. 24): The rear and front opening Guglielmettic Ipsoclips CM 783 and 784 are small spring-loaded ball retentive units that can be incorporated in C.S.P. attachments (after Steiger), telescopic crowns and milled bars to provide more positive retention. The smallest is only 2.60 mm in length with a maximum diameter of 2.90 mm which means that it can be accommodated in most situations very easily and without significant increase in bulk or contour.

Hinged Labial Retentive Units: Simmons[27] in 1963 first used a hinged cast labial retentive unit (Swing Lock)[28,29] as an alternative to an

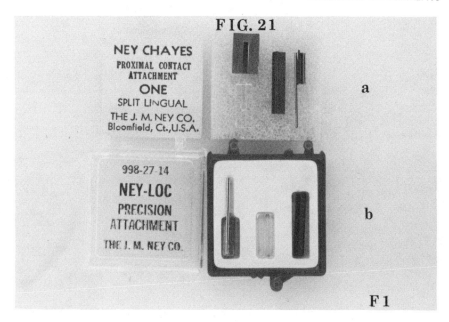

Fig. 21 Cross Arch Attachment—Rigid Retentive and Adjustable (F1.) **a.** Ney Chayes No. 9 split-lingual; matrix with wide proximal flange, carbon soldering patrix and patrix with temporary rod extension for indexing, investing and soldering; **b.** Ney Loc split lingual.

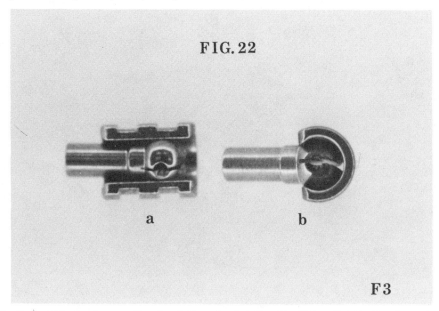

Fig. 22 Cross Arch Attachment—Rotational, Retentive & Adjustable (F3.) **a.** CM 613 Roach, patrix lying in matrix showing adjustable split-ball of patrix; **b.** CM 613 Roach, patrix in correct position in matrix showing soldering extension of patrix.

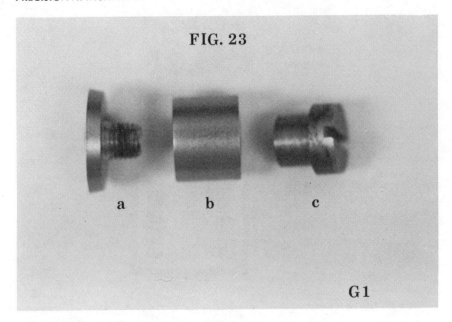

Fig. 23 Auxiliary Attachments—Screwblock Anchors (G1.) SCM 658 Schubiger anchor (3x mag.) **a.** patrix, soldering base with threaded post; **b.** matrix, ferrule with shoulder for locking screw; **c.** locking screw with female thread to engage male screw post.

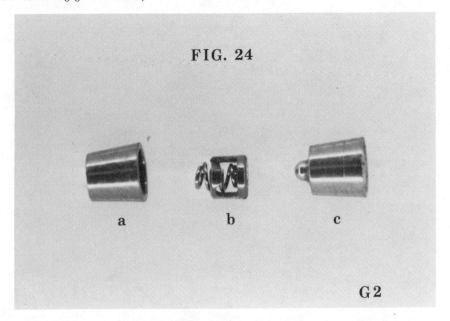

Fig. 24 Auxiliary Attachment—Retentive Anchor (G2.) CM 783 Ipsoclip, rear opening **a.** attachment housing; **b.** spring with locking base; **c.** Ipsoclip assembled—spring loaded ball engages dimple in associated casting.

immediate complete lower denture (Fig. 25). The hinged-unit is opened to allow insertion of the partial denture and is closed following insertion, enabling use of the labial surfaces on the anterior teeth for retention. Additionally, it is possible with "I" bar like fingers from the labial bar to hold the anterior teeth firmly against the rigid lingual metal flange of the partial denture. Swing-Lock and Nobil-Latch[30] (Fig. 26) are two of the patented attachments that incorporate the principle of the hinged labial retentive unit.

AVAILABLE PRODUCTS:

APM-Sterngold G/A Attachment, APM Sterngold Div. of Sterndent Corp.

APM-Sterngold G/L Attachment, APM-Sterngold Div. of Sterndent Corp.

APM-Sterngold Type 7 Attachment, APM-Sterngold Div. of Sterndent Corp.

Attachment Devices-Positioning Tools, Charles Development Co.

Beyeler Attachment, APM-Sterngold Div. of Sterndent Corp.

Brown Precision Attachment, Columbia Dentoform Corp.

Conex, APM-Sterngold Div. of Sterndent Corp.

Crismani Attachment, APM-Sterngold Div. of Sterndent Corp.

Cross Arch Roach Attachment, APM-Sterngold Div. of Sterndent Corp.

Dalbo Extracoronal Precision Attachment, APM-Sterngold Div. of Sterndent Corp.

Distal Extension Roach, APM-Sterngold Div. of Sterndent Corp.

Dolder Bar, APM-Sterngold Div. of Sterndent Corp.

Fusion, George Taub Products Inc.

Gerber Stud, APM-Sterngold Div. of Sterndent Corp.

Hader Bar & Rider, APM-Sterngold Div. of Sterndent Corp.

Huser Hook, APM-Sterngold Div. of Sterndent Corp.

Interlock Slide, APM-Sterngold Div. of Sterndent Corp.

Ipso-Clip, APM-Sterngold Div. of Sterndent Corp.

Iridio-Platinum Shoe, Williams Gold Refining Co. Inc.

McCollum Attachment, APM-Sterngold Div. of Sterndent Corp.

Ney-Loc Precision Attachment, J. M. Ney Co.

Ney Min-Rest, J. M. Ney Co.

Ney Mortice Rest, J. M. Ney Co.

Ney M. S. Attachment, J. M. Ney Co.

Ney #9 Precision Attachment, J. M. Ney Co.

Ney Stress Breaker, J. M. Ney Co.

Octolink Anchor, APM-Sterngold Div. of Sterndent Corp.

Octolink Bridge, APM-Sterngold Div. of Sterndent Corp.

Plastic Connector Patterns, APM-Sterngold Div. of Sterndent Corp.

Pin Des Marts, APM-Sterngold Div. of Sterndent Corp.

Precision Rest Attachment, APM-Sterngold Div. of Sterndent Corp.

Rothermann Stud, APM-Sterngold Div. of Sterndent Corp.

Round Bar & Rider, APM-Sterngold Div. of Sterndent Corp.

Schatzmann Intracoronal Attachment, APM-Sterngold Div. of Sterndent Corp.

Schubinger Screw Anchor, APM-Sterngold Div. of Sterndent Corp.

Shade-A-Guide, George Taub Products Inc.

Stainless Steel Clasps, Williams Gold Refining Co., Inc.

Stainless Steel Lingual Bars, Williams Gold Refining Co., Inc.

Strauss Ceramic Cores, APM-Sterngold Div. of Sterndent Corp.

Wilkinson Torque Eliminator, Wilkinson Co.

Zest Anchor, APM-Sterngold Div. of Sterndent Corp.

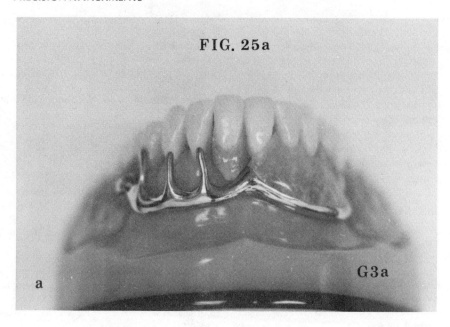

Fig. 25   Hinged Labial Retentive Unit (G3.a) Swing-Lock mandibular partial denture **a.** labial view; **b.** plastic patterns for hinge & lock; **c.** labial section open—incisal view; **d.** labial section hinged open showing lock.

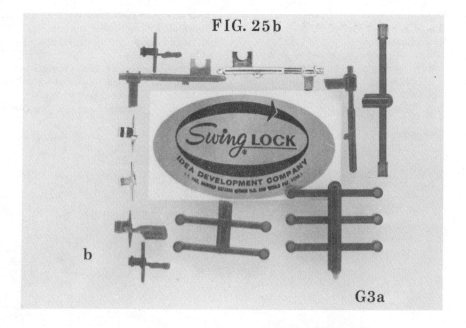

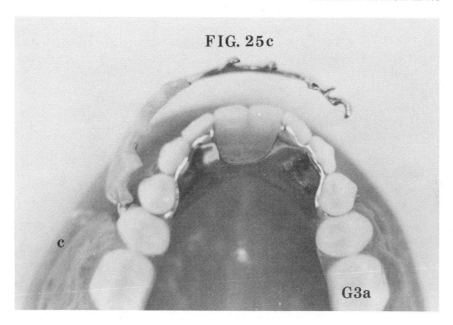

FIG. 25 c

c

G3a

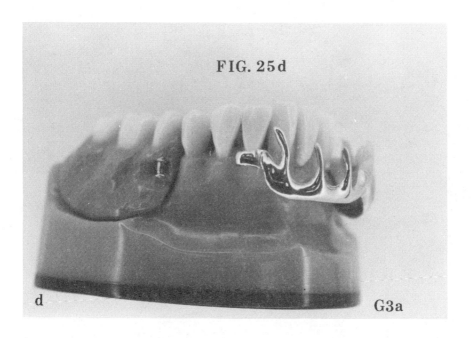

FIG. 25 d

d

G3a

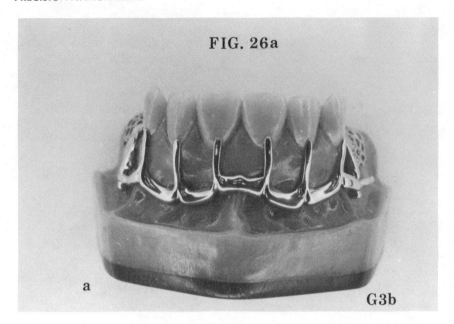

FIG. 26a

a

G3b

Fig. 26   Hinged Labial Retentive Unit (G3.b) Nobilium Latch maxillary partial denture **a.** labial view; **b.** patterns for hinge-post; **c.** labial section open—incisal view; **d.** labial section hinged open showing latch.

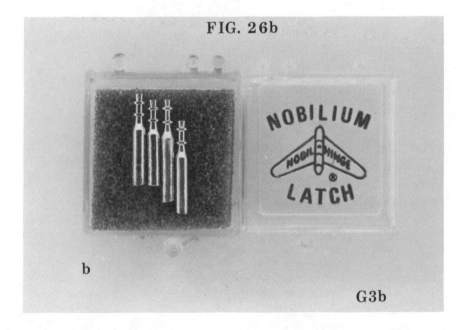

FIG. 26b

b

G3b

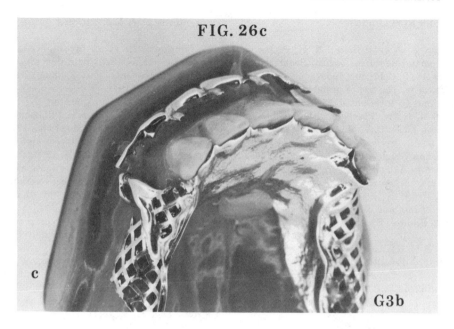

FIG. 26c

c

G3b

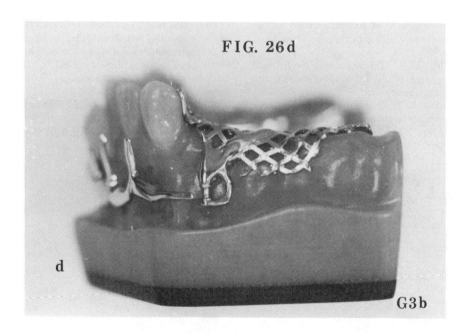

FIG. 26d

d

G3b

LITERATURE REFERENCES

1. Steiger, A. A., and Boitel, R. H. Precision work for partial dentures. Zurich, Switzerland, Buchdruckerie Berichthaus, 1959.

2. Nally, J. N. The use of prefabricated precision attachments. Int. Dent. J. 11:196, 1961.

3. Preiskel, H. W. Precision attachments in dentistry. St. Louis, C. V. Mosby Co., 1973.

4. Ray, G. E. Precision attachments. Bristol, England, John Wright, 1969.

5. Nakazawa, I., and Amemori, H. A new classification of attachments. Bull. Tokyo Med. Dent. Univ. 17:227, 1970.

6. Attachments and components for prosthetic dentistry. Bienne, Switzerland, Cendres and Metaux SA, 1970.

7. Mensor, M. C. Classification and selection of attachments. J. Prosthet. Dent. 29:494, 1973.

8. A.P.M.—Sterngold A procedure manual. San Mateo, California, A.P.M.—Sterngold, 1973.

9. Matsuo, E. The ASC-52 attachment. Kanagawa, Japan, 1970.

10. Mensor, M. C. The EM attachment selector. San Mateo, California, Bell International, 1971.

11. Cecconi, B. T. Rest design and force transmission. J. Prosthet. Dent. 32:141, 1974.

12. Miller, C. J. Intracoronal attachments for removable partial dentures. Dent. Clin. N. Am. 8:779, 1963.

13. Cunningham, D. M. Indications and contraindications for precision attachments. Dent. Clin. N. Am. 14:595, 1970.

14. Taylor, R. L.; Duckmanton, N. A.; and Boyks, G. Overlay dentures. Philosophy and practice. Part I. Aust. Dent. J. 21:430, 1976.

15. Preiskel, H. Prefabricated attachments for complete overlay dentures. Br. Dent. J. 123:161, 1967.

16. Mensor, M. C. Attachments fixation for overdentures. Part I. J. Prosthet. Dent. 37:366, 1977.

17. Rantanen, T., et al. Investigations of the therapeutic success with dentures retained by precision attachments. Part I. Suom, Hammaslaak Toim. p. 356, 1971.

18. Taylor, R. L.; Duckmanton, N. A.; and Boyks, G. Overlay dentures. Philosophy and practice. Part II. Aust. Dent. J. 21:495, 1976.

19. Waltz, M. E. Ceka extracoronal attachments. J. Prosthet. Dent. 29:167, 1973.

20. Rantanen, T., et al. Investigations of the therapeutic success with dentures retained by precision attachments. Proc. Finn. Dent. Soc. 68:73, 1972.

21. Overdenture attachment—Sandri pressure button. Burlingame, California, Bell International Inc., 1977.

22. Andrews, J. A., and Carlson, A. F. The Andrews bridge—A clinical guide. Amite, Louisiana, Institute of Cosmetic Dentistry, 1976.

23. Andrews, J. A., and Carlson, A. F. The Andrews bridge—a laboratory manual. Amite, Louisiana, Institute of Cosmetic Dentistry, 1976.

24. Dolder, E. J. The bar joint mandibular denture. J. Prosthet. Dent. 11:689, 1961.

25. Mensor, M. C. The rationale of resilient hinge-action stress breakers. J. Prosthet. Dent. 20:204, 1968.

26. Mensor, M. C. Attachments for free-end partial dentures. A rational approach with the ASC-52. Qunit. Dent. Tech. No. 1, p. 19, 1976.

27. Simmons, J. J. Swing-lock stabilization and retention. Tex. Dent. J., p. 10, 1963.

28. Swing-lock—Clinical manual. Dallas, Idea Development Co., 1968.

29. Swing-lock—Design and technique manual, Dallas, Idea Development Co., 1968.

30. The Nobil-hinge latch—Instruction sheet. Chicago, American Gold Co.

SPECIAL PURPOSE RESINS

COLD CURE REPAIR RESINS

Cold cure repair resins (also called curing or auto polymerizing resins) are methyl methacrylate polymers similar in composition and manipulation to cold cure denture resins. (See also monograph on cold cure resins on page 92.)

COMPOSITION: The repair resins usually are supplied in the form of a powder containing poly-(methyl methacrylate) with a polymerization initiator and a liquid containing methyl methacrylate monomer, a crosslinking monomer and a polymerization promoter. The materials may be pigmented or clear. While similar to cold cure denture base resins, the repair resins generally polymerize more rapidly because of the relatively simpler manipulations involved in repair as compared to fabrication.

USES: Cold cure repair resins are used to achieve rapid repair of fractured dentures.

DIRECTIONS FOR USE: In performing a repair, the fractured pieces are luted together with sticky wax and a model is poured of the tissue surface. The fractured surfaces are then relieved from 1.5 to 3 mm. Two frequently used techniques involve either the preparation of a rabbetted channel extending halfway through the base towards the tissue surface or beveling and rounding all surfaces of the enlarged fracture.[1] A separating medium (tinfoil substitute) is applied to the cast. Monomer and powder are then applied alternately to the assembled pieces on the cast filling the defect, with slight overfilling to allow for finishing. The repair may be bench cured in warm water although greater strength and lower porosities result when a pressure pot is used.

LIMITATIONS OF USE: The principal limitations of the repair materials involve the reduced strength in comparison with heat-cured denture base resins and possible problems with color match and stability. Depending on the method of application, repairs have transverse strengths of about 50 to 70 percent of those of heat-cured denture base resin.[1-4] If the original base frac-

129

tures in function rather than from abuse there is little likelihood that a repair will be successful. Because the eye is much more sensitive to color differences at a sharp interface between two materials than to differences between separate samples, any color mismatch or color instability of the repair material will be emphasized.

EVALUATION PROGRAM: Cold cure repair resins are covered by American Dental Association Specification No. 13. The general methods and requirements are the same as those of Specification No. 12 for denture base polymer except that packing and plasticity tests are begun earlier and loads and deflection limits for the transverse test are altered.

AVAILABLE PRODUCTS

BINDIT PINK; powder/liquid, Moyco Industries, Inc.
Biofast Cold Cure Repair Resin, B. L. Dental Co., Inc.
CAULK REPAIR MATERIAL PINK; PINK FIBERED; LIGHT FIBERED; PINK FREE FLOW; powder/liquid. L. D. Caulk Co., Div. of Dentsply International, Inc.
COE CURE LIGHT; DARK, Coe Laboratories, Inc.
COE CURE LIGHT FIBERED; DARK FIBERED, Coe Laboratories, Inc.
FASTCURE, CLEAR; TRANSVEINED; LIGHT VEINED, VEINED; PINK; PINK FINE, Kerr Mfg. Co., Div. of Sybron Corp.
HYGIENIC PERM REPAIR MATERIALS CLEAR; VEINED; HEAVY VEINED; HEAVY VEINED "B"; PLAIN PINK; PINK NO. 53, Hygienic Dental Mfg. Co.
Minit-Weld, Teledyne Dental Products
Nu-Weld, L. D. Caulk Co., Div. of Dentsply International, Inc.
No. 7 Fast Setting Repair Liquid, Teledyne Dental Products
PERFEX REPAIR RESIN, International Dental Products, Inc.
Re-store Denture Relining Material, L. D. Caulk Co., Div. of Dentsply International, Inc.
Sur-Weld, Modern Materials Mfg. Co.
Seta-Cure Cold Curing Denture Repair Resins, Accurate Set, Inc.

COLD CURE REPAIR RESINS

Do:

1. Determine the cause of fracture to rule out faults in the existing prosthesis or changes in the oral tissues as causes of fracture.
2. Accurately position and reassemble the fractured pieces prior to pouring the model.
3. Clean all parts thoroughly prior to repair.
4. Insure absolute immobility of fragments during processing.
5. Apply separating media to all areas of the cast which may be contacted by monomer.
6. Apply the monomer carefully with a brush (not a dropper); monomer is a solvent for the cured acrylic resin base material.
7. Cure the repair in a pressure-pot if possible.

Don't:

1. Repair dentures which have failed from design and construction errors in the original prosthesis (e.g., porcelain teeth set too close to the residual ridge or porcelain teeth ground too thin).
2. Repair dentures which have failed from fatigue resulting from poor fit.
3. Heat the denture excessively during curing or finishing of the repair as stress relief and warping will result.

CROWN AND BRIDGE RESINS

Crown and bridge resins are of two general types: temporary and permanent.

Temporary Crown and Bridge Resins

USES: Temporary crown and bridge resins are primarily used as an interim treatment during the fabrication of permanent prostheses. They are also used in splinting and in the fabrication of interarch records. In addition to the techniques for temporary crown fabrication which result in a crown made entirely of resin, the resins are often used to adapt commercial metal and plastic preformed crowns to the prepared tooth.

COMPOSITION: The three major categories of temporary crown and bridge resins are those based on methyl methacrylate, higher methacrylates and epimine resins. The methyl methacrylate resins are similar in composition and manipulation to unfilled restorative resins and cold cure repair resins. Like these resins, the crown and bridge resins are supplied as a powder containing poly(methyl methacrylate) with a polymerization initiator and a liquid which contains methyl methacrylate monomer with a polymerization promoter. The powder is pigmented to yield a resultant resin with reasonable color match to tooth material. Manipulation is similar to the other cold cure resins in that the two components are mixed and allowed to enter the dough stage before forming. Systems based on higher methacrylates are also powder-liquid systems, except that the powder is typically poly(ethyl methacrylate) and the liquid monomer is typically n-butyl methacrylate.[5] Manipulation is similar to the conventional methyl methacrylate based resins.

The epimine material is supplied as a two component system comprising a paste containing a difunctional epimine-terminated high molecular weight monomer with a polyamide filler and a liquid containing a benzene sulphonate ester catalyst. In appearance and manipulation, the epimine material is similar to the paste-liquid composite resins. (See also monograph on composite resins on page 46.)

DIRECTIONS FOR USE: Any of the three types of temporary crown and bridge materials may be conveniently molded while in the dough stage in rigid silicone rubber, vacuum or pressure formed thermoplastic matrices or polymeric crown forms. The matrix and resin are removed from the mouth while the resin is still in the "rubbery" stage to allow removal from undercuts and facilitate gross trimming.

LIMITATIONS OF USE: The methyl methacrylate based materials suffer from high polymerization shrinkage, a high exotherm (high temperature reached during curing) and the tendency of the methyl methacrylate monomer to irritate soft tissues. The higher powder-to-liquid ratios normally used with the higher methacrylate based materials reduce both the polymerization shrinkage and exotherm. In addition, flow is

---

TEMPORARY CROWN AND BRIDGE RESINS

Do:
1. Mix the material according to manufacturer's directions.
2. Insert the matrix and resin while the resin is in the early dough stage.
3. Use water spray to minimize temperature rise where required (particularly with the methyl methacrylate based resins).
4. Remove the matrix and resin while the resin is still rubbery.
5. Trim gross flash and undercuts before complete cure.
6. Complete cure in mouth, on bench, or in warm water, according to manufacturer's directions.
7. Final trim, open embrasures and shape pontic on fully cured resin.
8. Adjust occlusion prior to final finishing and polishing.

Don't:
1. Leave flash or rough resin surface in areas of soft tissue contact.

generally better with less tendency for the monomer to irritate soft tissues. The epimine material exhibits good flow, very low exotherm and very low setting shrinkage. However, the catalyst has the potential for tissue irritation and may be a sensitizing agent for the dentist. In addition, the epimines are not as strong as the acrylics.[5]

Permanent Crown and Bridge Resins

USES: The resins are used to provide permanent facings and veneers on crowns and bridges.

COMPOSITION: Permanent crown and bridge resins are available in a number of different compositions with differing recommended processing methods. The principal resins include acrylics, vinyl-acrylics and dimethacrylates. The acrylics and vinyl-acrylics are powder-liquid systems similar in composition and manipulation to the related denture base resins. (See monograph on denture resins and attachment devices on page 91.) There is no adhesion between the resins and castings; therefore, adequate retention must be designed into the casting. The surface of the gold alloy to be in contact with resin can be gold plated to minimize the tarnish of the alloy and subsequent discoloration of the resin should leakage at that interface occur. Walls of the recessed area in the casting are normally made to provide a slightly undercut butt joint. In addition, the facing surface of the wax pattern is covered with plastic beads, spurs, loops or nailhead buttons to yield adequate retention.

DIRECTIONS FOR USE: Manufacturers' directions for placement and curing of the resins differ markedly. Many vinyl-acrylic resins are packed in flasked cases and cured in water baths by procedures not unlike those used for denture base resins. Dry heat curing is also used in which the flasked crowns are placed in an oven at about 600 to 800°C (1,112 to 1,472°F) for about 15 minutes.[6,7] Residual water in the plaster mold prevents the actual internal mold temperature from exceeding 100°C (212°F).

The high molecular weights and consequent low vapor pressures of the dimethacrylate based resins allows them to be dry heat cured without flasking. Typical dimethacrylates used include diethylene glycol dimethacrylate and the adduct of bisphenol-A and hydroxy ethyl methacrylate. The materials may be built up stepwise on the crowns or pontics and each layer dry heat cured (e.g., 10 minutes at 275°F).[8] To improve the color, the crowns are often gold plated prior to facing. However, at least one manufacturer supplies a special alloy for use with its resin and does not recommend gold plating because the alloy is designed to be more readily wetted by the resin. In any case, the metal is usually masked with an opaquing resin prior to application of the esthetic veneering resin.

PERMANENT CROWN AND BRIDGE RESINS

Do:

1. Evaluate the merits of other esthetic materials and techniques (e.g., porcelain veneer, ground denture teeth).
2. Provide sufficient reduction for adequate thickness of the metal casting and veneer.
3. Provide adequate retention for the veneer.
4. Avoid occlusal or incisal contact at the veneer-metal interface.
5. Apply and cure the resins according to the manufacturer's directions.

If the veneer is to be placed by a technician:

Do:

1. Provide adequate guidance on shade selection and contour; a selected plastic denture tooth is a helpful guide.

LIMITATIONS OF USE: Limitations of the crown and bridge resins are related to their poorer abrasion resistance, stain resistance, strength and color stability in comparison with porcelain facings and veneers. Casting design, personal habits of the patient and economics must be included in any consideration of the relative merits of resin veneering.

EVALUATION PROGRAM: The physical and mechanical requirements of crown and bridge resins have never been set forth in formal guidelines under the Certification Program of the Council on Dental Materials, Instruments and Equipment; however, an Acceptance Program is under development.

AVAILABLE PRODUCTS

Biofil Cold Cure Crown & Bridge Resins, B.L. Dental Co., Inc.
Biolon, L.D. Caulk Co.
Biotone, L.D. Caulk Co.
Caulk Crown & Bridge Stains, L.D. Caulk Co.
Caulk Temporary Bridge Resin, L.D. Caulk Co.
Ceramco Liquid Medium, Ceramco, Inc.
Dominite, Nu-Dent Research Co., Inc.
Hue-Lon, L.D. Caulk Co.
Justi Opaquer, H.D. Justi Co.
Lactona/Universal Crown & Bridge Resin, Lactona/Universal
New Hue-Lon, L.D. Caulk Co.
Porcelain Repair Kit, Den-Mat, Inc.
Pyroplast, H.D. Justi Co., Div. of Williams Gold Refining Co, Inc.
Thermo-Jel Thermosetting Resin, L.D. Caulk Co.
Vita K & B Acrylics, Unitek Corp.

MOUTH PROTECTOR MATERIALS

USES: The widespread use of mouth protectors in organized sports is a preventive measure. Mounting evidence suggests that mouth protectors are effective in reducing sports related injuries other than those to the oral tissues. In one study, bone deformation and intracranial pressure induced by a blow to the chin were reduced.[9] In another, retrospective evaluations of football injuries indicated that the use of mouth protectors was associated with lower incidences of neck injuries and concussions.[10]

COMPOSITION: Mouth protector materials are available in three general forms: stock protectors, mouth-formed protectors and custom fabricated protectors. The stock protectors are used "off the shelf" and generally exhibit poorest fit and player acceptance. Custom fabricated protectors are available as a unit which can be molded intraorally or as a preformed tray which is filled with a thermoplastic or chemically gelling polymer prior to initial seating in the player's mouth. Commercial stock protectors are made of natural rubber, poly(vinyl chloride), poly(vinyl acetate-ethylene) copolymer, or polyurethane. The homogeneous mouth form-

---

MOUTH PROTECTOR MATERIALS

Do:
1. Evaluate the patient's involvement or potential involvement in sports.
2. Determine the patient's present use or lack of use of mouth protection.
3. Educate the patient on the benefits of mouth protection.
4. Be prepared to provide protectors upon request.

Don't:
1. Assume that any organized sport is already covered by mandatory mouth guard rules.
2. Overlook the need for mouth protectors in unorganized (sandlot) team sports.
3. Overlook the need for mouth protectors in individual hazardous athletic activities (e.g., wrestling, racing, skiing, skateboarding, karate, parachuting).

ed protectors are generally poly(vinyl acetate-ethylene) while the two component protectors generally use a poly(vinyl chloride) tray with a soft liner similar to materials used as denture soft liners. Custom protectors are fabricated from poly(vinyl acetate-ethylene) blanks and preforms, soft acrylic doughs or liquid rubber latex.[11]

LIMITATIONS OF USE: A major limitation of mouth protectors, particularly the stock and mouth formed types, is disuse traceable to discomfort, bulk, poor fit, poor hygiene, interference with speech, gagging and poor durability.[11] Also, inadequate coverage of all athletes may result in part from the confusing overlap of responsibility between the dentist and the athletic coach or trainer.

EVALUATION PROGRAM: No specifications currently exist which cover the physical, mechanical or performance properties of mouth protector materials.

AVAILABLE PRODUCTS

Dentsply Vacu-Press Day Guard-Perio Glove, Dentsply International Inc.
Dentsply Vacu-Press Mouth-Night Guard, Dentsply International Inc.
Lip Retractor, Zirc Dental Products
Oryl-Gard Mouth Protectors, Teledyne Dental Products
Vanguard Vinyl Blanks, Teledyne Dental Products

RESILIENT AND TREATMENT RELINERS

Resilient Liners

USES: Resilient liners are elastomeric materials used to form a portion or all of the tissue bearing surface of dentures. The most common indication for the use of soft liners is the presence of thin, narrow spiny or irregular ridges, particularly when the overlaying mucosa is thin and non-resilient. Additionally, resilient liners have been used in selected cases of chronic irritation

of the mucosa, bilateral undercuts not subject to surgical reduction, acquired and congenital oral defects and psychological aversion to rigid denture bases.[12,13]

COMPOSITION: The earliest resilient liners were natural rubber. The first synthetic materials were plasticized poly(vinyl chloride). Current materials generally include silicone elastomers, polymers based on the higher methacrylate homologs and hydrophilic acrylics.[14-18] Resilient liners of the higher methacrylate type are usually supplied as two components: a powder containing the higher methacrylate polymer or copolymer and a liquid. The liquid may contain ethyl alcohol, ethyl acetate and an aromatic plasticizer (e.g., butyl phthalyl butyl glycolate). In addition, a polymerizable monomer may or may not be present. When no monomer is present, mixing of the two components results in formation of an elastomeric soft liner because of the solvent and plasticizing effect of the liquid on the polymer powder. These materials are very similar in composition to the major class of tissue conditioners and no clear delineation can be made between the function of these liners and the related conditioners. Silicone materials may be heat or cold curing and are supplied as one component (which cures on exposure to atmospheric moisture) or two components (base and catalyst). (See also monograph on elastomeric impression materials on page 185.)

DIRECTIONS FOR USE: Each material is tailored for a specific mode of application and may be heat cured along with the denture base or applied to a tissue surface relieved denture as an alternative to rigid reline.

LIMITATIONS OF USE: A principal limitation to the more widespread use of resilient liners is their lack of permanence. Most materials suffer deleterious changes in their elastic properties, often becoming essentially rigid in periods ranging from months to years. Other shortcomings include weakening of the denture, loss of adhesion between denture base and lining, difficulty in adjustment and finishing, excessive water absorption, support of growth of microorganisms and poor abrasion resistance. Together, these limitations make the currently available resilient liners temporary expedients when compared with the expected service life of conventional rigid denture bases.

EVALUATION PROGRAM: Resilient and treatment reliners are covered under an Acceptance Program.

RESILIENT LINERS

Do:

1. Evaluate all possible alternatives for suitability (e.g., surgical modification of the supporting bony structures, polishing the surface of a conventional rigid base).
2. Prepare and apply the materials in accordance with the manufacturer's directions.
3. Prepare the tissue surface carefully to minimize subsequent adjustment and polishing.
4. Use a butt joint between liner and rigid resin; avoid feather edging.

AVAILABLE PRODUCTS

Adjusto, Teledyne Dental Products
COE SOFT, Coe Laboratories, Inc.
COE SUPER SOFT, Coe Laboratories, Inc.
PROLASTIC #1, #2, 35, Prolastic Company, Inc.
Soft Oryl, Teledyne Dental Products
Veltec, Teledyne Dental Products

Treatment Liners

USES: In many cases it is necessary to give the oral soft tissues an opportunity to recover before constructing a new denture, or rebasing or relining an existing denture. Withholding the offending denture for a period of 48 to 72 hours is an effective means of regaining support tissue health;[19] however, this method is generally not acceptable to the patient. Consequently, treatment liners are frequently used. Treatment liner resins remain soft for periods usually ranging up to several days. There is some question as to the desired balance between plasticity and elasticity in treatment reliners. If the material is completely plastic, flow under masticatory stresses will result in rapid loss of material. Conversely, completely elastic materials offer resistance to, and consequently hinder, the tissue remodeling. In either case, frequent replacement of the conditioning material is required. For tissue conditioning, the softest materials which retain good elastic recovery offer the advantage of longer intervals between replacements.[20,21]

Tissue conditioners may also be used as functional impression materials. For this purpose, good flow with minimal elastic recovery is desirable. The flow ensures continual adaptation of the material to the soft tissues as they are altered in response to functional stresses. Even though elastic recovery is minimized, the model must be poured immediately on removal of the denture from the mouth to ensure accuracy.

Besides their use as treatment materials prior to remaking a denture, these materials also are used in immediate denture construction, cleft palate speech aids and immediate surgical splints and stents for hemophiliacs.[22]

COMPOSITION: Most tissue conditioners are two component systems consisting of a higher methacrylate polymer (principally ethyl methacrylate) and a liquid consisting of ethyl alcohol, ethyl acetate and an aromatic plasticizer. The alcohol and ester are solvents for the polymer beads, swelling the beads and allowing the plasticizer to diffuse in. As a rule, with higher concentration of volatile solvents, the gel is formed more rapidly and is initially softer. However, leaching and evaporation of these components leads to rapid hardening of the material in the mouth.

DIRECTIONS FOR USE: If tissue conditioning and functional impression taking are both to be performed on the same patient, it may be advantageous to use two different materials in succession for optimal performance of the two different functions.

TREATMENT RELINERS

Do:

1. Allow for sufficient thickness to accommodate the anticipated alterations in the soft tissue and in no case less than 0.5 mm.
2. Maintain a frequent recall schedule.
3. Adjust occlusion and vertical dimension at each reline.
4. Emphasize to the patient the necessity of frequent replacement of the reliner.
5. Inform the patient of any special cleaning and handling procedures.

Don't:

1. Schedule intermediate replacements so infrequently that the material becomes hard between replacements.

In utilizing reliners as functional impressions,

Do:

1. Select a material with good flow and low elastic recovery.
2. Pour the model immediately after final removal of the functional impression from the mouth.

AVAILABLE PRODUCTS

COE-COMFORT, Coe Laboratories, Inc.
F. I. T. T., Kerr Mfg. Co., Div. of Sybron Dental Products
LYNAL-TREATMENT RELINER MATERIALS, L.D. Caulk Co., Div. of Dentsply International, Inc.

Opotow Triplastic, Teledyne Dental Products
VISCO-GEL TREATMENT RELINER MATERIAL, Ransom and Randolph Co.

SELF ADMINISTERED RELINING AND REPAIR MATERIALS

USES: Numerous materials are available on an over-the-counter basis which purportedly allow the denture wearer to adjust the fit of his own dentures or repair fractures.

COMPOSITION: Reline materials are available in the form of preformed thermoplastic pads (e.g., wax impregnated gauze, resin gels and strips) and powder-liquid materials somewhat similar in composition and manipulation to the acceptable treatment lining materials, except that a much wider range of polymers, solvents and plasticizers has been reported.[23] In addition, some denture "adhesives" are capable of being retained in such bulk as to constitute a reline. Repair materials are generally cold curing acrylic powder-liquid systems resembling the acceptable products.

DIRECTIONS FOR USE: The thermoplastic reline materials are typically softened in warm water, placed in the denture and seated in the mouth to achieve tissue adaptation. Powder-liquid reliners are mixed, poured into the denture and then seated in the mouth until gelation is achieved.

LIMITATIONS OF USE: The principal limitation of the reline and repair materials is their potential for misuse. Both may be used without serious consequence if used for their sole legitimate purpose as short-term emergency expedients only until a dentist can be seen. However, there is ample literature documenting the serious consequence of long term use of the products in lieu of professional consultation.[24-34] The solvents and plasticizers in the reline materials have weakened denture base material and, more importantly, caused lesions and irritation. Extended use has been associated with soreness, soft tissue hyperplasia, massive hard tissue resorption and the development of carcinomas.

Since 1969, the Food and Drug Administration of the Department of Health, Education and Welfare has required that all over-the-counter reliners, pads, cushions and repair kits include a label warning which emphasizes the limitations of use to temporary and emergency purposes.[35]

The use of the self administered repair and reline materials is beyond the dentist's direct control; his primary responsibility is in patient education.

SELF ADMINISTERED RELINING AND REPAIRING MATERIALS

Do:[36]

1. Warn the patient against self-adjustment, self-repair or self-relining of the denture.
2. Explain the reasons for the possible future need for adjustment in the dental office.
3. Explain the importance of adjusting occlusion and vertical dimension in addition to the soft tissue fit.
4. Explain the possible causes of fracture and the reasons why simply repairing the fracture may be contraindicated.
5. Establish a sequence of recall visits including regular visits during the adjustment period, followed by periodic recall as deemed advisable.
6. Emphasize the need for continuing dental attention.

OTHER AVAILABLE RESIN PRODUCTS

DENTURE BASE TEMPORARY RELINING RESINS

Biokwik Cold Cure Relining Material, B.L. Dental Co., Inc.

Denturelyne, Teledyne Dental Products

HARD ORYL RELINING RESIN, Teledyne Dental Products

Kerr Luralite, Kerr Mfg. Co., Div. of Sybron Corp.

New Truplastic, Teledyne Dental Products

RE-STOR, L.D. Caulk Co., Div. of Dentsply International, Inc.

Solitine, Kerr Mfg. Co. (for use as solvent with Luralite)

Super-Oryl, Teledyne Dental Products

ACRYLIC RESIN TEETH
ADA SPECIFICATION NO. 15

TYPE I, ANTERIOR

DENTORIUM, Dentorium Products Co., Inc.

DURA-BLEND; DURA-BLEND CHARACTERIZED; DURA-BLEND SPECIAL, Myerson Tooth Corp.

DYMON-HUE PLASTIC TEETH, Regal Dental Corp.

JUSTI IMPERIAL PLASTIC TEETH, H.D. Justi Co., Div. of Williams Gold Refining Co., Inc.

KENSON CAMBRIDGE ANTERIORS, Kenson Mfg. Co.

LUMIN ACRYL V ANTERIORS, Unitek Corp.

MAJOR SUPER G, ACRYLIC RESIN TEETH, Bruno Pozzi Dental Products

NEW HUE PLASTIC ANTERIORS, Dentsply International, Inc.

NEW MAJOR DENT ACRYLIC RESIN TEETH, American Tooth Mfg. Co.

NEW MAJOR SUPERLUX ACRYLIC RESIN TEETH, American Tooth Mfg. Co.

ORTOLUX-F ANTERIORS, N. Uhler Co.

TRUBYTE BIOTONE; BIOBLEND; BIOFORM; PRIMARY, Dentsply International, Inc.

VERIDENT; VERIDENT POLYCHROME, Lactona Corp., Subsidiary Warner-Lambert Co.

TYPE II, POSTERIOR-ANATOMIC

DENTORIUM, Dentorium Products Co., Inc.

DURA-BLEND FLX; SYNCHRONIZED (DURA-BLEND), Myerson Tooth Corp.

DURATOMIC POSTERIORS, Myerson Tooth Corp.

DYMON-HUE PLASTIC TEETH, Regal Dental Corp.

EXACTONE, Bruno Pozzi Dental Products

JUSTI IMPERIAL PLASTIC TEETH, H.D. Justi Co., Div. of Williams Gold Refining Co., Inc.

Kenson 30° Teeth, Kenson Mfg. Co.

KENSON CAMBRIDGE, Kenson Mfg. Corp.

KENSON POSTERIORS, Kenson Mfg. Corp.

ORTOLUX-F POSTERIORS, N. Uhler Co.

NEW HUE 33° PLASTIC POSTERIORS, Dentsply International, Inc.

Pilkington-Turner 30°, Dentsply International, Inc.

SUPER LINCOLN TEETH 20°, 30°, Lincoln Dental Supply Co.

TRUBYTE BIOFORM 20° PLASTIC POSTERIORS, Dentsply International, Inc.

TRUBYTE BIOTONE BLENDED 33° POSTERIORS; PILKINGTON TURNER: DENTRON 20°, Dentsply International, Inc.

VERIDENT NIC POSTERIORS, Lactona Corp., Subsidiary Warner-Lambert Co.

VIVOSTAR PE POSTERIOR TEETH, Williams Gold Refining Co., Inc.

TYPE III, POSTERIOR-NONANATOMIC

BIOTONE RATIONAL BLOCK, Dentsply International, Inc.

DYMON-HUE PLASTIC TEETH, Regal Dental Corp.

JUSTI IMPERIAL PLASTIC TEETH, H. D. Justi Co., Div. of Williams Gold Refining Co., Inc.

Kenson 0° Teeth, Kenson Mfg. Co.

MYERSON AND SEARS (DURA-BLEND): SHEAR KUSP (DURA-BLEND), Myerson Tooth Corp.

NEW HUE 0° PLASTIC POSTERIORS, Dentsply International, Inc.

ORTOLUX-F POSTERIOR-NONANATOMIC, N. Uhler Co.

SUPER LINCOLN FUNCTIONAL ZERO DEGREE, Lincoln Dental Supply Co.

TRUBYTE BIOTONE FUNCTIONAL POSTERIORS; RATIONAL, Dentsply International, Inc.

Universal, Lactona Corp.

VERIDENT BIO-MECHANICAL POSTERIORS, Lactona Corp., Subsidiary Warner-Lambert Co.

LITERATURE REFERENCES

1. Ware, A. L., and Docking, A. R. The strength of acrylic repairs. Austral. Dent. J. 54:27 Feb. 1950.

2. Stanford, J. W.; Burns, C. L.; and Paffenbarger, G. C. Self-curing resins for repairing dentures: some physical properties. JADA 61:307 Sept. 1955.

3. McCrorie, J. W., and Anderson, J. N. Transverse strength of repairs with self-curing resins. Br. Dent. J. 109:364 Nov. 1960.

4. Leong, A., and Grant, A. A. The transverse strength of repairs in polymethyl methacrylate. Austral. Dent. J. 16:232 Aug. 1971.

5. von Fraunhofer, J. A. Scientific aspects of dental materials. Boston, Butterworths, pp. 439-448, 1975.

6. Pincus, C. L. New concepts in model techniques and high temperature processing of acrylic resins for maximum esthetics. J. South. Calif. Dent. Assoc. 24:19 Feb. 1956.

7. Ryge, G., and Forley, D. E. Effect of dry heat processing on the physical properties of acrylic crowns. JADA 66:672 May 1963.

8. Nienabar, W. B. Preliminary report on a new veneering material, Pyroplast. Minneapolis Dent. J. 51:3 Mar. 1967.

9. Hickey, J. C., et al. The relation of mouth protectors to cranial pressure and deformation. JADA 74:735 Mar. 1967.

10. Stenger, J. M., et al. Mouthguards: protection against shock to head, neck and teeth. JADA 69:273 Sept. 1964.

11. Going, R. E.; Loehman, R. E.; and Chan, M. S. Mouthguard materials: their physical and mechanical properties. JADA 89:132 July 1947.

12. Laney, W. R. Processed resilient denture liners. Dent. Clin. N. Am. 14:531 July 1970.

13. Suchatlampong, C.; Davies, E. H.; and von Fraunhofer, J. A. Some physical properties of four resilient lining materials. J. Dentistry 4:19 Jan. 1976.

14. Eick, J. D.; Craig, R. G.; and Peyton, F. A. Properties of resilient denture liners in simulated mouth conditions. J. Prosthet. Dent. 12:1043 Nov.-Dec. 1962.

15. Wilson, J. R., and Tomlin, H. R. Soft lining materials. Some relevant properties and their determination. J. Prosthet. Dent. 21:244 Mar. 1969.

16. Wright, P. S. Soft lining materials: their status and prospects. J. Dentistry 4:247 Nov. 1976.

17. O'Brien, W. J.; Herman, J.; and Shepherd, J. H. Mechanical properties of hydrophilic acrylic polymer. J. Bio. Med. Mat. Res. 6:15 Mar. 1972.

18. McCabe, J. F. Soft lining materials: Composition and structure. J. Oral Rehab. 3:273 July 1976.

19. Lytle, R. B. Complete denture construction based on a study of the deformation of the underlying soft tissue. J. Prosthet. Dent. 9:539 July-Aug. 1959.

20. Wilson, H. J.; Tomlin, H. R.; and Osborne, J. Tissue conditioners and functional impression materials. Br. Dent. J. 121:9 July 1966.

21. Wilson, H. J.; Tomlin, H. R.; and Osborne, J. The assessment of temporary soft materials used on prosthetics. Br. Dent. J. 126:303 Apr. 1969.

22. George, W. A., and Aramany, M. E. Treatment materials for edentulous tissues. Penn. Dent. J. 32:3 Jan. 1965.

23. Caul, H. J., and Stanford, J. W. Composition of denture reliners used by the public. J. Dent. Res. 37:87 Feb. 1968 (abs.).

24. Denture relining materials for home use. Council on Dental Research—Council on Dental Therapeutics. JADA 47:214 Aug. 1953.

25. Lytle, R. B. Do it yourself prosthodontics. Dent. Prog. 1:221 Apr. 1961.

26. Larkin, J. D. Injury caused by denture reliner and adhesives self-administered by a patient. Texas Dent. J. 82:9 Nov. 1964.

27. Woelfel, J. B.; Kreider, J. A.; and Berg, T. Deformed lower ridge caused by the relining of a denture by a patient. JADA 64:753 June 1962.

28. Woelfel, J. B., et al. Documented reports of bone loss caused by use of denture liners. JADA 71:23 July 1965.

29. Woelfel, J. B.; Winter, C. M.; and Curry, R. L. Additives sold over the counter dangerously prolong wearing period of ill-fitting dentures. JADA 71:603 Sept. 1965.

30. Parker, E. M. Personal communication to the Council on Dental Trade and Laboratory Relations. Aug. 1954.

31. Smith, W. C. Report on injury resulting from use of a home reliner kit. Personal communication to Council on Dental Research of the American Dental Association.

32. Means, C. R. A study of the use of home reliners in dentures. J. Prosthet. Dent. 14:623 July-Aug. 1964.

33. Means, C. R. A report of a user of home reliner materials. J. Prosthet. Dent. 14:935 Sept.-Oct. 1964.

34. Means, C. R. The home reliner materials: The significance of the problem. J. Prosthet. Dent. 14:1086 Nov.-Dec. 1964.

35. Federal Register, Vol. 34, No. 172, Sept. 9, 1969.

36. Guidelines on after care for denture patients. Council on Dental Health. JADA 94:1187 June 1977.

ORTHODONTIC APPLIANCES, DEVICES AND MATERIALS

Orthodontics, as defined by the Council on Dental Education of the American Dental Association, is that area of dentistry concerned with the supervision and guidance of the growing dentition and correction of the mature dentofacial structures, and includes those conditions that require movement of teeth and/or correction of malrelationships of jaws and teeth and malformations of their related structures.

Major responsibilities of orthodontic practice include the diagnosis, prevention, interception and treatment of all forms of malocclusion of the teeth and associated alterations in their surrounding structures; the design, application, and control of functional and corrective appliances; and the guidance of the dentition and its supporting structures to attain and maintain optimum occlusal relations in physiologic and esthetic harmony among facial and cranial structures.

There are five possible tooth movements, namely tipping, rotation, bodily movements or translation, extrusion, and intrusion, which can achieve these orthodontic objectives. All of these movements can be effected by the utilization of removable or fixed orthodontic appliances.

REMOVABLE ORTHODONTIC APPLIANCES

Removable appliances are orthodontic devices which may be removed and re-inserted by the patient. There are a large number of removable appliances employed today and these include the Hawley appliance with its many modifications, bite plates, removable retainers of many varieties, the Frankel appliance, the Crozat appliance, the activators and many others. Some removable appliances are used in conjunction with fixed appliances.

COMPOSITION: Removable orthodontic appliances are either all metal, such as precious metal parts (gold) soldered together and stainless steel welded or soldered, or acrylic with or without various stainless steel wire attachments, e.g. clasps, springs, and labial arches. The active part of the removable appliance (springs, screws, rubber bands) is that portion which will deliver the force to the teeth. The framework of the acrylic appliance which is usually constructed of heat or cold cured, pink or clear resins is the support for the active part. The removable appliance is held in place by incorporating in its design a palatal section of acrylic resins, a labial bow and clasps designed to engage undercut areas on selected teeth.

USES: Removable orthodontic appliances, if myofunctional appliances are excluded, are effective primarily in tipping teeth. Proponents of the Crozat appliance claim that more extensive tooth movements are possible but its complexity of design and fabrication requires a comprehensive appreciation of its potentials prior to its application.

Springs: Springs incorporated into removable appliances, in effect, only tip teeth. A helix is frequently incorporated in the spring design since this allows for a more gentle force to be applied to the tooth and also increases the range of activation of the spring. The force in the spring is obtained by elastically deforming the spring. Springs used to move incisor teeth are fabricated from .016 or .018 inch stainless steel wire and should be activated no more than 2 to 3 mm. Springs used to apply force to premolar teeth are generally fabricated from larger diameter stainless steel wires, e.g. .020 or .022 inch. There are numerous spring designs and each should be fabricated according to the preference of the operator.

Expansion Screws: Expansion screws of various designs are available and these may be employed for moving a single tooth or a group of teeth. Expansion screws operate by the two halves moving apart when the central screw is turned in an opening direction. The amount of activation depends on the pitch of the thread of the screw and the frequency of activation.

Labial Bows: Labial bows or labial archwires of various designs are incorporated in removable appliances. Some labial bows, as employed in the Hawley retainer, serve to hold the removable appliance in place whereas others are designed to move teeth. Labial bows are probably most commonly fabricated from .028 inch stainless steel wires but some designs require other gauges depending on the application of the bow.

Clasps: Many clasp designs are available and selection depends on the indications of the particular case. Commonly employed clasps include the Adam's clasp, the arrowhead clasp (Schwartz), the ball clasp, the arrow pin clasp, the triangular clasp and the Duyzing's clasp.[1] These are fabricated from stainless steel wire of sizes ranging approximately from .024 to .032 inch in diameter.

Myofunctional Appliances: These appliances include the Andresen (activator), bite plates, oral screen and many others. The theory of these appliances is to alter muscular function and cause tooth and/or skeletal changes.[2] They operate by activating neuromuscular tissues and reflexes to guide the erupting teeth of child-

---

REMOVABLE APPLIANCES

Do:

1. Select and design the appliance that will most satisfactorily and easily achieve the objectives.
2. Insure patient comfort, understanding and co-operation.

Don't:

1. Attempt too complex tooth movements with a removable appliance.
2. Expect the appliance to replace a correct diagnosis and treatment plan.

ren with malocclusions into more acceptable relationships.[2] An understanding of growth and development is essential when use of these appliances is contemplated.

Retention Appliances: Removable appliances are often designed to retain tooth positions after fixed orthodontic appliance mechanotherapy. Retainers do not have active components.

FIXED ORTHODONTIC APPLIANCES

Fixed appliances are anchored to the teeth by means of orthodontic bands or bonds and cannot be removed and re-inserted by the patient. Components of fixed appliances include: bands which are cemented to the crowns of teeth; brackets which are welded to the bands or bonded directly to tooth enamel; archwires which are ligated to the brackets with wire or rubber ligatures; miscellaneous attachments welded to bands or bonded to enamel, such as lingual buttons, cleats, or tubes; and miscellaneous accessories such as hooks, springs of varying design, coil springs, elastic thread, elastic rings, palatal bars and lingual arches.

Fixed appliances effect tooth movement by elastic deformation of fabricated archwires and also by forces exerted by springs, coils and elastics.

Bands

An orthodontic band is a flattened continuous circumferential metallic ring which is constructed to fit and be cemented around the clinical crown of a tooth. Bands may be purchased prefabricated for each tooth in a wide range of sizes. The operator then merely selects a band for optimal size and fit. Alternatively, bands may be hand formed by the operator from strips of stainless steel band material. Previously, gold alloys had been employed but these have been replaced by stainless steel due largely to the cost factor. Operator hand fabricated bands are custom made for each tooth and this method of fitting orthodontic bands has given way to the use of prefabricated bands.

Bands are of varying widths (occluso-gingivally), thicknesses and diameters and are manufactured from various hardnesses of metal. To an orthodontic band are welded various brackets and orthodontic auxiliaries. Prefabricated bands may be ordered from the manufacturer with brackets already welded into position according to the operator's prescription.

A number of requirements of the material should be examined before selecting a particular band. It should be sufficiently soft and ductile to be adaptable to crown contours and allow burnishing of edges yet be sufficiently strong and stiff to maintain its shape under stresses placed upon it in the oral cavity, i.e., orthodontic and functional. The material should be sufficiently "springy" to pass over maximum tooth contours and return to original shape. It is essential that the materials be compatible with the oral tissues and be as esthetically pleasing as possible. Of importance is the ability of the material to be joined to other metal attachments by welding or soldering and present a smooth final finish.

The recommended sizes of stainless steel band material are presented in Table I.

Table I.

Type of Tooth	Thickness of Band Material
Molars	.006 x .220 inches
Cuspids and Bicuspids	.004 x .150-.180 inches
Incisors	.003-.004 x .125-.150 inches

Band Construction: Bands may be fabricated by the "pinch band" technique in stainless steel. Band material in roll form or prefabricated "blanks" may be used. Band forming pliers of varying designs are available; however, some operators prefer to use the "Howe" plier. Bands, after being "pulled up," are welded at their joint and folded over. Because the band material is not excessively thick the ends may be folded over and welded, thus forming a band. Contouring and adaptation is carried out as necessary both gingivally and occlusally.

Since molar bands are fabricated from thicker band material, some operators prefer to modify their construction in such a manner as to avoid excessive thickness at their seam or joint. This is achieved by having a thin band material insert welded in at the seam to join the two ends together. Where gold is used the joints are soldered. Other instruments which may be useful to aid in band fabrication include band stretchers, contouring pliers, amalgam pluggers, scalers, band pushers and automatic mallets.

Preformed bands: Thurow[3] considers it a distinct advantage to use preformed bands that are fully annealed. In orthodontic practice where multiband techniques are used, preformed bands are routinely employed. However, occasions occur where a preformed band may not adequately fit a particular tooth and the fabrication of a "custom built" band is desirable. Also, general practitioners who only occasionally use bands may fabricate these in order to avoid purchasing large inventories of preformed bands.

Most orthodontic commercial companies produce preformed bands for each tooth in the arch. In addition, certain "general purpose" bands for groups of certain teeth are available. The shape, design and contour of the bands vary according to the manufacturer. Bands may also be obtained with brackets or attachments prewelded to prescription or according to a predetermined technique.

BANDS

Do:

1. Insure correct fit.

Don't:

1. Overextend to irritate the periodontium.
2. Interfere with the occlusal surface of the tooth.
3. Place ill-fitted bands.

AVAILABLE PRODUCTS

Bands, Unitek Corp.
Williams #1 Plain; Contoured Bands, Williams Gold Refining Co., Inc.
Williams Paloy Band, Williams Gold Refining Co., Inc.
Williams Stainless Steel Whitman Bands, Williams Gold Refining Co., Inc.

Brackets and Tubes

An orthodontic bracket or tube is a device which projects horizontally from the orthodontic band (or directly from the tooth enamel in the case of direct bonding) to support an archwire.

USES: Brackets and tubes are used to attach archwires to the teeth so as to transmit forces from the archwire and any other force-delivering auxiliaries, e.g., elastics and coil springs, to the teeth in order to effect orthodontic tooth movements. They can also, because of their design, effect torque, tipping, bodily movement, intrusion, extrusion and rotation depending on the design of the archwire and the auxiliaries employed in the fixed appliance. Of vital importance in any fixed orthodontic appliance is the correct position of the brackets and tubes on the teeth.

TYPES: Numerous types of brackets and tubes have been developed over the years. These have undergone changes in shape, size, composition, and configuration. The two most widely used fixed appliances are the edgewise appliance, with its many variations, and the Begg appliance.[4,5] The essential difference between the edgewise and Begg appliances lies in the basic philosophy of treatment and bracket design. The edgewise appliance also employs rectangular archwires at some phase of the treatment. Other infrequently used fixed appliances include the labio-lingual and twin wire appliance. In all of these fixed appliances, the brackets and tubes may be angulated, torqued and also have other components attached, for example rotation arms and hooks. Various bracket and tube combinations are also manufactured. Examples with diagrams of the various brackets commercially available today may be seen in the catalogues printed by the supply houses. The vast majority of brackets and tubes manufactured today are produced from stainless steel.

DIRECTIONS FOR USE: In recent years many techniques have been developed for the direct bonding of orthodontic brackets to tooth enamel.[6-8] This procedure is dependent on the prior acid etching of enamel and then bonding specially manufactured brackets onto the etched enamel. Bonding relies on mechanical retention. The bonding material must be mechanically retained on the tooth via the etched enamel and on the bracket via a mesh on the undersurface of the bracket or retentive holes on the stainless steel bracket base. Again, numerous metal brackets have been designed for bonding purposes. Plastic brackets are available for use on anterior teeth but have not as yet been universally accepted since many have proven to be clinically unsatisfactory over periods of time. Orthodontic bonding materials are composite materials and these together with acid etching are described elsewhere in this book.

AVAILABLE PRODUCTS

Brackets & Tubes, Unitek Corp.
Lee-Fisher Plastic Brackets, Lee Pharmaceuticals
Lee Metal Mesh Edgewise Brackets, Lee Pharmaceuticals
Lee Metal Mesh Lingual Buttons, Lee Pharmaceuticals
Saif-Springs System, Northwest Orthodontics

ORTHODONTIC RESINS:

Caulk Orthodontic Resin, L.D. Caulk Co.
Concise Brand, 3M Company
Enamel Coat, Den-Mat, Inc.
Genie; Genie II, Lee Pharmaceuticals
Lee-Bond, Lee Pharmaceuticals
Lee Orthodontic Self-Curing Resin, Lee Pharmaceuticals
Once Orthodontic Polymeric Cement, Lee Pharmaceuticals

Protecto, Lee Pharmaceuticals

SPLINTING RESINS:

Lee Splinting Resin, Lee Pharmaceuticals

Other Orthodontic Attachments

Various other attachments which are welded (or, in case of gold alloys, soldered) to bands are available. These attachments include lingual and palatal sheaths, cleats, buttons, hooks, and eyelets. A complete list of attachments is available in commercial catalogues.

FIXED ORTHODONTIC APPLIANCES

Do:
1. Insure correct bracket and tube position on the tooth.

Don't:
1. Expect appliances to replace detailed diagnosis and treatment planning.

ORTHODONTIC AUXILIARIES

Extra-oral appliances such as headgear and chin caps are those devices which have their source of anchorage outside the mouth.

Headgear

Headgear includes all extra-oral orthodontic appliances which have as their anchor site the head or the neck. Headgears may be used to move teeth, reinforce anchorage or act as orthopedic appliances. Because headgear use causes no demonstrable change at its source of force, the neck or cranium, it is considered to be a relatively stable form of anchorage in orthodontics. Headgears of many varieties are used.

COMPOSITION: There are a number of major components of headgear appliances. The headcap and neckstrap have their anchor source on the head and neck, respectively, and are fabricated from a variety of materials, most commonly cloth covered plastic, elasticized straps or soft plastic strapping.

The extra-oral force facial bow is a common means of connecting the headcap or neckstrap to the intra-oral dental archwire directly or via a soldered joint to the removable intra-oral archwire. The facebow is often fabricated from .059 inch diameter stainless steel wire. The arms of the facebow vary in direction and length depending on the design. The facebow is adapted to follow the external contours of the cheeks but not be in contact with them.

The removable intra-oral archwire, when employed, is U-shaped and usually fabricated from .045 to .051 inch diameter stainless steel wire designed to pass from the lip commissures, about 3 mm ahead of the labial surface of the maxillary incisors into the buccal sulcus at approximately the occlusal plane level, and to fit into tubes attached to the buccal surface of the first molar teeth, most commonly the maxillary first molar teeth. Stops, soldered or bent, are placed approximately 7 to 10 mm from each of the two distal ends of the archwire. When this type of appliance is used, the removable extra-oral archwire is soldered to the extra-oral facial bow in the incisor area.

The force delivery system which connects the headcap to the distal end of the extra-oral facial bow may consist of either rubber bands, springs of varying design or elasticized strapping.

In the case of the chincup, a cup made of a variety of materials such as rubber or soft plastic is fashioned to fit over the chin and force is delivered to it from the headcap via rubber bands, coil springs or elasticized strapping.

DESIGNS: Numerous headgears are available with respect to both the inner arch and extra-oral facial bow design and the cranial and cervical attachment design. The selection of the correct headgear design depends on the effects desired.

USES: Headgear appliances are used for anchorage reinforcement, correction of Angle Class II malocclusions by controlling maxillary growth while permitting the mandible to express its growth, increasing arch length by moving molars distally, and retention of post-orthodontic treatment. Chincups are of value in controlling mandibular growth.

DIRECTIONS FOR USE: The effect of the headgear upon the dentition depends on the direction of the force delivered from the headgear assembly and the center of resistance of the tooth (or arch) to which the force is applied. Based on mechanical principles teeth may be intruded, extruded, moved bodily, tipped, or rotated in three planes of space by means of a headgear. For this reason, careful headgear selection is imperative.

Use of headgear should follow careful diagnosis and treatment planning. Predominant growth trends in the growing patient should also be anticipated prior to headgear use.

AVAILABLE PRODUCTS

Contour Stop Facebows, Northwest Orthodontics
Elastic Ligature Thread, Lee Pharmaceuticals
Orthodontic Auxillary Products, Unitek Corp.
Orthodontic Extra-Oral Appliances–Correction of Malocclusion, orpen bite cases, Prognathic Jaws, and Orthopedic correction, Orthoband Co.
Snap-way Safety Headcap, Northwest Orthodontics
Snap-way Safety J Hook Headgear, Northwest Orthodontics
Snap-way Safety Neckstrap, Northwest Orthodontics

Orthopedic Appliances

Dentofacial orthopedics is concerned with correction of abnormalities and deviations from the range of normality in the facial and oral tissues. Whereas classical orthodontic therapy is limited to correction of alveodental abnormalities, dentofacial orthopedics includes the treatment of changes in the jaws.[9] Rapid palatal expansion appliances, headgears and chincups are often referred to as orthopedic appliances since they tend to or attempt to orthopedically alter skeletal components of the stomatognathic system. The rapid palatal expansion appliance is cemented to the maxillary arch via bands on selected molar and premolar teeth and has an expansion screw in the midline. Opening of the screw over a period of 14 to 21 days splits the midpalatal suture. The appliance is left in place a number of months afterwards in order to allow reorganization of the tissues to insure maintenance of the expansion. Appliances such as the headgear and chincup have been designed to apply orthopedic forces of approximately 3 to 4 pounds to the maxilla and mandible, respectively. These appliances attempt to control growth in amount and/or direction in order to improve maxillomandibular relationships. The utilization of orthopedic appliances in particular requires a complete orthodontic diagnosis and treatment plan and a sound knowledge of growth and development.

ORTHODONTIC MATERIALS

Orthodontic Elastics

A number of elastic materials are employed in orthodontic mechanotherapy. For use with headgear, elastic rubber bands of various sizes and strengths are available to deliver the desired forces. In addition, elasticized strapping is also employed extra-orally for use as force delivery system with headgears.

Intra-orally, rubber bands of various sizes and strengths are employed to exert forces upon the teeth. Elastic material in the form of thread also may be selectively tied in place so as to exert forces on the teeth. Ligatures used to ligate archwires to brackets are often made of elastic materials in ring form. Very small rubber elastic rings are also available to separate teeth to allow for banding space.

The variety of elastic materials used in orthodontics is vast and reference to the commercial catalogues is advisable.

Orthodontic Wire

COMPOSITION: Stainless steel is by far the most widely used material for orthodontic wire. The stainless steel alloys are usually standard formulae based on specification of the American Iron and Steel Institute. Gold alloys used in orthodontics are usually manufactured by the suppliers, each to his own specifications thus resulting in much wider variation in gold alloys than in stainless steel wires. Gold alloys, in the form of bands or wires, are not commonly employed today.

Orthodontic appliances are largely fabricated from the Austentic Stainless Steel 300 series. These alloys contain iron, chromium and significant quantities of nickel for metal stability at high heat treatment temperatures. The chromium content greatly increases the room temperature strength and aids in corrosion resistance. Stainless steel orthodontic wire may be of the round or rectangular varieties.

USES: Orthodontic wires are the primary mechanism for force application to teeth.

DIRECTIONS FOR USE: The orthodontic appliance depends largely upon the physical properties and mechanical behavior of the metals employed. The selection of a particular archwire to improve one property of the appliance may adversely affect another. The appliance design must be carefully considered and the appropriate wire selected. Table II depicts the appropriate type and size of orthodontic wire for each use. Braided wires ("twistflex" or "wildcat") consist of strands of thin wire braided together to achieve flexibility. Rectangular wires, when in place in rectangular brackets or tubes, have the ability to apply torque forces to teeth. In round wire techniques, torque force is achieved by employing specially designed auxiliaries.

The ideal orthodontic archwire or spring should be one that will release a constant force throughout the entire range of spring activation. This should not imply that force levels must remain constant during a given type of tooth movement but rather that sudden change in force magnitude should be eliminated. Since Hooke's Law states that no spring can be completely constant in its action, the aim is to utilize springs with low load deflection rates. However, the spring or wire must be strong enough to withstand most normal usage.

Table II.

Orthodontic Wires

Type of Wire	Use	Range of Wire Diameter (in inches)
Round	Ligatures	.007-.012
	Fixed appliances	.014-.022
	Removable appliances	.016-.036
	Lingual arches	.036
	Headgear	
	inner arch	.045-.051
	facial bow	.060
Braided	Archwires	.015-.020
Rectangular	Edgewise fixed appliances	.016 x .016- .022 x .028

ORTHODONTIC WIRE

Do:

1. Select wire sized correctly.
2. Employ loops and helices to increase wire length and flexibility.
3. Bend archwires slowly to minimize stresses in the wire.
4. Insure light forces by careful appliance design.
5. Activate loops in the same direction as the original bend.

Don't:

1. Make sharp bends in wires.
2. Bend wire repeatedly in the same place.
3. Burn archwire when soldering.

EVALUATION PROGRAM: Recently the Council on Dental Materials, Instruments and Equipment of the American Dental Association approved the new Specification No. 32 for orthodontic wires not containing precious metals.[10] This specification is for straight orthodontic wires not containing gold and platinum group metals and covers Type I–low resilience and Type II–high resilience wires. Reference to this specification will insure a complete understanding of requirements.

AVAILABLE PRODUCTS

Lee Super Resilient Arch Wire-Tooth Colored, Lee Pharmaceuticals

Lok-Tite Ortho Wire, Williams Gold Refining Co., Inc.

Paloy Ortho Wire, Williams Gold Refining Co., Inc.

Qwik Tie Ligature Instrument and Wire, Lee Pharmaceuticals

Unitek Nitinol Activ-Arch Wire, Unitek Corp.

Unitek HI-T II Wire, Unitek Corp.

Unitek Permachrome Wire, Unitek Corp.

Unitek Permachrome Resilient Wire, Unitek Corp.

Unitek Permachrome Unisil Wire, Unitek Corp.

Williams Stainless Steel Ligature Wire, Williams Gold Refining Co., Inc.

Williams #2 Ortho Wire, Williams Gold Refining Co., Inc.

Wilkinson H. S. Wire, Wilkinson Co.

Wilkinson Ortholux Wire, Wilkinson Co.

ORTHODONTIC INSTRUMENTS

Many of the instruments employed in general dental practice are also used in orthodontic practice. These include x-ray equipment, office equipment, chairs and sterilization equipment. Hand instruments are used according to the preference of the operator.

As in other dental disciplines, diagnosis is the key to successful mechanotherapy. Specialized orthodontic diagnostic aids include study casts, panoramic and/or full mouth intra-oral radiographs and clinical photographs of the full face, profile and intra-oral view. In addition to the equipment required to perform these diagnostic measures, specialized chairs and operatory equipment specifically suited to orthodontic needs should be considered. Items specifically designed for orthodontic use include the following.

Orthodontic pliers: Orthodontic pliers are manufactured in many designs and forms. Reference to commercial catalogues will indicate the wide variety of orthodontic pliers available.

Bracket gauges: These are instruments employed in marking bracket heights on orthodontic bands. Many different designs are available.

Turretts: Orthodontic turretts are designed instruments that aid in initial arch forming of orthodontic wires.

Welders: Welding is the joining of metals by means of heat without the addition of any other material. Numerous types of welders with many features are available. In orthodontics, welding is used primarily to affix brackets and other attachments to bands.

Soldering equipment and materials: Orthodontic blowpipes with many additional soldering aids are used to join brackets and attachments to bands. In addition, soldering is employed to attach hooks, stops, and other auxiliaries to archwires. Soldering requires the addition of another alloy to bind the two alloys being joined. Flux is required for soldering.

Electro soldering units, many manufactured in combination with welding units, are available. The source of heat for the soldering procedure is obtained electrically.

Available Products

E. A. Beck Orthodontic Pliers, E. A. Beck & Co.

Bar Stainless Pliers, Utility. Loop Forming, Band Removing, Unitek Corp.

Biostar Orthodontic Instruments: Retainers; Positioners; Model Duplications; Splints; Mouthguards; Chin Cups; Custom Impression Trays; Fluoride Trays, Great Lakes Orthodontic

Products

ETM Hand Instruments, Pliers, Cutters, Banding Instruments, Specialty Instruments, Unitek Corp.

Miltex Band Pushers, Miltex Instrument Co.

Miltex Pliers, Miltex Instrument Co.

Ortho Craft Stainless Steel Enamel Stripper, Ortho Craft Orthodontic Specialty Products

Ortho Craft Steel Abrasive Strips, Ortho Craft Orthodontic Specialty Products

Orthodontic Pliers, Lee Pharmaceuticals

Unitek Hand Instruments, Pliers, Cutters, Unitek Corp.

Literature References

1. Graber, T. M., and Neumann, B. Removable orthodontic appliances. Philadelphia, W. B. Saunders Co., 1977.

2. Woodside, D. G. The activator. in Salzmann, J. A. (ed.) Orthodontics in daily practice. Philadelphia, J. B. Lippincott Co., 1974.

3. Thurow, R. C. Edgewise orthodontics. ed. 3, St. Louis, C. V. Mosby Company, 1972.

4. Graber, T. M. Orthodontics: principles and practice. ed. 3, Philadelphia, W. B. Saunders Co., 1972.

5. Begg. P. R., and Kessling, P. C. Begg orthodontic theory and technique. ed. 2, Philadelphia, W. B. Saunders Co., 1971.

6. Retief, D. H.; Dreyer, C. J.; and Gavron, G. The direct bonding of orthodontic attachments to teeth by means of an epoxy resin adhesive. Am.J. Orthodont. 58:21, 1967.

7. Retief, D. H., and Sadowsky, P. L. Clinical experience with the acid etch technique in orthodontics. Am. J. Orthodont. 68:645, 1975.

8. Zachrisson, B. U. A post-treatment evaluation of direct bonding in orthodontics. Am. J. Orthodont. 71:173, 1977.

9. Salzmann, J. A. (ed.) Orthodontics in daily practice. Philadelphia, J. B. Lippincott Company, 1974.

10. New American Dental Association specification no. 32 for orthodontic wires not containing precious metals. JADA 95:1169, 1977.

DENTAL IMPLANTS

Dental implants consist of metallic, ceramic, or polymeric materials which are placed either on or within the mandibular or maxillary bone to support fixed or removable prostheses. The function of an implant is to provide an abutment to support and stabilize a prosthesis. Generally an implant is placed in an edentulous area after it is determined that a conventional restorative modality is not satisfactory.

The replacement of missing teeth using dental implants has been attempted since the early days of the Egyptians, and many different implant designs and materials have been used. Modern implant dentistry is noted by the development of the cast cobalt-chromium subperiosteal implant and full removable denture by Goldberg and Gershkoff.[1]

For the past 40 years, extensive work has been conducted improving the subperiosteal implant and developing endosseous and endodontic implants. The fundamental problems associated with implant design and application have been: (a) obtaining highly biocompatible materials which withstand the adverse oral environment without corrosion and loss of mechanical properties; (b) designing implant shapes and restorations which provide mechanical support and stabilization for the prosthesis without causing extensive bone resorption; and (c) developing an interlocking between the gingival and mucosal tissues and the implant to prevent bacterial penetration and infection in sites where the implant extends into the oral cavity.

Dental implants have had a controversial history. Surveys conducted five years ago indicated that as high as 60 percent of the endosseous and unilateral subperiosteal implants failed after only two years or less.[2] At times the failure resulted in infection and extensive bone resorption. As a result of this history, these procedures have found little acceptance in the mainstream of the restorative dental practice.

In the past five years, great advances have occurred. The profound need for a series of safe dental implant procedures to aid in the restorative process has spurred a strong push with respect to the research regarding these procedures. With more cautious patient selection and better materials and techniques, the degree of success and safety has progressively increased. In the hands of the experienced dentist, dental implants can now hold the promise of enduring as effectively as other contemporary restorative procedures.

Today, several biocompatible materials having adequate mechanical properties are in use. A variety of dental implant designs have been developed to meet anatomical, surgical and restorative requirements as well as oral hygiene needs, and minimize bone resorption around the implant.

No one implant technique or material can suffice to fulfill all of the restorative needs of the various dental situations. Many failures have occurred in the past because attempts were made to make one particular implant design or technique function for all situations. Greater success can result where the dentist is familiar with all implant materials and techniques, and then uses the type of implant which can best fit into the given restorative situation.

In general, where patients have adequate bone, one of a variety of endosseous implant designs should be utilized. The subperiosteal implant design should be limited to those areas where most or all of the alveolar bone has resorbed. In some situations, combinations of endosseous and subperiosteal implants must be utilized to satisfy the needs of the patient.

The critical factors in performing implant dentistry are: 1) careful patient diagnosis including a detailed health history, panoramic and periapical x-rays, oral examination and a clear demonstration of the need for a dental implant; 2) the use of surgical procedures which minimize infection and trauma to the bone and patient; 3) careful surgical techniques which fit the implant into close contact with the supporting bone; 4) restoration design which minimizes stresses on the bone supporting the implant and prevents lateral stresses from occurring; 5) careful patient hygiene; and 6) continuing maintenance.

The patient must be informed in detail about the implant procedure and all of the potential complications. The patient must be further informed why an implant is being considered in place of a conventional restorative procedure. Because the functional life of the implant is so interdependent with the systemic health of the patient, it becomes more difficult to predict the term of life of the implant than it is to predict the life of other restorative procedures. It is necessary to obtain informed consent for the benefit of the practitioner as well as the patient.

In order to have more successful results with dental implants, the dentist must pay special attention to these areas: 1) health history, 2) patient selection, 3) treatment planning, 4) presurgical treatment, 5) surgical procedures, 6) splinting techniques, 7) postoperative care and maintenance, 8) restorative techniques, and 9) occlusion. Most implant dentists feel that the greatest attention must be applied to the areas of patient selection, oral hygiene or preventative maintenance, and occlusion.

PATIENT SELECTION

Patient selection is probably the most important aspect of the implant procedure. Although some rigid guidelines may be set for evaluating the patient, there is much subjectivity involved, and the dentist must often draw from experience to assess the systemic makeup of the patient. The health of the gingival tissues is dependent upon a balanced body chemistry. Systemic disorders of a metabolic nature, (diabetes, liver and kidney function), will affect the health of the attachment mechanism around the functioning tooth, and therefore the implant. The implant dentist must evaluate the past and present health and dental history of the patient and related family, and then attempt to predict the future health of the patient.

The adaptation of the tissues surrounding the implant, the bone or gingival tissues, is basically of mechanical form. To date no commercial implant is available for which there is a direct attachment of connective tissue from bone or gingiva into the surface of the implant.

Grooves, undercuts, holes or texturing on the surface of the implant tend to allow a mechanical tissue interlock onto the surface of the implant. This interlock helps to retain the implant in place and prevent bacteria and oral fluids from penetrating along the body of the implant.

In order for this tissue interlock to occur and be maintained, a balanced body chemistry is necessary. Generally, patients with a history of diabetic disorders, kidney or liver malfunction and other systemic problems of metabolic origin do not provide circumstances in which good tissue growth and maintenance is optimal.

In order to evaluate the systemic health, not only a detailed health history should be obtained, but also a thorough examination of the mouth should be conducted. The color, tone and surface characteristics of the gingival tissues should be noted. If these tissues are in good health and the attachment apparatus is good around the existing teeth, then it is likely that the response to the dental implant will be good. On the other hand, if the periodontal condition is poor or questionable, the response to an implant will be poor and early failure can readily occur.

Wherever possible, laboratory studies should be conducted to verify or determine the body chemistry of the individual. Blood chemistry studies such as the SMA-12 and CBC can help to discover imbalances in the metabolism. Treatable conditions should be corrected prior to the institution of any surgical procedures. Particular attention should be given to cholesterol, glucose and triglyceride levels, as these are indicators of sugar metabolism difficulties. Patients who display either hypoglycemic or hyperglycemic conditions are, on the whole, relatively poor implant candidates.

PREVENTATIVE MAINTENANCE

Proper oral hygiene is imperative around dental implants. Because there is no direct connective tissue attachment into the implant surface, the union of the gingival tissues to the

implant is more precarious than that around a natural tooth. Gingival conditions will more readily result in pocket formation around a dental implant than around a natural tooth. Invagination of the epithelium can often occur around implants where chronic periodontal conditions exist. Prior to the implant surgery, the patient must demonstrate the ability to provide the necessary maintenance. The practice of brushing, flossing and other preventive measures must be carried out enthusiastically. This, in addition to periodic examinations and prophylaxis will ensure long-term life to the implant.

OCCLUSION

Many implant failures can be attributed to improper occlusal design. Forces which are applied to the implant in lateral directions can be highly destructive to the surrounding tissues around the implant. Around a natural tooth the supporting apparatus, namely, the periodontal membrane with its arrangement of connective tissue fibers, distributes occlusal stresses evenly to the bone supporting the tooth. Although there is usually a connective tissue interface between the implant and bone, it does provide a shock-absorbing or stress-distributing quality.

Poor occlusal design can result in concentrated stresses in the bone which can lead to rapid bone resorption. The following rules should be followed with respect to occlusal design:

1. Cusp designs and crown alignment should be made so that stresses are directed along the long axis of the implant. Designs which tend to impart lateral stresses should be avoided or at least minimized.

2. The width of the occlusal table of the implant crown should be minimal. Wherever possible, the occlusal table should be no wider than the width of the implant root. With tooth-shaped implant designs, this may be accomplished prac-

tically, whereas with blade and subperiosteal designs, the table should only be wide enough to provide centric function.

3. Cusp height should be minimized, again, to decrease the lateral stresses that may be applied to the implant. The occlusal table should be relatively flat, providing only centric function.

IMPLANT STABILIZATION (SPLINTING)

The implant must be stabilized immediately after placement and free of any movement. Movement causes formation of connective tissue in the interface between bone and implant. This connective tissue provides a flexible cushion and subsequent mobility. Where there is implant mobility, epithelial invagination and implant failure often occur.

Fixation or splinting may be accomplished by one or more methods:

1. The implant may be placed so the top is near the crest of the bone, allowing the gingival tissues to be sutured over the top of the implant, sealing it from the oral cavity. After suitable healing, the implant may be uncovered and restored.

2. A provisional restoration may be placed on the implant, splinting it to adjacent natural teeth. This may be accomplished by making crown preparations on the adjacent teeth or by bonding the implant to adjacent teeth with an adhesive resin.

3. Screws may be used for fixation, thus anchoring the implant to the bone surface. Although some dentists feel this is not necessary, it has been demonstrated that, where screw fixation is not used in subperiosteal placement, a higher ratio of early failures occurs.

Any one or a combination of these splinting methods is necessary to have implant success. Certainly other fixation methods may be utilized; however, the methods mentioned above appear to be the most effective and safe.

If care is taken to provide optimal patient selection, proper implant design selection, good preventive maintenance, and correct occlusal design, then successful implant procedures can result.

DENTAL IMPLANT MATERIALS

There are several ceramic, metallic and polymeric materials which have adequate biocompatibility, mechanical properties, corrosion resistance and handling/fabrication properties for use as dental implant materials. Commercially available implants are currently fabricated from high purity aluminum oxide, vitreous carbon, surgical cast and wrought cobalt-chromium alloys, or chemically pure titanium. Each of these materials has features which make it suitable for implant design and application.

Aluminum Oxide

Aluminum oxide implants are made from high density, multicrystalline, high purity (99.8 percent) aluminum oxide fabricated by high temperature processes.[3] Aluminum oxide has a high compressive strength, but its brittleness reduces its tensile strength. The white color of aluminum oxide simplifies the esthetic problems of restorative dentistry. Table I compares the tensile strength and modulus of elasticity of aluminum oxide to other biomaterials discussed later. Aluminum oxide has the highest modulus of elasticity (stiffness) of the implant biomaterials and is very hard, like enamel and vitreous carbon. The material may be cut or adjusted using high speed diamond dental instruments.

Aluminum oxide is very inert, resistant to corrosion in the oral and physiological environments, and is, therefore, well tolerated by tissues. Bone forms in very close apposition to aluminum oxide when the implant is immobile.

The commercial forms of aluminum oxide endosseous implants include tooth-root shaped and blade-shaped implants. The implants have deep horizontal grooves into which bone can form to provide long-term stabilization. These

Table I.
Mechanical Properties of Dental Implant Materials

Material	Tensile Strength × 10⁸ dynes/cm²	Modulus of Elasticity × 10¹¹ dynes/cm²
Aluminum oxide[3,4]	17.2-34.5	34.5
Vitreous carbon[4]	17.0-24.0	2.1-2.8
Cast cobalt-chromium[5]	65.5	21.4
Wrought cobalt-chromium[5]	103.4-172.4	22.5
Titanium chemically pure[3,4]	23.4	12.0

deep grooves greatly increase the surface area of contact between the implant and supporting tissues reducing the stress transmitted to bone at the interface with the implant. These implants may be used either as abutments for fixed partial dentures or as single tooth replacements.

Carbon—Vitreous Carbon

Vitreous carbon is a glassy form of high purity carbon (99.9 percent) made by molding or casting a resin into the desired shape and thermally degrading the resin at high temperature under an inert atmosphere and then under vacuum.[4] The properties of vitreous carbon are similar to those of glassy materials. Although the compressive strength of this material is adequately high for use as a dental implant, the flexural and tensile strengths are low due to its brittleness. The vitreous carbon implants are therefore made sufficiently thick to overcome this potential difficulty.[6] Vitreous carbon is a hard biomaterial, but it can be cut and the implant adjusted in shape using high speed, diamond cutting instruments.

The modulus of elasticity of vitreous carbon is quite different from that of the other implant materials and is approximately in the same range as that of bone. Dental implant materials and ceramics are five to fifteen times stiffer than bone and vitreous carbon.

A significant feature of vitreous carbon is its translucency to x-rays. Usually, after the implant site has healed, the outline of the implant can be seen on an x-ray, but it is not possible to determine radiographically how near bone has formed to the implant surface or whether a layer of fibrous tissue exists around the carbon implant. The dentist must rely on mobility and percussion tests for this determination. The stainless steel post in the center of the implant identifies the location and orientation of the implant.

Vitreous carbon is highly resistant to environmental degradation in the mouth and is well tolerated by oral tissues. The material does not provoke inflammatory responses, and bone forms very near to the carbon implant surface as long as the implant is immobile. Bone formation within the circumferential grooves in the implant surface serves to stabilize the implant after healing.

A very low rate of infection occurs around vitreous carbon implant materials, apparently due to the close, tight adaptation of tissues which form around the implant where it protrudes through the gingiva.

Cobalt-Chromium Alloys

Cobalt-chromium alloys have had the longest period of function in humans; some of the early subperiosteal implants have been in function for as long as 20 to 25 years. There are several commercial surgical grade cobalt-chromium alloys for cast and wrought implant devices. Cobalt-chromium alloys are used in cast form for subperiosteal, endosseous blade, screw and other implant designs, and in its wrought form for endodontic pin stabilizer implants. Table II presents the composition ranges of cast and wrought surgical grade cobalt-chromium alloys.[5]

Surgical cobalt-chromium alloys have high corrosion resistance due to the formation of a chromium oxide layer on the surface. The corrosion rate of these implants is sufficiently slow

Table II.

Composition Ranges of Cast and Wrought Surgical Cobalt-Chromium Alloys[4]

Element	Cast Alloy (Weight percent)	Wrought Alloy (Weight percent)
Co	balance	balance
Cr	27-30	19-21
Mo	5-7	—
C	0.35 max	0.05-0.15 max
Mn	1.0 max	2.0 max
Si	1.0 max	1.0 max
Fe	0.75 max	3.0 max
Ni	2.5 max	9-11
W	—	14-16

that significant corrosion has not been observed on some implants which have been in function for over 20 years. Increased concentrations of cobalt and chromium ions have been observed in body tissues of patients wearing cobalt-chromium partial denture clasps[7] for a short term and in dog tissues surrounding endodontic pin implants,[8] but tissues adjacent to a 12-year old subperiosteal implant in a human have not shown high concentrations of these ions.[9] Thus, corrosion products are probably removed to other parts of the body or excreted.

Histologically, one generally sees encapsulation of cobalt-chromium alloy implants with a layer of fibrous tissues isolating the implant from the body. Regions which experience heavy force, such as beneath abutment posts in subperiosteal implants may show bone resorption with thickening of fibrous tissue. Gingival tissues surrounding cobalt-chromium posts occasionally show chronic irritation and require regular hygienic maintenance.

Although cobalt-chromium alloys are not as biocompatible as other implant materials, they have withstood the test of long periods of time in humans. The flexibility of use, the ability to cast a custom implant for a patient, the high values for mechanical properties and an acceptable level of tissue tolerance have made this

alloy the choice for subperiosteal implants. Some dentists use cobalt-chromium for endosseous implants as well.

Titanium (Chemically Pure Titanium)

Commercial titanium blade implants are fabricated by a coining process from chemically pure titanium; titanium cannot be cast in the manner of cobalt-chromium alloys. Thus, like aluminum oxide and vitreous carbon, titanium implants are prefabricated to various sizes and shapes and adjusted to fit the site.

Titanium forms a surface oxide layer extremely rapidly; the rapid formation and constant maintenance of this layer forms an interface with tissues, making titanium a highly biocompatible material. Titanium is well tolerated by oral tissues, and when held immobile, bone forms through the implant vents and over the shoulder.[10] In function, the implant often becomes encapsulated by a fibrous tissue layer.

The titanium blade implant is sufficiently ductile that the post may be bent or rotated to provide proper alignment for restoration. The primary design of titanium implants is the blade-shape with variations in length and height and with single or double abutment posts. There are, however, a wide variety of additional implant shapes and sizes for specific restorative functions.

New Implant Materials

There has long been a desire to create an artificial periodontal ligament around endosseous implants which attaches to the implant material. Growth of fibrous tissues into porous aluminum oxide, cobalt-chromium alloys, poly (methyl methacrylate) and carbon have been studied experimentally, but porosity has led to reduced mechanical properties and infection when exposed to the oral environment. It is possible that these problems may be overcome in the future. The vitreous carbon tooth-shaped implant and the titanium blade implant attempt to simulate the mechanical attachment concept by microscopically texturing the implant surface and by providing short range tissue ingrowth into the implant surface.

Encouraging work is being performed on bioglass materials which form chemical bonds to tissues. These materials may form the surface coating of implants and may achieve an intimate attachment of gingival tissues and periodontal tissues to implants in the future.

IMPLANT DESIGNS

Efforts should be made to distribute the occlusal stresses over as much of the bone surface area as possible. This minimizes concentrated stresses being applied to the supporting bone. Sharp edges on the implant surface can lead to the development of concentrated stresses in the bone and consequent bone resorption.

If considerable alveolar bone remains in the edentulous ridge, both in width and height, then a tooth-shaped endosseous implant should be utilized. If there is adequate height of alveolar bone but the ridge has narrowed through progressive bone resorption, then a blade design should be used. If alveolar bone resorption has decreased both the height and width of the bone so that endosseous implantation would encroach on vital anatomical structures, maxillary sinuses or the mandibular canal, then a subperiosteal implant design should be used.

Subperiosteal Implants

COMPOSITION: The subperiosteal implant (Fig. 1) is a framework, cast from surgical grade cobalt-chromium alloys, which rests precisely on the bone in the mandible or maxilla. (See the section on Cobalt-Chromium Alloys on page 153)

USES: Most subperiosteal implants are placed in edentulous areas which have suffered from extensive bone resorption, and restoration may be accomplished through a fixed partial denture attached to the implant and to natural abutment teeth. Although the use for support in a full mandibular denture has demonstrated the best success of all subperiosteal applications, uses in unilateral application as support for fixed appliances are gradually demonstrating better success than formerly. A more extensive knowledge of occlusal design in conjunction with implant procedures and improved implant design helps to account for these increasingly favorable results.

Fixed prostheses should only be utilized where there are some remaining natural teeth to bear the stresses of occlusal loading. Very little success has occurred with a fixed prosthesis used as a full arch subperiosteal implant. When a patient displays a fully edentulous ridge, the full subperiosteal implant may show good success when it is used as support and retention for a removable complete denture.

DIRECTIONS FOR USE: Placement generally involves two surgical procedures; one in which the gingiva is reflected and impressions taken of the edentulous boney ridge, and the second in which the implant is placed after fabrication.

It is necessary that all alveolar bone resorption has occurred prior to implantation; otherwise, subsequent bone resorption may result in exposure of the implant struts, leading to infection and potential failure.

The surgical procedure involves reflection of the gingival tissues from the edentulous ridges to expose a wide latitude of bone. It is important that the main framework be supported by highly stable basal bone, with minimal support being gained by contact with alveolar bone. The design of the framework should be as simple as possible with adequate strength to prevent distortion under forces of occlusion. There should be a minimal number of struts that cross over

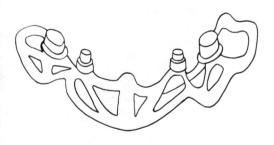

Fig. 1   Framework of the subperiosteal implant

the alveolar ridge to minimize the possibilities of penetration through the mucosal tissues. The extent of the soft tissue flap should be sufficient to allow access for an impression of the edentulous ridge.

After the tissues have been fully elevated, an impression is made of the bone using an elastic rubber or silicone impression material with a custom acrylic tray to carry the impression material to place. Thiosulfide rubbers seem to provide the best results. These materials allow the dentist some flexibility with regard to setting times and also have a rather long term semielastic state during which the impression material can be manipulated into the deep peripheral areas where the basal bone exists. Upon completion of the impression, the gingival tissues are returned over the bone and sutured.

A framework cast of cobalt-chromium alloy is fabricated to fit the stone model replica of the edentulous ridge. The framework should be designed with from one to several screw holes where the greatest amount of alveolar bone exists. Screws, cast of the same cobalt-chromium alloy as the implant framework, 5 to 7 mm in length, are used to gain the initial fixation of the implant framework to the supporting bone.

On a second appointment, the patient returns to have the framework installed. The interval between the impression surgery and the placement surgery may range from 24 hours to several weeks. Some implant dentists feel that by fabricating and placing the implant within 24 hours, the patient is required to go through only one recuperative period. Maximum postoperative swelling and pain seem to occur between 36 and 72 hours after the surgery for impression. Placement of the implant within the first 24 hours avoids the discomfort of a second period of swelling and pain.

On the second appointment, the implant is seated over the bone and at least one screw should be used to help stabilize the framework while the periosteal fibers are reattaching to the bone over the implant framework. It usually takes 2 to 6 months for these fibers to regenerate a firm attachment to the bone. If the framework is lifted from the bone in any way during this initial healing period, connective tissue will invade the area between the bone and framework, possibly leading to a slow, progressive breakdown, which may not be reversible. Usually nothing is done to the implant for the first 6 to 12 weeks after placement and it is allowed to remain in a static condition. This period of time is allowed to pass before any occlusal stresses are applied to the implant.

Again, the occlusal stresses should be directed along the long axis of the implant post, so stresses are centralized. Occlusion should be of a centric nature, with a minimizing of lateral stresses. This can be best accomplished by designing the implant crown with a narrow occlusal table and a relatively flat occlusal surface.

LIMITATIONS OF USE: The full subperiosteal implant is best used in the mandibular arch, with less success in the maxillary arch. The softer maxillary bone tends to resorb more readily when subjected to the forces of occlusion applied to the implant. The results in failure can be rather disasterous in that, if bone is lost and the implant has to be removed, there may not be enough remaining bone to support a complete maxillary denture. It is also seldom that patients cannot function with a complete maxillary denture. A high rate of success is demonstrated where a conventional maxillary removable denture opposes a mandibular implant denture.

The full subperiosteal framework may fail when opposing natural teeth. The implant attachment mechanism is not strong enough to act against the stresses of muscle function which can be applied via the firmly fixed natural teeth in the opposing arch. Appliances attached or supported by a full subperiosteal implant should be of a removable nature and not fixed. Where the implant is used to stabilize a removable appliance, long term success has usually resulted in a high percentage of the cases.

Endodontic Implants

COMPOSITION: These implants are fabricated from wrought surgical cobalt-chromium alloys and titanium.

USES: The endodontic stabilizer implant (Fig. 2) is utilized to stabilize excessively mobile teeth.[11] The implant is either a smooth-sided or threaded pin which is placed through the pulpal canal and through the alveolar bone to be anchored into the cortical bone at the inferior border of the mandible or floor of the nasal cavity. The implant improves the crown/root ratio of the tooth and thereby provides immobilization.

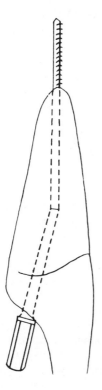

Fig. 2   Endodontic stabilizer implant

The endodontic implant has an advantage over other dental implants in that it does not communicate with the oral environment in healthy situations. Complications can occur if the implant is placed in a tooth having a periodontal defect communicating with the apex of the tooth. Cement is used to bond the implant into the tooth and, if expressed beyond the apex of the tooth, the cement can cause irritation. The use of the endodontic stabilizer is contraindicated where important anatomical structures exist near the apex of the tooth, e.g., the mandibular canal.

Endosseous Implants

Tooth-shaped implants

COMPOSITION: Several tooth-shaped implants are in use. Hodosh, Shklar and Povar[12] have conducted a lengthy series of investigations of tooth root replica implants fabricated from a mixture of methyl methacrylate, anorganic bone and a foaming agent (to add porosity to the implant). Although they have obtained excellent results in experimental usage, the material is not commercially available, and the methyl methacrylate presents potential problems unless processed properly.

A series of vitreous carbon tooth-shaped implants of varying sizes is available with a medical grade stainless steel sleeve and post and core to facilitate restoration. (Fig. 3) These implants may be placed below the gingiva for an extended healing period, during which bone forms within the grooves of the surface of the implant locking it into place. It is subsequently exposed for restoration. The implant may also be placed extending through the gingiva for immediate restoration. The implant is contoured by the dentist to fit the implant socket prior to placement, and great flexibility in implant size and shape can be achieved.

Tooth-shaped implants are also fabricated from high purity aluminum oxide.[13] The very high strength of this alumina enables the formation of implants with high surface area contact through the placement of deep grooves in the implant surface. Aluminum oxide also has the

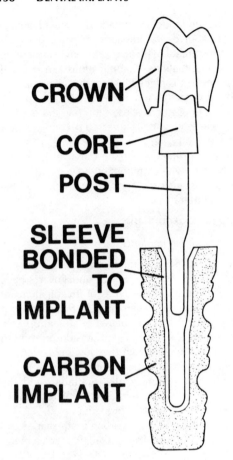

CROWN

CORE

POST

SLEEVE
BONDED
TO
IMPLANT

CARBON
IMPLANT

Fig. 3 Tooth-root shaped implant

unique advantage among implant materials of being creamy white in color and slightly translucent, enabling very esthetic anterior implant restorations which will not lose their esthetic quality if gingival recession occurs. The aluminum oxide implant can also be adjusted using a diamond bur at high speed rotation to place a finish line on the implant shoulder.

USES: The goal of tooth-shaped implants is to fit the natural tooth socket after extraction and to attempt to distribute stresses in a manner similar

to natural teeth. Tooth-shaped implants have the advantage that they can be placed into existing sockets, but they are generally too broad for placement in edentulous ridges which have been severely resorbed.

These implants achieve retention and stabilization through bone formation within grooves in the implant surface or channels cut through the implant apex.

Vitreous carbon endosseous implants are used as distal and anterior abutments for fixed partial dentures, for replacement of single teeth without permanent attachment to adjacent teeth and, in some cases, to support removable dentures. The use of vitreous carbon implants to reduce alveolar ridge resorption after tooth extraction is also being studied experimentally.

DIRECTIONS FOR USE: These implant designs require that a tooth-shaped socket be cut into the alveolar bone. This may be accomplished either in fresh extraction sites or in areas where long term healing has taken place provided enough bone remains. The socket should be made so that the implant fits as precisely as possible. Sized drills or burs and sized gauges (vitreous carbon) aid in providing this precision fit. The dentist can further modify the shape of the implant to allow it to closely fit the contoured socket. The final stabilization of the implant is dependent upon having bone grow close to the implant surface. If large spaces exist initially between bone and implant, these spaces may fill with a wide thickness of connective tissue. This can cause poor stability and possible failure of the implant.

During bone socket contouring, great care should be taken to avoid traumatizing the bone; this may lead to considerable postoperative bone resorption. Slow speed rotary instruments and fairly large diameter burs or drills are necessary to contour the socket and reduce heat production when cutting the bone. Along with this, a sterile water or saline wash should be used to minimize overheating the bone during cutting. The bone chips, removed during socket formation, may be salvaged and used to help fill the interface between the bone and implant.

There should be enough alveolar bone height so the implant root is well secured in the bone; support should be provided in at least a 1:1 crown to root ratio. Positive implant root support is necessary to minimize the effect of any lateral occlusal stresses. Implant positioning should be such that occlusal stresses will be directed along the long axis of the implant.

One of two surgical techniques may be utilized for tooth-shaped implants. The implant may be placed so it protrudes through the gingiva. With this procedure the implant must be splinted in some manner, attaching it to adjacent natural teeth. A second technique allows the implant dentist to place the top of the implant so it is near the crest of the alveolar ridge. After the implant is seated in the boney socket, the gingival tissues are returned back over the top of the implant, providing the necessary immobilization during healing.

Positive immobilization is essential to success with tooth-shaped implants. Bone ingrowth may require 6 to 12 months. Periodic x-rays allow the dentist to monitor this bone growth.

After adequate healing, the implant may be exposed by removing the gingival tissues that cover it, or the retaining splint may be removed and then conventional impression and restorative procedures may be instituted to complete the restoration. The implant may be restored with gold alloys, or porcelain in esthetic areas.

Blade Shaped Implants

Blade implants (Fig. 4) have been designed by Linkow, Chercheve and Jones,[14] Cranin, Dennison and Schnitman,[2] Driskell and Heller[13] and others. The blade implant can be placed on narrow alveolar ridges. A series of sizes and shapes are available for anatomical restrictions of the site. Final stabilization of the implant is achieved through mechanical interlocking with bone via the long lateral sides of the implant and bone growth through apical vents and over the implant shoulder. Some dental investigators believe that the fibrous encapsulation which develops around the implant serves as an artificial periodontal ligament;[15] others believe it is the result of mechanical irritation to the surrounding bone. The post(s) which extend through the gingiva are designed to be hygienic and to minimize infection.

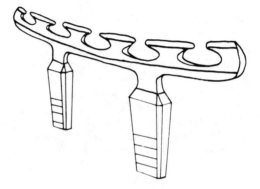

Fig. 4   Blade-shaped implant

COMPOSITION: The blade implants designed by Linkow[14] are manufactured from chemically pure titanium and utilize a series of ridges on the surface plus microscopic surface texturing to increase the surface area and interlocking with tissues. An aluminum oxide blade implant, designed by Driskell and Heller[13] is available and a variety of blade implants are fabricated from surgical cobalt-chromium alloys. A pyrolytic carbon blade implant is in experimental use.

USES: Blade implants have been utilized for a wide variety of applications, centering on providing abutments for fixed applications. The use of blade implants as stabilization for removable appliances has not shown good long term results.

Blade-shaped implants may be partially useful where adequate alveolar bone height exists and bur ridge width has narrowed due to progressive resorption.

DIRECTIONS FOR USE: In the latter procedure, a

narrow slot is prepared in the remaining alveolar bone, and the implant is fitted so that the base of the head portion of the implant is at the crest of the alveolar ridge and the shoulder of the substructure is well below the crest. Either the superstructure or substructure of the implant may be modified by grinding or bending to allow the implant framework to skirt around important anatomical structures or to gain proper direction to occlusal forces applied to the body of the implant.

Gingival tissues should be reapproximated around the implant head so that attached gingiva completely surrounds the head where it emerges into the oral cavity. Mucosal tissues cannot provide the necessary type of gingival seal. The gingival tissues must remain firmly adapted to the head of the implant in order to prevent the penetration of bacteria and oral fluids along the body of the implant.

Once placed, the blade implant should be splinted to adjacent natural teeth, usually by means of a provisional restoration. An acrylic temporary restoration usually functions best in this capacity. Optimum success is gained when final restorative procedures are instituted soon after the gingival tissues have healed from the implant surgery. This provides a more positive means of stabilization and insures the development of a positive bone support.

Because of the narrow dimension of the implant substructure, the following rules help to provide the most effective results:

1. Minimize lateral stresses. Keep occlusal forces directed along the long axis of the implant.
2. Keep the occlusal table of the implant crown narrow (4 to 5 mm maximum width).
3. Wherever possible, use a two-post implant. This, when attached to a natural tooth (teeth) will help to prevent any rotary forces from developing in the implant substructure as lateral forces are applied to the implant crown.
4. Try to use as many natural tooth abutments as possible to help bear the load of the occlusal stresses.

Once normal healing of the gingival tissues has taken place, conventional restorative procedures may be conducted. Crowns and fixed appliances may be fabricated of acrylic, gold or porcelain.

Screw-shaped Implants

COMPOSITION: Various attempts have been made over the years to produce screw-shaped implants of many designs and materials.[16] Today, implants of this design are fabricated of surgical cobalt-chromium alloys, titanium, or aluminum oxide (Fig. 5).

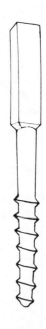

Fig. 5 Screw-shaped implant

USES: Results with this type of implant are best when it is used as an abutment for a fixed bridge either at the end of the span, or as an abutment somewhere in the center of a long span of a fixed prosthesis. The symmetrical round shape of the implant precludes its use as a single tooth replacement, because the implants have a tendency to rotate. Any movement, either in a lateral or rotary direction, tends to promote the formation of thickened fibrous tissue around the implant, leading to increased mobility and possible subsequent failure.

Another problem exists with this design. The normally sharp threads tend to produce areas of stress concentration in the bone around the threads. Because of the high elastic moduli of the implant materials, these stresses may be magnified as the occlusal stress is transmitted into the bone supporting the implant. Problems with screw-shaped implants include: excessive bone resorption and encapsulation with fibrous tissues, excessive mobility as bone resorption develops, mucosal invagination along the screw shaft, and infection.

This implant design, therefore, has some limited application. Crowns attached to this type of implant must be carefully designed to take into consideration the inherent stress factors. Unfortunately. bone resorption observed with this type of implant design can be rather severe, sometimes ranging 2 to 4 mm from the implant surface.

Applications of this type of implant should, therefore, be limited to those situations where the implant can be well stabilized and where occlusal forces can be centralized over the long axis of the implant.

DIRECTIONS FOR USE: The screw-shaped implant design offers a simple surgical technique with minimal surgical trauma since a sized hole is drilled into the alveolar bone. Then, threads are produced in the boney socket, either with a tap or with self-tapping threads on the implant itself.

The threads, produced in the boney socket, allow the implant to have a comparatively precise fit to the bone. They also allow the implant to be self-immobilized basically from the time of placement.

Pin-Shaped Implants

COMPOSITION: The Scialom tripodal pin implant[17] utilizes three pins which are placed at divergent angles, avoiding anatomical landmarks, and which are joined together at the ridge crest to form an abutment (Fig. 6). Substantial retention is achieved in this manner. The Scialom tripodal pin implant is fabricated from tantalum.

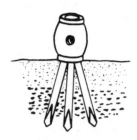

Fig. 6   Tripodal pin implant

USES: These pins may be utilized for areas where there is minimal bone over critical anatomical structures such as the maxillary sinuses and mandibular canal, the pins being placed into the bone so as to skirt around important structures. The pins may be used as an abutment to a fixed bridge, and, in limited and carefully selected situations, as a single tooth replacement. They also may be used as support in the center of an existing fixed prosthesis, where some of the natural tooth support has been lost. In this latter situation, the pins are placed into the bone through a hole made through one of the pontic areas of the fixed bridge. The pins are then placed into the bone and bonded to the bridge with an autopolymerizing resin.

DIRECTIONS FOR USE: The surgical technique for direct placement into the bone involves drilling three holes, 1.2 mm in diameter, in diverging angles from each other to form a tripodal convergence where the holes emerge from the crestal alveolar bone. Once the pins are placed into the drilled holes, they will converge somewhere slightly above the crest of the bone. At this point the pins are bent parallel to each other and perpendicular to the crest of the supporting bone. These pins are then bonded together with an autopolymerizing resin, forming the tripodal support for fixed or removable appliances.

LIMITATIONS OF USE: The main problem with this type of implant is that it is difficult to produce a maintainable, hygienically sound area where the pins are bonded together at the crest of the gingiva. Here one may see resorption and cupping, or saucerization, of the crestal bone which leads to a nonhygienic situation. This then becomes the focus of recurring periodontal problems.

Intramucosal Inserts

Occasionally the dentist has a patient in whom a conventional denture is difficult to tolerate due to physical or psychological problems or poor anatomical shape of the edentulous ridge. One potential solution is to use the small mushroom-shaped fasteners which are attached to the tissue bearing surface of the denture. Epithelialized holes in the soft tissues of the edentulous ridge accept these inserts and help retain the denture more firmly.

This technique involves only the soft tissues over the boney ridges, and is simple and effective. An autopolymerizing resin is used to attach 12 to 14 or more inserts into the denture surface in areas where the opposing soft tissue thickness is two or more millimeters thick. Once the inserts are attached into the denture, they are coated with indelible pencil, and the denture is seated firmly in the patient's mouth. This records the position of the opposing fasteners onto the soft tissues.

The gingival tissues in these areas are then anesthetized, and small holes are cut or drilled into the gingiva to provide receptor sites. The denture is seated and then temporarily sutured in place to maintain it firmly positioned.

The denture is kept in place for approximately 10 days. During this time the receptor holes epithelialize around the inserts and their undercuts. After 10 days the denture is removed and daily maintenance is instituted. The denture snaps in place and is retained by the elastic action of the soft tissues as they lock into the undercuts in the inserts.

Because this device involves only the soft tissues, there is little or none of the inherent problems that are encountered with other types of implantation procedures.

Other Endosseous Implant Designs

There have been many other endosseous implant designs which have been used at different times in the past. Many of the desirable features of these implants have been incorporated into the implant designs in current use, and some previous implant design concepts are being regenerated as improved biomaterials become available.

The transosseous implant technique has been revived recently. This implant uses rods or threaded pins which penetrate through the anterior portion of the mandible from the inferior border through to the alveolar crest. Recent work has shown this implant design to be acceptable when performed with new available materials.

THE FUTURE OF DENTAL IMPLANTS

With the use of new materials and techniques, dental implant procedures are gradually becoming more successful. A better understanding of the physiological responses to the implant and better means for patient selection have promoted the development of more refined procedures that allow dental implantation to become more safe and effective.

Much research has been directed toward this area of restorative dentistry. The fruits of this research will soon be available to the profession and passed on to the patient as highly effective procedures to reconstruct the oral health of the patient.

Do:

1. Take a health history that includes the patient's history plus the family history.
2. Include in the health history questions to gain information of a physical, metabolic and psychological nature.
3. Review the health history with the patient.
4. Ask specific questions to determine if the patient has systemic problems of a metabolic nature.
5. Inspect the condition of the gingival tissues with respect to tone, color and surface characteristics.
6. Note the condition of the attachment around the teeth.
7. Note occlusal disharmonies or other abnormal conditions.
8. Evaluate oral hygiene.
9. Examine edentulous or implant site, noting size of the edentulous ridge.
10. Determine the thickness of the soft tissues covering the edentulous ridge.
11. Take periapical and panoramic diagnostic radiographs.
12. Whenever possible, perform blood laboratory studies.
13. Mount the models on an articulator and wherever possible in complex cases, do pantograph tracings to determine jaw movements.
14. Select healthy patients for implant procedures. When in doubt, use conventional restorative techniques.
15. Select patients who have a healthy periodontal condition.
16. Evaluate occlusal makeup of the patient.
17. Select the proper implant design to fit into the edentulous ridge.
18. Observe ridge size—width and height.
19. Observe the alignment of the teeth adjacent to the implant site.
20. Determine the implant size to be used prior to the surgery.
21. Determine if the implant must be modified to skirt around existing anatomical structures.
22. Select an implant size that will give the best crown:root ratio.
23. Use antibiotics to control and minimize the possibility of infection.
24. Use sterile techniques.
25. Cool bone with sterile water wash while cutting.
26. Design a surgical flap to expose the implant site adequately.
27. Use anesthetics with vasoconstrictors to control bleeding.
28. Exercise care in handling soft tissues.
29. Design the surgical flap so that when repositioned, there will be attached gingiva completely around the implant post.
30. Line up the implant to receive occlusal forces through the center of the long axis of the implant.
31. Carefully line up the direction of the bur as the socket is prepared to avoid perforation through the wall of supporting bone.
32. Always immobilize the implant in some manner at the time of the surgery.
33. Select a splinting technique that will allow the patient to maintain oral hygiene.
34. Fix the splint rigidly in place.
35. Place the final restoration as soon after the surgery as possible when using the implant as an abutment for a fixed partial denture.
36. Avoid application of dislodging forces to the implant within the first several months after placement.

37. Avoid lateral stresses on the implant.
38. Avoid heavy occlusion on the implant initially.
39. Instruct the patient in good oral hygiene procedures.
40. Use conventional impression procedures.
41. Allow some form of splinting to remain in place while the bone is remodeling around the implant, either a temporary or a permanent fixation.
42. Establish crown contours that will allow the patient to maintain oral hygiene.
43. Correct occlusal disharmonies before final restorative techniques are instituted.
44. Direct occlusal forces along the long axis of the implant.
45. Use a narrow, flat occlusal table on the implant crown.
46. Incorporate cuspid lift or protection in the occlusion wherever possible.
47. Use implants with double posts wherever possible with blade and subperiosteal implants.
48. Always try to use multiple natural tooth abutments as support against occlusal stresses.
49. Always obtain informed consent.
50. Inform the patient of all of the potential problems connected with the implant procedure.
51. Justify the selection of an implant procedure over conventional restorative techniques to the patient.
52. Inform the patient of the potential chance of failure due to the problems in predicting the future health of the patient.
53. Record all information related to the implant procedure.

Don't:

1. Assume the patient will relate or remember all of the important facts related to his health history.
2. Accept that the ridge size on the study model indicates the actual bone size. Determine the soft tissue thickness.
3. Perform implants on patients with uncontrolled systemic disorders.
4. Do implants on patients with existing periodontal conditions.
5. Do implants on patients with known diabetic conditions. Be suspect of patients where there is a family history of diabetes.
6. Do implant procedures on patients with uncorrectable occlusal problems, especially heavy bruxism.
7. Do implant procedures if contraindicated by any physical or psychological problems.
8. Try to make one implant type or design conform to all of the restorative situations.
9. Place the implant until all occlusal problems and other significant dental problems have been corrected.
10. Select surgical sites where four good walls of bone do not exist.
11. Contaminate the surgical site.
12. Overheat the bone during the cutting procedure.
13. Use high speed cutting instruments.
14. Attempt to bend the implant once it is seated in the bone.
15. Leave the implant unsplinted.
16. Ever place a single unit free standing implant where centric occlusion is nonexistent.
17. Ever use a full subperiosteal implant opposing natural tooth occlusion.
18. Use endosseous implants to support and stabilize full denture prostheses.

Available Products

Denserts, Denserts

Dentatus Screw Posts, Charles B. Schwed Co., Inc.

Jermym Paralaid, Prolastic Co., Inc.

Plastic Endodontic Posts, APM-Sterngold Div. of Sterndent Corp.

Schenker Stepped Pivot, APM-Sterngold Div. of Sterndent Corp.

Stutz Pivot with Shell, APM-Sterngold Div. of Sterndent Corp.

Literature References

1. Goldbert, N. I., and Gershkoff, A. Implant dentures. Philadelphia, J. B. Lippincott, 1957.

2. Cranin, A. N.; Dennison, T. A.; and Schnitman, P. The present status of endosteal oral implants. J. Bio. Med., Mat. Res. Symposium No. 5, (part 2), p. 385, 1974.

3. Niesz, D. E., and Tennery, V. J. Ceramics for prosthetic application—orthopedic, dental and cardiovascular. MCIC Report 74-21, Columbus, Ohio, Battelle Columbus Laboratories, 1974.

4. Von Fraunhoffer, J.A.; L'Estrange, P. R.; and Mack, A. O. Materials science in dental implantation and a promising new material: vitreous carbon. Bio. Med. Eng. p. 114, 1971.

5. Weisman, S. The skeletal structure of metal implants. Oral Implant. 1:69, 1970.

6. Grenoble, D. E., and Voss, R. Design of the vitreous carbon tooth root replacement system. JADA, to be published.

7. Soremark, R., et al. Penetration of metallic ions from restorations into teeth. J. Prosthet. Dent. 20:431, 1968.

8. Seltzer, S., et al. Vitallium endodontic implants: A scanning electron microscope, electron microscope, electron microprobe and histological study. Oral Surg. 35:828, 1973.

9. Bodine, R. L.; Melrose, R. J.; and Grenoble, D. E. Long term implant denture histology and comparison with previous reports. J. Prosthet. Dent. 35:665, 1976.

10. Armitage, J. E., et al. An evaluation of early bone changes after the insertion of metal endosseous implants in the jaws of rhesus monkeys. Oral Surg., Oral Med., Oral Path. 32:558, 1971.

11. Frank, A. L. The endodontic endosseous implant. in Cranin, A. N. (ed.) Oral implantology. Springfield, C. C. Thomas, p. 215, 1970.

12. Hodosh, M.; Shklar, G.; and Povar, M. Current status of the polymer tooth implant concept. Dent. Clin. N. Am. 14:103, 1970.

13. Driskell, T. D., and Heller, A. L. Clinical use of aluminum oxide endosseous implants. Oral Implant. 7:53, 1977.

14. Linkow, L. I.; Chercheve, R.; and Jones, M. (eds.) Theories and techniques of oral implantology. St. Louis, C. V. Mosby, Vols. I and II, 1970.

15. James, R. A. A histopathological study of the nature of the epithelium surrounding implant posts II. Oral Implant. 3:139, 1973.

16. Sandhaus, S. Nouveau aspects de l'implantologie, l'implant. Suisse, C. B. C., 1969.

17. Scialom, J. Tripodal pin implants. in Cranin, A. N. (ed.) Oral Implantology. Springfield, C. C. Thomas, p. 143, 1970.

ENDODONTIC MATERIALS

Several types of materials are used to fill and seal the root canal system of a tooth once it has been cleansed of tissue and/or debris and shaped to receive the root canal filling. The relationship between the cleansing and shaping, or root canal preparation, procedures is an intimate one, influencing the selection of root canal filling material as well as the technique of application (Table I).

The most widely accepted root canal filling materials today can be broadly classified as either root canal filling points (core materials), root canal sealer cements, or root canal filling pastes. Neither root canal filling points nor root canal sealer cements are advocated for independent use to seal a root canal system, due to recognized problems of material adaptation or dimensional stability. When root canal filling pastes are used as the sole material for sealing a root canal, they require special instrumentation for proper placement in the tooth.[1,2]

ROOT CANAL FILLING POINTS

Root canal filling points are usually cemented into the prepared root canal space with root canal sealer cements. These points are manufactured of silver or gutta percha, and can be added to insure complete lateral and vertical seal of the root canal system.

Silver

COMPOSITION AND PROPERTIES: As used in endodontic practice, silver is manufactured into tapering points or cones designed to correspond to root canal instrument size and taper and hence intraradicular tooth preparation.[3] The surface texture and physical shape of silver points vary considerably among manufacturers. The preciseness of shape affects the accuracy of fit while the surface texture affects both cement adherence and corrosion potential. The chemical composition of commercially available brands was found to be similar and potentiostatic investigation showed no significant differences in corrosion potential.[4]

The corrosion behavior of silver points has been observed in clinical cases, investigated by SEM techniques, and examined by potentiostatic methods. The corrosion films formed were non-continuous, non-passivating, and allowed corrosion to continue at high current densities. Root canal sealer cements protect the silver

Table I.

Selection of Root Canal Filling Material for Core and Sealer Techniques

Core Material	Silver Point	Gutta Percha Cone
1. Type of root canal preparation best seated	Resistance form not essential. Retention form well defined with precise apical collar. Little flare to convenience form.	Resistance form essential. Retention form rudimentary with minimal apical collar. Much flare to convenience form to allow for apical compaction.
2. Types of root canals most suited	Uncomplicated mature roots. Narrow, with straight or gradual curves. Complicated mature roots with curved, dilacerated, or bifurcated apical canals. Mature roots with calcified canals and loss of apical constriction.	Uncomplicated mature roots of most sizes with straight or gradual curves. Complicated mature roots with auxiliary, lateral, or accessory canals. Immature roots with flaring apical foramen.
3. Optimal size of instrument finishing apical collar.*	20–60	40–100
4. Primary advantages or disadvantages.	Ease of manipulation and control of material. Requires precise preparation and fit.	Adaptability to irregularities in preparation when used with compaction techniques. Not as readily controllable during manipulation.

*For apical collars prepared of necessity by instruments smaller than 20 or larger than 100 paste filling techniques without cores should be considered.

points which are embedded in apical tissues from corrosion until the properties of the sealer cement are altered by biologic activity. Eugenol, a common ingredient of root canal sealer cements, is noncorrosive to silver points. Corrosion of a silver point can be limited by sealing the point entirely within the root canal and insuring that it is protected by sealer cement from interaction with apical tissues or fluids.[5]

USES: One of the reasons for the selection of silver in deference to other metals as a root canal filler aside from its availability and physical properties, is undoubtedly its bacteriocidal effect, referred to as its "oligodynamic" property.[4]

DIRECTIONS FOR USE: The single silver cone cemented into place with a root canal sealer cement enjoys limited popularity today and has undergone several modifications. The central core of silver is not infrequently surrounded by laterally compacted gutta percha points in the most common modification, although laterally placed silver points have been used in one technique variant. A second major technique modification, when using silver points, involves sectioning the point in such a way that in the completed root canal filling it will obturate the apical one-third of the root only, the middle and cervical thirds of the root being filled with gutta percha or utilized for gold cores or dowels in conjunction with coronal restorations. Usually this sectioning is accomplished by "notching" the point at the level where segmentation is to occur, strain hardening the circumferentially weakened area after cementation of the point in the root apex, and subsequently removing the occlusal or incisal portion after fracture although there are other methods.[6]

SILVER ROOT CANAL FILLING POINTS

Do:

1. Store endodontic silver points in sealed containers or vials.
2. Use only corrosion-free endodontic silver points for root canal obturation.
3. Place endodontic silver points into dry root canals only when seating for trial measure.
4. Coat the endodontic silver point thoroughly with root canal sealer when cementing to place within the tooth.
5. Use standardized endodontic silver points in root canals prepared with appropriate apical collars by means of standardized instruments.

Gutta Percha

COMPOSITION AND PROPERTIES: At ordinary temperatures, gutta percha is 60 percent crystalline, the remainder being amorphous in nature. It exhibits a property common to polymers: viscoelasticity, that is, elastic properties and the properties of a viscous liquid simultaneously. Routine, rapid cooling of an amorphous melt of gutta percha results in crystallization of the "beta" form of transpolyisoprene which occurs as the predominant form in most commercially available gutta percha. There is evidence that the slow, gradual transformation of commercially available gutta percha from the "beta" form to the more brittle naturally occurring "alpha" form accounts for the shelf life and deterioration of the material as used in dentistry.[7] Since information concerning the nature and sources of the base materials or procedures used in processing dental gutta percha are proprietory secrets, most investigations of the complex composite as used in dentistry are neither uniform nor comparable. It is however reasonable to assume that gutta percha root canal filling points are composed of approximately 20 percent gutta percha, 66 percent zinc oxide filler, 11 percent heavy metal radiopacifier, and 3 percent plasticizer.[8] The ratio of the organic components (gutta percha and waxes or resins) to the inorganic components (zinc oxide and heavy metal sulfates) in commercially available endodontic points appears to be a fairly constant one despite variations in the organic or inorganic components. The appearance of these points under SEM examination tends to collaborate the chemical analysis in that "jelly bean" shaped particles of inorganic material are interspersed between amorphous masses of organic resin.

The mechanical properties ascertained by the deformation of gutta percha points in tension correspond to those of a typical viscoelastic, partially crystalline material.[9] Compressibility values reported for gutta percha in triaxial testing proved to be less than that of water, which is, for all practical purposes, noncompressible. Below these levels of pressure, there occurred the compaction of the material due to consolidation and the collapse of internal voids which could have been predicted from SEM examinations. Contrary to empirical claims, no molecular "spring back" of the material can be expected to assist the clinician in sealing the dentin-gutta percha interface by the compaction techniques advocated for gutta percha root canal fillings. Several other physical properties of gutta percha have been reported.[10] Penetration of gutta percha by a modified Gilmore needle shows a continuous distortion of the material under a constant pressure expressed over a period of time. There is an increase in resistance to penetration, as well as an increase in hardness and/or stiffness with decreases in temperature at a fairly uniform rate. Gutta percha undergoes linear expansion with increases in temperature. Since gutta percha remains solid at temperatures higher than body temperature by 10°C or more, alterations of temperature within the root canal by insertion of heated instruments during root canal filling are most likely insignificant in clinical practice.

Alterations of dental gutta percha by the use of chemical solvents has had a long history in endodontics, and there can be little doubt as to the effectiveness of root canal filling techniques using solvents in duplicating the intricate internal anatomy of root canal systems.[11] The lack of dimensional stability of this form of root canal filling material once the solvent is lost and the material solidifies is also well known.[12] The physical properties of gutta percha required for filling a root canal are contrary to those required for the compaction of the material into the root canal filling point or a paste made with chloroform or eucalyptol. The stiffer the filling point, the less compactible it will be. The more fluid the paste, the higher the potential for dimensional changes and shrinkage it will have. As the chemically plasticized gutta percha solidifies, a surface film sets first followed by gradual internal setting with porosity. It was in response to these problems that the root canal sealer cements were developed in the late 1920's.

USES: As a pure substance, gutta percha was at first found to be useless in dentistry, but the discovery that its innate hardness and other physical properties could be altered by the addition of zinc oxide, zinc sulfate, alumina, whiting, precipitated chalk, lime, or silex in various combinations increased its potential as a restorative material.[13] Attempts to use the polymer with various inert fillers as a permanent restorative material proved futile by the middle of the 19th century, but its use in temporary restorations continued unabated for over a hundred years.

GUTTA PERCHA ROOT CANAL FILLING POINTS

Do:

1. Store gutta percha endodontic cones in closed packages in cool or preferably refrigerated storage.
2. Recrystallize brittle gutta percha endodontic cones by immersion in hot tap water until flexibility returns prior to use.
3. Disinfect gutta percha endodontic cones by immersion in alcohol.
4. Remove excess gutta percha from a root canal filling by application of hot instruments as soon as feasible following root canal obturation.
5. Use standardized gutta percha cones with techniques employing either vertical or lateral condensation and a suitable root canal sealer in a properly flared root canal preparation.

Don't

1. Expose gutta percha endodontic cones to air, heat or room temperature for extended periods of time.
2. Use endodontic gutta percha cones that have become brittle due to progressive recrystallization.
3. Attempt to sterilize gutta percha endodontic cones by heat sterilization, autoclaving, or immersion in topical disinfectants containing organic solvents.
4. Remove excess gutta percha from root canal fillings following root canal obturation by means of burs or solvents alone.
5. Use tapered gutta percha cones without sealer, or without condensation, or in a root canal preparation not flared sufficiently to permit condensation in the apical portion of the root.

At the present time, gutta percha is a widely used root canal filling material. It can be used in the form of a filling cone cemented into the root canal in the manner described for a silver cone or it can be used as a cemented master cone surrounded by laterally condensed accessory cones. It also can be fitted to the canal, sectioned, and condensed apically as a series of segments in conjunction with heated pluggers, a root canal sealer, or any one of several solvents.

The injection of molten gutta percha as a means of root canal filling has recently been reported; however, the dimensional changes upon cooling to body temperature appear to indicate contraction of the material with this procedure.

ROOT CANAL SEALER CEMENTS

COMPOSITION: Whether the root canal filling point is made of silver or gutta percha, under the majority of clinical circumstances, it will be used with a root canal sealer cement. Several types of root canal sealer cements have been formulated; most are available. The most common type of root canal sealer cement in current usage is based upon zinc oxide-eugenol. These include sealer cements such as those formulated by Rickert (Kerr), Grossman (Procosol), and Wachs (Pulpdent). The Rickert formula (1931) has a relatively rapid setting time, and as a consequence presents some problems in clinical practice.[14] The original Grossman formula (1936) was developed in order to overcome this feature. The two products do not differ in essential composition. In the Rickert formula the powder consists of zinc oxide, silver (precipitated molecular), oleoresins, and dithymol iodide, and the liquid contains oil of cloves and Canada balsam. The Grossman formula powder contains zinc oxide, silver (precipitated molecular), hydrogenated resin, and magnesium oxide, and the liquid contains eugenol and Canada balsam. The percentage of each ingredient varies somewhat between the formulations. A criticism of both the Rickert and original Grossman formulas lies in their use of precipitated silver as an agent for radiopacity. Such an ingredient tends to stain dentin and thereby compromises the esthetics of an endodontically treated tooth. Grossman revised his sealer cement formula in 1958 to counter this second criticism by using bismuth subcarbonate and barium sulfate as the radiopaque ingredients.[15] The formulation has been revised more recently by the addition of sodium borate to the powder component and the elimination of all ingredients save eugenol from the liquid component. This is essentially how the Grossman non-staining root canal cement is marketed today whereas the Rickert root canal sealer remains largely unaltered since its introduction nearly fifty years ago. This family of sealer cements enjoys the most widespread popularity among the zinc oxide type cements today.

Wachs paste, a similar zinc oxide-eugenol formulation, was originally compounded in 1925 but did not receive widespread attention until publication of its use and reintroduction of the material occurred circa 1955. In addition to zinc oxide and oil of cloves, it contains calcium phosphate tribasic, bismuth subnitrate and subiodide, and magnesium oxide in the powder and Canada balsam, eucalyptol and beechwood creosote in the liquid. The addition of eucalyptol and beechwood creosote (2 percent each) to the liquid accounts for its particular effectiveness when used with gutta percha or in infected cases. It is now marketed under several commercial labels with minor formulation changes.

Tubliseal (1961) was introduced by the Kerr Manufacturing Company as an alternative to the Rickert formula. It is a two-tube paste system, as contrasted to the powder-liquid systems of the other zinc oxide sealer cements. The exact formulation remains a trade secret, but from available sources in the literature, the base appears to contain zinc oxide, oleo resins, bismuth trioxide, thymoliodide, oils and waxes, and the catalyst contains eugenol, polymerized resin, and annidalin.

Free eugenol remains in freshly mixed zinc oxide-eugenol sealer cements and persists after the setting of these materials. This has been demonstrated by investigations showing that the comparative hardness of fresh dentin exposed to zinc oxide-eugenol root canal sealers is increased in direct proportion to the amount of free eugenol available.[16] A more significant effect of free eugenol lies in increased cytotoxicity and in the demonstrated high degree of antigenic potential of the substance in living tissue. Zinc oxide-eugenol cements have been shown to disintegrate over extended periods of time in the oral cavity, but the effects of this process on the efficacy of root canal fillings has not as yet been demonstrated in vivo. For these reasons alternatives to the zinc oxide-eugenol formulations have been advocated.[17]

Chloropercha (Moyco) is a direct descendant, relatively unaltered, of gutta percha based root canal sealers in use for over a century. Kloropercha N-Ø was introduced circa 1939 from Norway, and is similar to several empiric gutta percha based formulas dating to the early 1900's. The powder is stated to contain, in addition to gutta percha (20 percent), rosin, Canada balsam, and zinc oxide, with the liquid solvent being chloroform. The addition of 80 percent fillers and rosins no doubt accounts for its superior physical properties in comparison to gutta percha alone dissolved in chloroform.

Two polymer materials that were introduced in the 1950's for use as root canal sealer cements enjoy limited popularity. Diaket (1951) is an organic polyketone.[18,19] The material consists of a very fine powder containing zinc oxide and bismuth phosphate and a thick viscous liquid 2.2'-dihydroxy-5.5'-dichlorodiphenyl methane propionylacethophenone, triethanolamine, caproic acid, and copolymers of vinyl acetate, chloride, and isobutyl ether. The resin resulting from mixing the components is very tacky in texture, adheres readily to tooth structures and can be difficult to manipulate. A polyvinyl resin, Diaket is essentially a ketocomplex in which basic salts and metal oxides react with neutral organic agents, forming polyketones which in turn unite with the metallic substances

in the material to form cyclic complexes which are insoluble in water but dissolve in chloroform or organic solvents. AH-26 (1957) is an epoxy type resin adopted for use in endodontics. It is an araldite epoxy, used commercially as an industrial adhesive and insulator with the addition of a hardener, hexamethycine tetramine, making the polymerized resin chemically and biologically inert.[20]

A noneugenol containing root canal sealer cement No-genol (Coe Laboratories) has been developed recently which appears to retain the physical properties and handling characteristics of the more familiar zinc oxide-eugenol root canal sealers without the immediate effects of eugenol cytotoxicity. It is a two tube paste system said to contain zinc oxide, barium sulfate, natural resins, salicylic acid, vegetable oil. and fatty acids in the mixed formulation.[17.]

PHYSICAL PROPERTIES: There have been relatively few investigations of the physical properties of root canal filling materials. Data from studies of other types of dental cements are reported in Table II.[21-26] Each investigator used an individualized set of experimental conditions; hence, the studies are not directly comparable, but do offer some insights into the physical characteristics of these materials.

The setting times in minutes, recorded by various investigators at differing temperatures and a relative humidity (RH) of 100 percent, are summarized in the first column of Table II. Since most of the sealers investigated are zinc oxide-eugenol types, the data reported is not unexpected. The increased setting times for the Grossman formulations contrasted to the Rickert formula are apparent. The surface film set of chloropercha without internal setting of the mass can also be noted. Setting times can be related to handling properties and tissue irritation potentials.

Compressive strength was measured by crushing a specimen after the specimen had been in 37°C water for seven days. The low values obtained are indicative of the weakness of these materials under these experimental circumstances.

Table II.
Physical Properties of Root Canal Sealer Cements

Investigator	Setting Time (Min at 100% RH)				Compressive Strength (Kg/cm²)	Flow		Film Thickness (μm)	Solubility %			Water Absorption (% increase)	Volume Change			Radio-opacity	
	A	B	C	D	D	(mm/sec) E	(mm) D	B	(H₂O) B	(HAc) B	(Sample) D	C	(7 day) A	(30 day) A	(90 day) A	B	D
Kerr (Rickert)																	
22°C	50	21	30	59	180	0.51	44.0	21.7	0.48	0.32	3.96	0.99	1.28	2.98	2.98	0.55	0.09
28°C	21																
37°C																	
Kerr (Tubliseal)																	
22°C	44	23.5		17	65	1.2	43.5	8.3	0.39	7.84	1.48	NA	1.59	3.26	4.95	0.67	0.22
28°C	12																
37°C																	
Procosol Ag (Grossman)																	
22°C	5892	None	240	360	NA	0.36	39	13.3	0.40	0.29	2.77	2.78	1.28	1.99	3.26	0.98	0.34
28°C	329																
37°C																	
Procosol Nonstain (Grossman)																	
22°C	362		70		220	NA	31	NA	NA	NA	1.24	NA	No set	No set	No set	NA	0.28
28°C	520																
37°C																	
AH 26 (Schroeder)																	
37°C				630	490	0.49	44.5	NA	NA	NA	1.69	NA	0.00	1.28	No set	NA	0.10
Diaket (Schmitt)																	
37°C		22.5		210	340	0.37	20	43.3	0.16	4.26	0.43	NA	NA	NA	NA	0.75	0.31
Kloropercha (Ostby)																	
37°C	None				NA	0.64	NA	16.7	0.72	1.11	NA	NA	NA	NA	NA	1.17	NA

A. Weiner and Schilder
B. Higginbotham
C. Isamendi
D. McComb and Smith
E. Weisman

Flow rates have been measured by either aspiration of the sealer into a pipette under a vacuum or the application of a weight onto a specimen placed upon a glass slab three minutes after mixing. Other methods have been used, ranging from sophisticated rheologic techniques to simply allowing the freshly mixed material to flow down the surface, but are not included in Table II. Flow rates can be related to the ability of the root canal sealer to penetrate crevices and irregularities of the root canal system prior to setting. Viscosity studies indicate that some root canal sealers are pressure rate sensitive and behave like pseudoplastic materials.

The film thickness as measured by a modification of American Dental Association Specification No. 8 for dental zinc phosphate cements is shown in Table II. It is worthy of note that the maximum allowable film thickness for fine grain (Type 1) zinc phosphate cement is 25 μm. Diaket exceeds this value, and the Rickert formula approaches it. The film thickness of an endodontic sealer may be of considerable importance in gutta percha condensation techniques.

The solubility of root canal sealers in distilled water and buffered acetic acid has been determined by suspending tablets of the set material in crucibles containing the solvent. It has also been determined by storing specimens of known weight in 37°C water in sealed vessels for several days. Water absorption as determined by immersion in distilled water for 48 hours has also been reported.

Volume changes of root canal sealers at seven, thirty and ninety days following the insertion of fresh mixes into micropipettes is shown in Table II. The relative stability of the Rickert formula at thirty days and thereafter when compared to other root canal sealers is apparent, as is the failure of the non-staining Grossman formula to set at all under these conditions. Ideally, a root canal sealer should expand slightly and remain dimensionally stable following set, or at the very least remain dimensionally stable once set.

The index of the radiopacity as shown in Table II of the various root canal sealers was obtained by radiographing a specimen of known thickness at 65 kVp and 10 mA for a predetermined length of time, using a film of known value. The resultant images were then measured by a reflection-transmission densitometer. By this method an equivalent value of gutta percha (1.1 mm thick) would be 0.34 and silver (1.1 mm thick) 0.78. The higher the value, the more radiopaque is the material.

DIRECTIONS FOR USE: With the exception of those sealer cements which contain gutta percha solvents (such as eucapercha or chloropercha and their variants) which result in a chemical bonding of gutta percha points and sealer cement, the bond between root canal filling points and sealer cement is a nonadhesive one. Root canal filling point and root canal filling techniques using cement involve an interface between the filling point and the sealer cement, and a second interface between sealer cement and the surrounding dentin walls of the root canal. With these techniques, it is doubtful that the use of accessory points in any way alters this relationship. Hence, the mass of root canal filling consists of the central point, or core, and surrounding accessory points separated from each other and the surface of the dentin by a thin film of sealer. One of the objectives of these techniques is to achieve dimensional stability by minimizing the amount of core material. This critical relationship has been repeatedly demonstrated not only by investigations of the efficacy of root canal sealing techniques, but also upon those occasions in which the degree of adherence of sealer cement to tooth structure was found to be at variance with that to core material.[27-31]

EVALUATION PROGRAM: There are no current specifications that are applicable to the root canal sealers used in endodontics, although such specifications dealing with the physical properties of these materials are currently under development at both the national and international levels.

ROOT CANAL SEALER CEMENTS

Do:

1. Select a root canal sealer and mix it to a consistency compatible with the technique of root canal filling being used.
2. Recognize that room temperature, humidity, and time of spatulation affect the setting time of most root canal sealers.
3. Coat the walls of dry root canal systems with root canal sealers when filling root canals.
4. Confine the root canal sealer to the root canal system.
5. Remove root canal sealer from the coronal portion of the tooth following root canal filling by means of a suitable solvent so as to avoid staining tooth structures.
6. Minimize the amount of manipulation of sealer within the root canal once inserted since body temperature and manipulation combine to accelerate set.
7. Use as thick a mix as possible with as short a setting time as possible to minimize hazards of extrusion and toxicity and maximize dimensional stability when using a root canal sealer without silver or gutta percha cones to seal a root canal.
8. Use zinc-free amalgam to seal effectively the root canal in conjunction with retrograde endodontic procedures.

Don't:

1. Assume that any one root canal sealer mixed to any single consistency is applicable to all root canal filling circumstances or methods.
2. Rely entirely on manufacturers' directions in using prepackaged components if you desire consistent mixes of root canal sealers.
3. Attempt to insert root canal sealers into moist or hemorrhagic root canals as nonadherence to the dentinal surfaces and/or accelerated setting will occur.
4. Extrude root canal sealers beyond the confines of the tooth into the surrounding tissues as all root canal sealers are cytotoxic to one degree or another.
5. Leave root canal sealer in the coronal portion of the tooth following root canal filling.
6. Engage in prolonged adjustments of master cones or manipulation of accessory cones in root canals in which root canal sealers are used.
7. Use thin mixes or sealers with prolonged setting times when using root canal sealers as the sole material to obturate a root canal system.
8. Use zinc-containing amalgam root canal sealers, or dental cements to seal root canals in conjunction with retrograde endodontic procedures.

Tissue Toxicity of Endodontic Materials

Of concern to dentistry for many decades has been the tissue toxicity of many of the materials used clinically in endodontic procedures as they are placed in apposition to viable connective tissues such as the pulp or periodontal ligament.[31-39]

Among the many methods used to determine the tissue toxicity of dental materials, several have been adopted specifically for endodontic materials. The most notable techniques include the refined methods of implantation in bone and connective tissue using teflon tube containers and cell culture techniques based upon the release of chromium ions.[40] Recently, the potential immunological consequences of the use of various types of root canal sealer cements, most notably those containing eugenol or paraformaldehyde, has also been reported.[41,42]

While comparisons of reports are extremely tenuous due to experimental differences from the mass of seemingly disjointed data available in the literature, some broad general conclusions can be drawn. All endodontic filling materials are cytotoxic when freshly mixed, including the zinc-free dental amalgam used for retrograde root canal fillings. The degree of cytotoxicity is directly related to the ingredients or components of the material. For example, eugenol, eucalyptol, chloroform, iodoform, paraformaldehyde and acids are all very tissue toxic, and this is reflected in the biologic evaluations of those materials which contain them. The faster and more completely the endodontic material sets and/or becomes chemically stable, the higher is its biocompatibility. Endodontic sealers having large eugenol components which can result in the presence of free eugenol not only have retarded setting times, but the leaching of eugenol from the set material into the surrounding tissue results in a prolonged low grade irritation. Therapeutic cements containing paraformaldehyde can be deceptive in this regard, as the initial reversible inflammatory response expected from the eugenol component appears to be delayed, due to either the more rapid set of the material or the fixation of the surrounding tissues, but is followed by a steadily increasing tissue reaction as therapeutic agents leach out or the cellular reaction to the surrounding fixed and necrotized tissues becomes more apparent with the passage of time. The reaction of the body to a toxic root canal filling material need not be confined to circumscribed local lesions but can also affect remote target organs if heavy metal components such as mercury or lead are present.[43]

AVAILABLE PRODUCTS

Anteaus-Silver Points, Charles B. Schwed Co., Inc.

Caulk Absorbent Points, L. D. Caulk Co.

Dent-O-Lux Absorbent Points, Charles B. Schwed Co., Inc.

Dent-O-Lux Gutta Percha Points and Accessory Points, Charles P. Schwed Co., Inc.

Gutta Percha Points, Pulpdent Corp. of America

Gutta Percha Points and Accessory Points, Midwest American

Healthco Absorbent Points, Healthco Inc.

Healthco Endodontic Paste Fillers, Healthco Inc.

Hydron Anterior Root Canal Filling System, NPD Dental Systems, Inc.

Hydron Root Canal Filling System, NPD Dental Systems, Inc.

Johnson & Johnson Absorbent Sterile Points, Johnson & Johnson Dental Products Co.

Kerr Guttapercha Points, Kerr Mfg. Co., Div. of Sybron Corp.

Kerr Silver Points, Kerr Mfg. Co., Div. of Sybron Corp.

Lentulo Paste Fillers, Pulpdent Corp. of America

PCA Root Canal Sealer, Pulpdent Corp. of America

Premier Cavit ESPE, Premier Dental Products Co.

Premier Cavit-G ESPE, Premier Dental Products Co.

Premier Gutta Percha Points, Premier Dental Products Co.

Premier Diaket ESPE, Premier Dental Products Co.

Premier Paper Points, Premier Dental Products Co.

Premier Silver Points, Premier Dental Products Co.

Pulp Canal Sealer, Kerr Mfg. Co., Div. of Sybron Corp.

Pulpdent Paste, Pulpdent Corp. of America

R & R Absorbent Points, Ransom & Randolph Co.

R & R Gutta Percha Points, Ransom & Randolph Co.

R & R Silver Points, Ransom & Randolph Co.

Root Canal Filling Points & Sealer Cement, Unitek Corp.

Root Canal Liquid (non-staining), Moyco Industries Inc.

Root Canal Points (gutta percha), Moyco Industries Inc.

Root Canal Powder (non-staining), Moyco Industries Inc.
Silver Points, Pulpdent Corp. of America
Sterile Paper Points, Pulpdent Corp. of America
Tubli-Seal, Kerr Mfg. Co., Div. of Sybron Corp.
Unitek Gutta Percha Points, Unitek Corp.
Unitek Super-Absorbant Paper, Unitek Corp.

LITERATURE REFERENCES

1. Heuer, M. A. Instruments and materials, in Cohen, S., and Burns, R. (eds.) Pathways of the pulp. ed. 1. St. Louis, C. V. Mosby, 1976.

2. Heuer, M. A. Endodontic materials, in Craig, R. G. (ed.) Dental materials a problem oriented approach. ed. 1, St. Louis, C.V. Mosby, 1978.

3. Jasper, E. A. Root canal therapy in modern dentistry. Dent. Cosmos. 75:823, 1933.

4. Tayler, R. L., et al. Characterization of endodontic silver points. J. Dent. Res. 54(A):175, 1975.

5. Tayler, R. L., et al. Anodic polarization of endodontic silver points. J. Dent. Res. 54(A):175, 1975.

6. Messing, J. J. Precision apical silver cones. Br. Endod. Soc. J. 3:22 Apr.-June 1969.

7. Oliet, S., and Sorin, S. M. Effect of aging on the mechanical properties of hand rolled gutta percha endodontic cones. Oral Surg., Oral Med., Oral Path. 43:954 Jan. 1977.

8. Friedman, C. M., et al. Composition and mechanical properties of gutta percha endodontic points. J. Dent. Res. 54:921 Sept.-Oct. 1975.

9. Schilder, H.; Goodman, A.; and Aldrick, W. The thermomechanical properties of gutta percha I. The compressibility of gutta percha. Oral Surg., Oral Med., Oral Path. 37:946 June 1974.

10. Gurney, B. F.; Best, E. J.; and Gervascio, G. Physical measurements on gutta percha. Oral Surg., Oral Med., Oral Path. 32:260, 1971.

11. Goldman, M. Evaluation of two filling methods for root canals. J. Endod. 1:69 Feb. 1975.

12. McElroy, D. L. Physical properties of root canal filling materials. JADA 50:433, 1955.

13. Goodman, A.; Schilder, H.; and Aldrich, W. The thermomechanical properties of gutta percha II. The history and molecular chemistry of gutta percha. Oral Surg., Oral Med., Oral Path. 37:954 June 1974.

14. Dixon, C. M., and Rickert, U. G. Histologic verification of results of root canal therapy in experimental animals. JADA 25:1781, 1938.

15. Grossman, L. I. An improved root canal cement. JADA 56:381, 1958.

16. Biven, G. M.; Bapna, R. J.; and Heuer, M. A. Effect of eugenol and eugenol containing root canal sealers on the microhardness of human dentin. J. Dent. Res. 51:1602 Nov.-Dec. 1972.

17. Crane, D., et al. Biological and physical properties of an experimental non-eugenol endodontic sealer. J. Dent. Res. 54(A):L40, 1975.

18. Stewart, G. C. Comparative study of three root canal sealing agents. Oral Surg., Oral Med., Oral Path. 1:1029, 1958.

19. Bjorndal, M. A. A critique of new and improved materials for root canal filling. Iowa Dent. J. 46:67, 1960.

20. Keresztesi, K., and Kellner, G. The biologic effect of root filling materials. Int. Dent. J. 16:222 June 1966.

21. Weiner, B. H., and Schilder, A. A comparative study of important physical properties of various root canal sealers. I. Evaluation of setting time. Oral Surg., Oral Med., Oral Path. 32:768 Nov. 1971.

22. Weiner, B. H., and Schilder, H. A comparative study of important physical properties of various root canal sealers. II. Evaluation of dimensional changes. Oral Surg., Oral Med., Oral Path. 32:928 Dec. 1971.

23. Higginbotham, T. L. A comparative study of physical properties of five commonly used root canal sealers. Oral Surg., Oral Med., Oral Path. 24:89, 1967.

24. Isomendi, F. A. Etude comparative des cements de Rickert et de Grossman. Rev. Franc. Odontostomat. 14:1187 Aug.-Sept. 1967.

25. Weisman, M. I. A study of the flow rate of ten root canal sealers. Oral Surg., Oral Med., Oral Path. 29:255 Feb. 1970.

26. McComb, D., and Smith, D. C. Comparison of physical properties of polycarboxylate based and conventional root canal sealers. J. Endod. 2:228 Aug. 1976.

27. Marshall, F. J., and Massler, M. The sealing of pulpless teeth evaluated with radioisotopes. J. Dent. Med. 16:172, 1961.

28. Kapsimalis, P., and Evans, R. Sealing properties of endodontic filling materials using radioactive polar and non-polar isotopes. Oral Surg., Oral Med., Oral Path. 22:386, 1966.

29. Grieve, A. R., and Parkholm, J. D. O. The sealing properties of root canal filling cements, further studies. Br. Dent. J. 135:327 Oct. 1973.

30. Sanders, S. H., and Dooley, R. J. A compar-

ative evaluation of polycarboxylate cement as a root canal sealer. Oral Surg., Oral Med., Oral Path. 37:629 Apr. 1974.

31. Wollard, R. R., et al. Scanning electron microscope examination of root canal filling materials. J. Endod. 2:98 Apr. 1976.

32. Dixon, C. M., and Rickert, U. G. Tissue tolerance to foreign materials. JADA 20:1458 Aug. 1933.

33. Mitchell, D. F. Irritational qualities of dental materials. JADA 59:954, 1959.

34. Guttuso, J. Histopathologic study of rat connective tissue response to endodontic materials. Oral Surg., Oral Med., Oral Path. 16:713 June 1963.

35. Feldman, G.; Nyborg, H; and Conrado, C. A. Tissue reactions to root filling materials. III. A comparison between implants of root filling material N2 and silver in jaws of rabbits. Odont. Revy. 18:387, 1967.

36. Friend, L. A., and Browne, R. J. Tissue reactions to some root canal filling materials in the bone of rabbits. Arch. Oral Biol. 14:629, 1969.

37. Spangberg, L. Biological effects of root canal filling materials. Odont. Revy. 20: Sup. 16, 1969.

38. Langeland, K. Root canal sealants and pastes. Dent. Clin. N. Am. 18:309 Apr. 1974.

39. Recommended standard practices for biological and clinical evaluations, in Guide to dental materials and devices. ed. 8. Chicago, Council on Dental Materials and Devices, American Dental Association, Ch. 16, 1976.

40. Spangberg, L. Kinetic and quantitative evaluation of material cytotoxicity in vitro. Oral Surg., Oral Med., Oral Path. 35:389 Mar. 1973.

41. Block, R. M., et al. Cell mediated immune response to dog pulp tissue altered by N2 paste within the root canal. Oral Surg., Oral Med., Oral Path. 45:131 Jan. 1978.

42. Block, R. M., et al. Antibody formation to dog pulp tissue altered by eugenol within the root canal. J. Endod. 4:53 Feb. 1978.

43. Oswald, R. J., and Cohen, S. A. Systemic distribution of lead from root canal fillings. J. Endod. 1:59 Feb. 1975.

IMPRESSION MATERIALS

Impression materials are used in dentistry to register or reproduce the form and relationship of the teeth and oral tissues. The earliest dental impression materials were waxes used in the 18th and 19th centuries, and plaster, used from the mid 19th century to the present. Both exhibit qualities that significantly limit their effective use as dental impression materials.

There are seven basic categories of impression materials. Each type possesses characteristics which influence the purpose to which it is best suited (Table I). As the purpose varies, so does the relative importance of these characteristics. The judgment of the dentist determines which of the available materials is best suited to any specific case. Chemical composition and physical properties of the impression materials may be found in dental materials texts.[1-6]

AGAR

COMPOSITION: Agar impression materials are compounded from thermally reversible agar gels. They liquify when heated (the sol state) and return to the solid state (gel) when cooled, a property which distinguishes them from the thermally irreversible alginate gels.

USES: Reversible agar hydrocolloid materials have been used as dental impression materials since about 1925, and were the first of the satisfactory elastic impression materials. Their principal uses are in partial denture prostheses, fixed prosthetic and restorative procedures, and laboratory duplication techniques.

DIRECTIONS FOR USE: The material is packaged in plastic jackets and poly tubes. The injectable material is available in sticks for use in a reusable syringe, or pre-packaged in disposable syringes. Both the tray and syringe materials are manufactured in regular or heavy-bodied types.

The material is liquified by immersion in boiling water for varying periods of time according to the manufacturer's directions, up to 10 minutes. The tray and injection material may be stored at 145 to 150°F (63 to 66°C) for indefinite periods of time. Prior to use, the material is placed in an appropriate water-cooler tray and

Table I.

Characteristics of Dental Impression Materials

	Agar	Alginate	Plaster	Zinc Oxide	Compound	Polysulfide	Silicone	Polyether
Non-irritating	+	+	+	0	+	0	0	−
Esthetic & pleasant to use	+	+	−	0	0	−	0	−
Stable in storage	−	−	+	0	0	+	+	+
Elasticity	0	0	−	−	−	+	+	+
Rigidity	0	0	+	+	+	+	+	+
Consistency suited to technique	+	0	+	+	0	+	0	0
Economically practical	+	+	+	+	+	0	0	0
Convenient to use	+	+	0	0	0	0	0	0
Ability to withstand tearing and distortion	0	0	−	−	−	+	+	+
Dimensional stability of impression	0	0	+	+	0	+	+	+
Accuracy of impression	+	0	+	+	−	+	+	+
Working and setting time	+	+	+	+	+	+	+	0
Metal die or plating	−	−	−	−	+	+	+	+
Use with minimal equipment	−	+	0	0	0	0	0	0
Casts allowed to set vertically vs. inverted	+	+	+	0	0	+	+	+

Key: + = Relatively superior;   0 = Average;   − = Relatively inferior

tempered at 110 to 115°F (43 to 46°C) for 3 to 5 minutes according to the manufacturer's directions. Injectable material used for restorative impressions is used at the storage temperature.

Once in the mouth, the material is cooled for 5 minutes by 55°F (13°C) water circulating through tubes incorporated in the tray. When set, the tray is removed from the mouth with a snapping action; it is important that the tray not be rocked or "teased" out of the mouth, as this will increase the chance of discrepancies in the impression.

Hydrocolloid impressions are the least dimensionally stable of the elastic impression materials; they lose moisture and shrink when exposed to air. They should be poured immediately.[7] If this is not possible, they may be stored for a short time in 100 percent relative humidity humidors or wrapped in wet towels.

Poured impressions should set in a 100 percent relative humidity humidor. Casts poured from hydrocolloid impressions exhibit the most bubble-free surfaces.[8]

LIMITATIONS OF USE: Agar impression materials are not recommended for procedures requiring a long delay in pouring such as removable prosthetic techniques or fixed or restorative techniques. Teeth that have extremely deep gingival extensions or severe undercuts in their contour or preparations also preclude the use of agar materials.

EVALUATION PROGRAM: Physical and laboratory quality specifications for agar hydrocolloid impression materials are delineated in American Dental Association Specification No. 11.[3]

AGAR

Do:

1. Frequently check accuracy of temperatures of boiling, tempering and holding water baths.
2. Follow package instructions meticulously.
3. Pour impression in stone immediately.
4. Remove impression from mouth with snapping action.

Don't:

1. Rock or tease impression when removing from mouth.
2. Let impression sit in air before pouring.

AVAILABLE PRODUCTS

AGARLOID REVERSIBLE HYDROCOLLOID IMPRESSION MATERIAL, Cadco Products
RUBBERLOID HEAVY BODY, Van R Dental Products, Inc.

RUBBERLOID REGULAR, Van R Dental Products, Inc.
RUBBERLOID SYRINGE MATERIAL, Van R Dental Products, Inc.
SURGIDENT HYDROCOLLOID IMPRESSION MATERIAL, Lactona Corp., Subsidiary Warner-Lambert Co.
SURGIDENT HEAVY BODY, Lactona Corp., Subsidiary Warner-Lambert Co.
SURGIDENT HEAVY BODY II, Lactona Corp., Subsidiary Warner-Lambert Co.
Surgident Syringe, Lactona Corp., Subsidiary Warner-Lambert Co.
THOMPSON HEAVY BODY II, Lactona Corp., Subsidiary Warner-Lambert Co.
THOMPSON SUPER-STRENGTH, Lactona Corp., Subsidiary Warner-Lambert Co.

ALGINATE

COMPOSITION: Alginate impression material is an irreversible hydrocolloid based on salts of alginic acid, a derivative of marine kelp.[5] Alginates change from the sol to the gel state by an irreversible chemical action.

USES: The alginate impression materials are used in full and partial denture prostheses and in orthodontics. They may also be used in making impressions for study casts and in limited cases of fixed partial prostheses. Considering all available elastic impression materials, alginate is the least accurate.[9]

DIRECTIONS FOR USE: Alginate impression materials are packaged in powder form and are mixed with water. Correct measuring, proportioning and mixing are required, as inaccuracies in these procedures can affect working and setting times as well as the strength and accuracy of the impression. Variations in the temperature of water used in the mix affect the setting time; high temperatures shorten the time and cool temperatures lengthen it.[5] Alginate impression materials continue to gain strength and increased properties for ten minutes after their initial set. They should be left in the mouth for a minimum of two minutes after the initial set.[10]

Like agar hydrocolloid materials, alginate impressions lose water when exposed to air and will shrink and eventually harden. They should therefore be poured in stone as soon as possible. If storage of the impression is necessary, it should be in a humidor at 100 percent humidity or wrapped in wet towels.

EVALUATION PROGRAM: American Dental Association Specification No. 18[3] for dental alginate impression materials defines two types: (1) fast set which must gel in 1 to 2 minutes after beginning of mix, and (2) normal set which must gel in 2 to 4½ minutes after beginning of mix.

ALGINATE

Do:
1. Store in an airtight container.
2. Follow manufacturer's instructions for measuring and mixing.
3. Use the correct impression tray.
4. Rinse and clean the mouth before taking the impression.
5. Rinse and dry the impression before pouring.
6. Pour immediately in stone.
7. Check setting time by observing material remaining in mixing bowl.
8. Remove the impression with a snapping motion.

Don't:
1. Leave the impression exposed to air before pouring.
2. Rock or tease the impression when removing it from the mouth.

AVAILABLE PRODUCTS

TYPE I, FAST SETTING

Algee Alginate, Accurate Set, Inc.
ALGITEC ALGINATE, Doric Corp.
CODESCO ALGINATE IMPRESSION MATERIAL, Codesco, Inc.

COE ALGINATE, Coe Laboratories, Inc.
CUTTER JEL, TYPE I, FAST SET IMPRESSION MATERIAL, Cutter Laboratories
D-P KEY TO ALGINATES, Teledyne Dental Products
D-P KEY TO ALGINATES HEAVY BODY, Teledyne Dental Products
HYDRO-JEL FAST SETTING ALGINATE, Professional Products Co.
Jelset, Teledyne Dental Products
JELTRATE, FAST SET, L. D. Caulk Co., Div. of Dentsply International, Inc.
KALGINATE ALGINATE IMPRESSION POWDER, Teledyne Dental, Getz-Opotow Division
KERR ALGINATE FAST SET, Kerr Mfg. Co., Div. of Sybron Corp.
Key-to-Alginate, Teledyne Dental Products
NU-GEL ALGINATE IMPRESSION MATERIAL, Teledyne Dental Products Co.
OPOTOW JELSET, Teledyne Dental Products Co.
PLASTODENT ELASTIC IMPRESSION POWDER, Plastodent, Inc.
S. S. WHITE ALGINATE IMPRESSION MATERIAL, S. S. White Div. of Pennwalt Corp.
SUPER GEL FAST SET IMPRESSION MATERIAL, Harry J. Bosworth Co.
SURGIDENT ALGINATE, Lactona Corp., Subsidiary Warner-Lambert Co.
UNIJEL II, Unitek Corp.
VERNOGEL, Vernon Benshoff Co.

TYPE II, NORMAL SETTING

Algee Alginate, Accurate Set, Inc.
Algisol, Teledyne Dental Products
CODESCO ALGINATE IMPRESSION MATERIAL, Codesco, Inc.
COE ALGINATE, Coe Laboratories, Inc.
D-P ELASTIC IMPRESSION COMPOUND, Teledyne Dental Products Co.
HYDRO-JEL NORMAL SETTING, Professional Products Co.
JELTRATE NORMAL SET; HEAVY BODY, L. D. Caulk Co., Div. of Dentsply International Inc.
Jelset, Teledyne Dental Products
KALGINATE NORMAL SETTING, Teledyne Dental Products Co.
KERR ALGINATE NORMAL, Kerr Mfg. Co., Div. of Sybron Corp.

LD-21 ALGINOID, Lang Dental Mfg. Co., Inc.

NU-GEL, Teledyne Dental Products Co.

OPOTOW JELSET, Teledyne Dental Products Co.

PALGINEX '75' ALGINATE IMPRESSION MATERIAL, REGULAR SET, International Dental Products

PLASTODENT IMPRESSION POWDER, Plastodent, Inc.

S. S. WHITE ALGINATE IMPRESSION MATERIAL, S. S. White Div. of Pennwalt Corp.

SUPERGEL ALGINATE IMPRESSION POWDER, Harry J. Bosworth Co.

SURGIDENT ALGINATE, Lactona Corp.

UNIJEL II ALGINATE IMPRESSION MATERIAL, Unitek Corp.

PLASTER

COMPOSITION: Plaster impression materials consist of dental plaster plus various additives such as flavoring, gums, and chemicals to enhance handling characteristics. Since plaster is a rigid material in its set state, it breaks before bending or distorting; therefore if teeth or undercut areas are included in the impression, the impression must be broken before it can be withdrawn.

USES: Plaster is used for making impressions for complete dentures, crown and bridge procedures, and the recording of jaw relations. It is also used as "wash" liner for final impressions.

DIRECTIONS FOR USE: Plaster impression material is a powder which when mixed with water hardens. Regular set and modified fast set materials are available for dental use. There are several factors which further affect the setting time, including the ratio of powder to water, time and rate of spatulation and temperature of the mix.[5]

Sealing the impression before pouring the stone cast prevents adherence and allows easier, more accurate separation. Several products may be used for this purpose: varnish, lacquer, sodium silicate, soap or alginate solutions.

When used as wash liners for final impressions, plaster materials retain dimension only if the tray materials retain stability. Because tray materials may distort to release stresses on standing, it is best to pour impressions as soon as possible.

EVALUATION PROGRAM: American Dental Association Specification No. 25 has been developed for dental gypsum products.[3]

PLASTER

Do:

1. Store in an airtight container to prevent changes in properties.
2. Use the recommended water/powder ratio.
3. Spatulate under vacuum.
4. Use a separating medium before pouring the cast.

Don't:

1. Use excess separating medium that may obliterate surface detail.

AVAILABLE PRODUCTS

TYPE I, PLASTER IMPRESSION

Cloverleaf XX Quickset, J. E. Healy Co.
Impression Plaster, Modern Materials Mfg. Co.
Impressotex, Whip-Mix Corp.
Microtrue, Whip-Mix Corp.
R&R Orthodontic Plaster, Ransom and Randolph Company
Snow White Plaster #2, Kerr Mfg. Co., Div. of Sybron Corp.
Solutex, Whip-Mix Corp.
True Plastic, Special Formula True Plastic, Teledyne Dental Products

TYPE II, PLASTER, MODEL

CLOVERLEAF LABORATORY PLASTER, J. E. Healy Co.
Easycut Plaster, Modern Materials Mfg. Co.
KERR SNOW WHITE PLASTER NO. 1, Kerr Mfg. Co., Div. of Sybron Corp.
Lab Plaster, Modern Materials Mfg.Co.
LABORATORY PLASTER, Whip-Mix Corp.
MODEL PLASTER, GRADE A, Whip-Mix Corp.

Orthodontic Plaster, White, Whip-Mix Corp.
Orthodontic Plaster, Modern Materials Mfg. Co.
Plaster, Pre-Vest, Inc.
R&R MODEL PLASTER, Ransom and Randolph Company

TYPE III, DENTAL STONE

Bitestone-White, Whip-Mix Corp.
CASTONE, Ransom and Randolph Company
COECAL BUFF, White, Coe Laboratories, Inc.
Denstone, Modern Materials Mfg. Co.
Die-Keen, Modern Materials Mfg. Co.
Die Stone, Modern Materials Mfg. Co.
Flasking Stone, Whip-Mix Corp.
Flasking Stone, Modern Materials Mfg. Co.
Hydrotex Dental Stone, Whip-Mix Corp.
India Die Stone, Lactona Corp., Div. Warner-Lambert Corp.
Laboratory Stone, Whip-Mix Corp.
Labstone, Modern Materials Mfg. Co.
MICROSTONE, Whip-Mix Corp.
Mounting Stone, White, Whip-Mix Corp.
Orthodontic Stone, Super White, Whip-Mix Corp.
O-67 Snow White Stone, Modern Materials Mfg. Co.
Pre-Vest Stone, Pre-Vest Inc.
QUICKSTONE, Whip-Mix Corp.
RAPID STONE, Kerr Mfg. Co., Div. of Sybron Dental Products
Surgident Functional Bite Stone, Sterndent Corp.

TYPE IV, DENTAL STONE HIGH STRENGTH

DIE ROCK, Whip-Mix Corp.
DUROC, Ransom and Randolph Company
Master Model Stone, Pre-Vest, Inc.
R&R Laboratory Stone, Ransom and Randolph Company
SILKY-ROCK, Whip-Mix Corp.
Super-Die (vivid yellow) Whip-Mix Corp.
Tru-Stone, True Stone Fast-Set, Modern Materials Mfg. Co.
UTK Blue Die Stone, Unitek Corp.
VEL MIX STONE, Kerr Mfg. Co., Div. of Sybron Corp.

ZINC OXIDE PASTES

COMPOSITION: Zinc oxide impression materials combine zinc oxide with one of three chemically related aromatic oils: eugenol, guaiacol, or methyl guaiacol. When combined, they set into a hardened mass. Eugenol is the most commonly used component.[5]

USES: Zinc oxide impression materials were introduced in the 1930's and are most often used as corrective impression materials in complete and partial denture prostheses. The zinc oxide pastes may be used in registering final impressions; for stabilizing base plates in bite registration; as temporary reline materials; and in bite registration procedures for inlay, crown and bridge techniques.

ZINC OXIDE PASTES

Do:

1. Select the product designed to provide characteristics in setting time and consistency compatible with the specific task.
2. Follow the manufacturer's recommendations and directions.
3. Mix on paper pad for easier clean up.

Don't:

1. Attempt to alter setting time or consistency beyond the manufacturer's recommendations.
2. Mix on glass slab, as material will adhere to glass and make clean up difficult.

DIRECTIONS FOR USE: Zinc oxide-eugenol impression materials are usually available as two homogenous pastes in collapsible metal tubes. The two pastes are of different colors so that thoroughness and homogeneity of the mix may be determined by visual inspection. The two pastes are measured by length onto a paper mixing pad and spatulated. Temperature, humidity, length of spatulation, and ratio of the two component pastes affect working time, setting time, consistency of the mix and flow properties, strength, and physical characteristics of the set impression.[5] Products are available which have been formulated to give specific working time and consistencies, and the clinician should choose the product designed to meet his needs, rather than attempt to modify the characteristics of an unsuitable material.

LIMITATIONS OF USE: Set material is rigid; therefore, it cannot be removed from undercuts without fracture.

EVALUATION PROGRAM: American Dental Association Specification No. 16 applies to impression pastes.[3]

AVAILABLE PRODUCTS

TYPE I, HARD

CAULK IMPRESSION PASTE, L. D. Caulk Co., Div. of Dentsply International, Inc.
COE-FLO, Coe Laboratories, Inc.
Hard Set Impression Paste, S. S. White Div., Pennwalt Corp.
Kelly's Paste, Teledyne Dental Products
KERR EQUALIZING PASTE, Kerr Mfg. Co., Div. of Sybron Corp.
OPOTOW LOWER; MANDIBULAR; STANDARD, Teledyne Dental Products
PLASTOPASTE, Harry J. Bosworth Co.
SUPERPASTE, Harry J. Bosworth Co.

TYPE II, SOFT

KREX IMPRESSION CORRECTIVE, Teledyne Dental Products
MULTI-FORM DUAL PURPOSE IMPRESSION PASTE, Lactona Corp., Subsidiary of Warner-Lambert Co.
S. S. WHITE IMPRESSION PASTE, S. S. White Div., Pennwalt Corp.

IMPRESSION COMPOUNDS

COMPOSITION: Impression compounds are thermoplastic materials, softened to working consistency by immersion in hot water or by heating over a flame. They set in the mouth to a hardened mass which bends or distorts when withdrawn from undercut areas.

USES: Impression compound is one of the oldest impression materials and is still widely used for complete edentulous mouth impressions.

DIRECTIONS FOR USE: The compound is heated and softened either by immersion in water or by exposure to an open flame. The compound should be heated carefully, as overheating can cause loss of the more volatile elements and alter the composition. Also, when heating, consideration must be given to the mass of the compound to ensure softening of the central portions of the mass. For edentulous impressions, cooling is accomplished by allowing the material to set in the mouth. Individual band impressions are cooled with a water spray.

In taking impressions of cavities prepared in the teeth, sticks or cones of compound are heated over a flame, taking care not to overheat the outside portion. The softened compound is placed in a metal band which has been adapted to the tooth.

When used to make impression trays, the softened compound is adapted to a study model and trimmed to the border of the denture area. Compound trays lack strength and dimensional stability, and have therefore been largely replaced by trays made from self-curing acrylic resins.

LIMITATIONS OF USE: Impression compound hardens to a rigid mass that distorts when removed from undercuts; therefore, it cannot be used where undercuts are present and accurate registration is required.

EVALUATION PROGRAM: There are two general types of compound, based upon American Dental Association Specification No. 3 for dental impression compounds.[3] Type I, impression compound, is used for sectional impressions of partially edentulous jaws, for certain types of individual tooth preparations and as backings for all types of matrices. Type II, tray compound, is used primarily to form impression trays. Within these general types, products are available which offer the clinician a wide range of characteristics such as softening temperature, plasticity and body, form of the product and hardness when set.

IMPRESSION COMPOUNDS

Do:

1. Follow the manufacturer's instructions.
2. Select the product whose characteristics are best suited to the intended purpose.
3. Pour models immediately to reduce distortion.
4. Use strong, rigid trays or bands for impressions.

Don't:

1. Use for procedures requiring accurate impressions of undercut areas.
2. Over-knead or water will be incorporated into the material.
3. Overheat, as volatile components will evaporate or ignite.
4. Leave immersed in hot water for too long or volatile components will leach out.

AVAILABLE PRODUCTS

TYPE I, IMPRESSION COMPOUND

KERR BLACK; GREY; PERFECTION; WHITE, Kerr Mfg. Co., Div. of Sybron Corp.
KERR GREEN IMPRESSION COMPOUND, Kerr Mfg. Co., Div. of Sybron Corp.
MIZZY LOW HEAT, Mizzy, Inc.
Mizzy Trolastic, Mizzy Inc.
Muco Seal 45; 54, H. D. Justi Co., Div. of Williams Gold Refining Co., Inc.
Vivostat, H. D. Justi Co., Div. of Williams Gold Refining Co., Inc.

ELASTOMERIC IMPRESSION MATERIALS

COMPOSITION: Elastomeric impression materials were originally developed for a variety of industrial purposes and have been adapted for use as dental impression materials. Mercaptan polysulfide, silicone, and polyether rubber materials are all essentially liquid polymers which can be converted to solid rubbers at room temperature when mixed with a suitable catalyst.[5] The materials exhibit a degree of accuracy comparable to alginate and agar hydrocolloid, and are more easily prepared for use and are more dimensionally stable over a period of time than the hydrocolloids. Also, rubber impression materials can be electroformed to give metal dies, an advantage over stone dies because of greater abrasion resistance.[11] When more than one die is indicated, two separate impressions should be taken, as second pour dies are inaccurate.

EVALUATION PROGRAM: American Dental Association Specification No. 19 for non-aqueous elastomeric impression materials contains a classification of materials into types according to elastic properties and dimensional changes after setting. Viscosity and intended use serve as further classification within the types of materials. Polysulfides, silicone base, and polyether materials are all described in the specifications. They are all used for similar purposes, but operators have various preferences for the materials because of differing physical properties.

Polysulfide

Polysulfides have been used as dental impression materials longer than the silicone or the polyether products, and have been found to be reliable clinically. They are strong, relatively stable, elastic, and accurate when used as recommended. The materials gain tear resistance in 10 to 15 minutes.

Tear resistance of polysulfides is significantly superior to silicones and slightly more than polyethers.[12] Use of the lead peroxide catalyst results in a brown color which some find unpleasant. The freshly mixed paste is sticky and will stain linen.

In dental procedures, the rubber base and catalyst are available as pastes in collapsible tubes. These are dispensed onto a paper pad and spatulated. The plastic thickens and forms a solid rubbery mass in a two stage process. The first stage (initial set) results in a stiffening of the paste without the appearance of elastic properties. The second stage (final set) begins with the appearance of elasticity and proceeds through a gradual change to solid rubber. Clinically, the material may be manipulated during the first stage only, and must be in place in the mouth before elastic properties start to develop.

The material is available in heavy, regular, and light-bodied forms. Usually, the light-bodied material is injected into the cavity preparation, then a tray of heavy-bodied material is carried to place in the mouth. The heavy-bodied material has less tendency to be displaced by gingival tissue or seepage.[13]

Mixing time and avoidance of contamination from handling are most important. Also, care during spatulation can eliminate small air bubbles that are normally present in the pastes; spatulation in a side-to-side motion, flattening the mix into a thin layer, is recommended .

Setting time is affected by temperature and humidity; a rise in temperature speeds the set. When using the light-bodied material in an injecting syringe technique, difficulty may be experienced in hot weather due to accelerated set.

Individual or custom trays formed from tray acrylic to limit the bulk of impression material are preferred over stock perforated trays. The advantage of individual trays, wherein a 2 mm thick bulk of material can be used, is their superior accuracy.[14] Impressions are stable and may be silverplated. Some products include an adhesive material used to bond the rubber base to the impression tray. These adhesives are solutions of rubber in volatile organic solvent which are painted onto the tray and allowed to dry. The surface of custom acrylic trays must be thoroughly cleaned and the adhesive should be allowed to dry for a minimum of 15 minutes.[15] As an alternative, use of perforated impression trays usually eliminates the need for this adhesive.

POLYSULFIDE IMPRESSION MATERIALS

Do:

1. Choose the product (heavy, regular, light) best suited to the intended purpose.
2. Mix carefully according to the time recommended by the manufacturer.
3. Avoid contamination by fingers during spatulation.
4. Spatulate with side-to-side motion to allow air bubbles to rise to surface.
5. Use the specified tray and, when applicable, adhesive recommended by the manufacturer.
6. Leave the impression in the mouth as long as clinically convenient for maximum elasticity (4 to 6 minutes).
7. Use a thin layer of rubber to reduce dimensional change.
8. Allow 10 to 20 minutes after removal from the mouth for recovery from elastic strain before pouring.[16]

Don't:

1. Over or undermix.
2. Attempt manipulation after the final set has begun and elastic properties are present.
3. Contaminate the product with water.
4. Cool below the dew point.

Silicone

The early silicone products exhibited a variety of defects such as poor elastic qualities, evolution of gas during polymerization, incomplete set with a tacky surface, short shelf life, and short working time. Many of these have been overcome, and the resulting products are both clinically acceptable and esthetically more pleasant than the polysulfide materials. They are also easier to mix.

Silicone impression material is available as two pastes in collapsible tubes, like the polysulfide materials, though some products supply the catalyst in liquid form. It is available as light, regular, and heavy-bodied material, as well as silicone putty. The proportioning and mixing of the silicone product is essentially the same as for polysulfides. Air bubbles are usually not present, so no special steps are required to counteract them.

The set for silicone materials occurs in two stages, as it does for polysulfides. The setting times of the silicone materials are generally shorter, and the point of initial set is not so easily detected. The working time for silicone products used in a syringe technique may not be sufficient for some clinical procedures, and this must be taken into account when selecting the impression material.

Significant setting shrinkage is a disadvantage of silicone impression materials; therefore, custom trays to limit the bulk of material are necessary. Shrinkage can be compensated for by utilizing the putty or the double mix technique; however, without spacing in the custom tray, distortion is increased.[17]

Silicone products are not as responsive to changes in temperature and humidity as are the polysulfide rubbers.[5] Retarded elastic deformation of silicones is less than the polysulfide impression materials.[18,19]

Another important limitation which must be considered when using silicone impression materials is the short working time. Also, cavity preparations must be dry and free of moisture contamination as water has been noted to alter the physical properties of the material.[20]

Polysiloxanes (Addition Reaction Silicones)

This type of rubber impression material was introduced in 1975. It is supplied as a two-paste system, with low molecular weight silicones in each paste. One contains terminal vinyl groups, the other terminal hydrogen groups. These terminal groups react with each other to polymerize the silicone, with no by-products being formed.

The manufactured products are available as light, regular, and heavy bodied materials. These are mixed as equal lengths of the base catalyst pastes. The regular paste can be used in both syringe and tray (custom made) for the complete impression. In the two-phase or "wash technique" the heavy bodied material can be applied over a spacer if a stock tray is preferred; then either the light bodied or regular bodied paste can be applied by the syringe for the final impression as a "wash" inside the heavy bodied material.

The working time is longer than the polyether and silicone materials, though not as long as some polysulfide materials. Like the polyethers it has relatively low flexibility when set, compared to silicones and polysulfides, yet has been found easier to separate from teeth and stone models than regular polyether impressions.

A recent survey[22] showed the polysiloxane to have the best elastic properties and lowest dimensional changes on setting of all the rubber impression materials tested.

The material is colorless and tasteless. Laundering removes staining on fabrics. It can be copper or silver plated.

Polysiloxane impression materials have a number of disadvantages. For example, the setting time is not adjustable by the catalyst/base

---

SILICONE IMPRESSION MATERIALS

Do:

1. Follow the manufacturer's recommendations for time and method of mix.
2. Moisten hands to prevent sticking of putty material.
3. Obtain a thorough incorporation of catalyst.
4. Pour model as soon as possible.[21]

Don't:

1. Take restorative impressions if hemorrhage or moisture is not controlled completely.
2. Use silicone impression materials in injectable techniques requiring a long working time.

ratio or by choice of body consistency; however, a retarder is available. In addition, the material has only a one year shelf life. An important concern for the light bodied type of material is its tendency to flow too much in some positions.

considerations related to custom trays, bulk, and adhesives apply. The impressions may be used in silver plating techniques. Allergic reactions have been reported; caution and discontinuance of use is indicated in suspected cases.[23] A status report on polyether materials may be found in the dental literature.[23]

POLYSILOXANE IMPRESSION MATERIALS

Do:

1. Follow the manufacturer's directions for time and method of mix.
2. Mix thoroughly.
3. Use adhesive on trays.

Don't:

1. Take restorative impressions in the presence of hemorrhage or moisture.
2. Attempt to remove spills on fabrics before setting is complete
3. Combine polysiloxane materials with condensation reaction silicones.

POLYETHER IMPRESSION MATERIALS

Do:

1. Follow the manufacturer's instructions.
2. Mix to a uniform color.
3. Exercise care in mixing and handling to prevent potential hypersensitivity reactions.
4. Delay pour for a minimum of 10 minutes to reduce deformation.[22]

Don't:

1. Store the impression in water.[20]
2. Permit unnecessary exposure to vapors of tray adhesive.

Polyethers

Polyether elastic impression materials are supplied in the form of two pastes, a base and a catalyst, with a thinner available to alter the physical properties.[5,23]

It is faster setting than the polysulfides, with low values of permanent deformation, flow and dimensional change upon polymerization and storage in air. Compared to silicone products, it shows similar tear properties, is relatively stiff, and has low values for strain in compression.[12] Water sorption values are about 14 percent at equilibrium in water, so it is *not* recommended to store impressions in that medium. Flow characteristics are poorer than silicones or polysulfide rubbers. Because of flow characteristics, polyether elastic impression materials have limitations in quadrant or full arch impressions.

Either custom or stock trays may be used in the impression technique. The aforementioned

AVAILABLE PRODUCTS

POLYSULFIDE BASE

ACCRALASTIC WASH, TYPE III, LOW VISCOSITY, Kerr Mfg. Co., Div. of Sybron Corp.
COE FLEX LIGHT: REGULAR; HEAVY, Coe Laboratories, Inc.
FORMTEX RUBBER BASE IMPRESSION MATERIAL, Nu-Dent Porcelain Studio, Inc.
Getz Rubber Base, Teledyne Dental Products
IMPREX LIGHT BODY, Cadco
KERR PERMLASTIC LIGHT BODIED; REGULAR BODIED; HEAVY BODIED, Kerr Mfg. Co., Div. of Sybron Corp.
KERR UNILASTIC, TYPE III, LOW VISCOSITY IMPRESSION MATERIAL, Kerr Mfg. Co., Div. of Sybron Corp.
MIRADENT 70 LIGHT BODY; REGULAR BODY, Miradent Corp.
MLM, S. S. White Dental Products International Div. Pennwalt Corp.

NEO-PLEX IMPRESSION MATERIAL REGULAR; LIGHT, Lactona Corp., Subsidiary Warner-Lambert Corp.

OMNIFLEX, Coe Laboratories, Inc.

PROFLEX LIGHT BODY; REGULAR BODY; HEAVY BODY, Professional Products Inc.

Rubberjel, L. D. Caulk Co., Div. of Dentsply International, Inc.

Set Lastic Heavy Body; Light Body; Regular, Accurate Set, Inc.

STA-TIC "X" REGULAR; STA-TIC HEAVY BODY, Buffalo Dental Mfg. Co., Inc.

SILICONE BASE

ACCOE SILICONE IMPRESSION MATERIAL, TYPE III, MEDIUM VISCOSITY, Coe Laboratories, Inc.

CITRICON (WASH), Kerr Mfg. Co., Div. of Sybron Corp.

ELASTICON SYRINGE; TRAY; HEAVY BODIED, Kerr Mfg. Co., Div. of Sybron Corp.

High Pute Body, H. P. Wash, Accurate Set, Inc.

JELCONE REGULAR BODY, L. D. Caulk Co., Div. of Dentsply International Inc.

KERR REFLECT, Kerr Mfg. Co., Div. of Sybron Corp.

KERR TRAYCON, Kerr Mfg. Co., Div. of Sybron Corp.

Leeform; Leeform II, Lee Pharmaceuticals

OPTOSIL — SILICONE PRELIMINARY IMPRESSION MATERIAL, Unitek Corp.

PERMAGUM WASH ELASTOMERIC VINYL POLYSILOXANE, TYPE I, LOW VISCOSITY, ESPE Dental Products Corp.

PERMAGUM, TYPE I, MEDIUM VISCOSITY (SYRINGE) ELASTOMERIC VINYL POLYSILOXANE IMPRESSION MATERIAL, ESPE Dental Products Corp.

PERMAGUM TRAY ELASTOMERIC VINYL POLYSILOXANE, TYPE I, HIGH VISCOSITY, ESPE Dental Products Corp.

PERMAGUM K TYPE PUTTY ELASTOMERIC VINYL POLYSILOXANE, TYPE I, VERY HIGH VISCOSITY, ESPE Dental Products Corp.

Polysil Putty; Heavy Body; Light Body, Accurate Set, Inc.

Polytrans, Teledyne Dental Products

R & R Silicone, Ransom and Randolph Company

REPRISOL HEAVY BODY VINYL POLYSILOXANE, TYPE I, HIGH VISCOSITY, L. D. Caulk Co., Div. of Dentsply International, Inc.

REPRISOL LIGHT BODY VINYL POLYSILOXANE, TYPE I, LOW VISCOSITY, L. D. Caulk Co., Div. of Dentsply International, Inc.

REPRISOL REGULAR BODY VINYL POLYSILOXANE, TYPE I, MEDIUM VISCOSITY, L. D. Caulk Co., Div. of Dentsply International, Inc.

Siccofrom Repro Elastomer, Pfingst and Co.

Silc, Teledyne Dental Products

XANTOPREN BLUE, LIGHT BODY; GREEN, REGULAR BODY, Unitek Corp.

ZYLOX IMPRESSION MATERIAL, TYPE I, LOW VISCOSITY, Premier Dental Products Co.

POLYETHER BASE

IMPREGUM IMPRESSION MATERIAL, TYPE I, MEDIUM VISCOSITY, Premier Dental Products Co.

POLYGEL, TYPE I, MEDIUM VISCOSITY, L. D. Caulk Co., Div. of Dentsply International, Inc.

DUPLICATING MATERIALS

COMPOSITION AND PROPERTIES: The most common duplicating material is based upon agar, and is therefore thermally reversible, can be stored as a sol, has adequate strength, can be used in undercut areas, and is satisfactorily accurate in recording detail. The agar material used for duplicating is similar to agar impression material but has a higher water content.[4]

Other duplicating materials include irreversible alginates and reversible plastic gels, basically polyvinyl chloride.

USES: The primary use for duplicating materials is for making copies of gypsum master casts of patients' dentition. They are also used to make the elastic denture-forming molds used in fluid resin techniques.

DIRECTIONS FOR USE: The reversible hydrocolloid and plastic materials may be reheated and reused in accordance with manufacturers' instructions. Most agar materials include a recommendation that the gypsum master cast be wet and at about 100 to 105°F (38 to 41°C) when the mold is poured. Regulated cooling to the gel state is also recommended to prevent development of stresses in the mold.

The same basic handling instructions and precautions given for the agar and alginate impression materials also apply to the duplicating materials.

EVALUATION PROGRAM: American Dental Association Specification No. 20 delineates the physical and chemical properties of duplicating materials.[3]

DUPLICATING COMPOUNDS

Do:

1. Remove master cast from mold with a snapping action.
2. Pour the mold immediately.
3. Wash the gel after each use to remove gypsum contaminants before reusing.
4. Store in a plastic bag or other environment that will provide 100 percent relative humidity.

Don't:

1. Reuse the reversible products beyond the manufacturer's recommendations.
2. Store in water.

AVAILABLE PRODUCTS

Duplicating Colloid, Teledyne Dental Products
DUPLI-COE-LOID, Coe Laboratories, Inc.
Duplitex, Whip-Mix Corp.
Korvel, Teledyne Dental Products
R & R Multi-Gel, Ransom and Randolph Company
Surgident Duplicating Compound, Lactona Corp., Subsidiary of Warner-Lambert Co.

LITERATURE REFERENCES

1. Anderson, J. N. Applied dental materials. ed. 5, Oxford, Blackwell Scientific, 1976.
2. Craig, R. G.; O'Brien, W. J.; and Powers, J. M. Dental materials: Properties and manipulation. St. Louis, C. V. Mosby, 1975.
3. Guide to dental materials and devices. ed. 7, Chicago, American Dental Association, 1974-75.
4. Guide to dental materials and devices. ed. 8, Chicago, American Dental Association, 1976.
5. Craig, R. G., and Peyton, F. A. Restorative dental materials. ed. 5, St. Louis, C. V. Mosby, 1975.
6. Phillips, R. W. Skinner's science of dental materials. ed. 7, Philadelphia, W. B. Saunders, 1973.
7. Stackhouse, J. A. A comparison of elastic impression materials. J. Prosthet. Dent. 34:305 Sept. 1975.
8. Lorren, R. A., et al. The contact angles of die stone in impression materials. J. Prosthet. Dent. 36:176 Aug. 1976.
9. Sawyer, H. F., et al. Accuracy of casts produced from three classes of elastomeric impression materials. JADA 89:644 Sept. 1974.
10. Jorgenson, K. D. A new method of recording the elastic recovery of dental impression materials. Scand. J. Dent. 84:175 May 1976.
11. Cooney, J. P. A comparison of silver-plated and stone dies from rubber base impressions. J. Prosthet. Dent. 32:262 Sept. 1974.
12. Herfort, T. W., et al. Tear strength of elastomeric impression materials. J. Prosthet. Dent. 39:59 Jan. 1978.
13. Herfort, T. W., et al. Viscosity of elastomeric impression materials. J. Prosthet. Dent. 38:396 Oct. 1977.
14. Sieweke, J. C.; Eames, W. B.; and Wallace, S. W. Elastomeric impression materials: effect of bulk on accuracy. J. Dent. Res. 56(B):B147, 1977.
15. Davis, G. B., et al. The bonding properties of elastomeric tray adhesives. J. Prosthet. Dent. 36:278 Sept. 1976.
16. Gunther, G., and Welsh, S. L. Evaluation of a rubber-base impression material. J. Prosthet. Dent. 39:95 Jan. 1978.
17. Fusayama, T., et al. Accuracy of the laminated single impression technique with silicone materials. J. Prosthet. Dent. 32:270 Sept. 1974.

18. Goldberg, A. J. Viscoelastic properties of silicone, polysulfide, and polyether impression materials. J. Dent. Res. 53:1033 Sept.-Oct. 1974.

19. Kaloyannides, T. M. Mixtures of elastomeric impression materials of the same group: II. Permanent deformation. J. Dent. Res. 53:1491 Nov.-Dec. 1974.

20. Hembree, J. H., Jr., et al. Effect of moisture on polyether impression materials. JADA 89:1134 Nov. 1974.

21. Luebke, R. J.; Scandrett, F. R.; and Kerber, P. E. The effect of delayed and second pours on the dimensional stability of elastomeric impression materials. J. Dent. Res. 56 (B):B148, 1977.

22. Craig, R. G. A review of properties of rubber impression materials. J. Mich. Dent. Assoc. 59:254 Apr. 1977.

23. Council on Dental Materials and Devices: Status report on polyether impression materials. JADA 95:126 July 1977.

WAXES

Waxes are among the oldest materials used in dentistry. Beeswax, for example, has been used to produce impressions of areas of the mouth for more than 200 years. A wax is a high molecular weight organic molecule. Dental waxes are mixtures of plant, animal, mineral, and synthetic waxes with resins and even metallic fillers. The physical and mechanical properties that characterize a dental wax are determined primarily by the amount of hydrocarbon and ester waxes present, by the molecular weight distribution of each component, and by the amount of impurities present.

Dental waxes are characterized by high coefficients of thermal expansion, by flow that may or may not be desirable depending on the use of the wax, and by a tendency for stress relaxation with accompanying dimensional changes and distortions.

INLAY CASTING WAX

COMPOSITION: The compositions of the commercial inlay waxes are not published but a survey of the literature shows that paraffin wax, carnauba wax, ceresin wax, beeswax, candelilla wax, and gum dammar have been used as constituents. Thermogravimetric and differential thermal analysis curves for three dental inlay waxes—Kerr hard, Kerr regular and Peck's purple hard—did, however, indicate the amount of carnauba wax present as well as the type of hydrocarbon wax used.[1] Coleman[2] reported a thermal expansion of 0.72 percent (an average coefficient of $600 \times 10^{-6}/°C$) between 28 and 40°C for an experimental wax consisting of 60 percent paraffin [55°C (131°F) melting point], 25 percent carnauba wax, 10 percent ceresin wax, 5 percent refined beeswax, and a very small amount of oil-soluble coloring material. The use of synthetic waxes in the formulation of dental inlay waxes is now permitted by the Specification Program of the Council on Dental Materials, Instruments and Equipment.

USES: Dental inlay casting waxes are divided into three types in the third revision of American Dental Association Specification No. 4. The intended uses for the three types are: Type A, a hard or low-flow wax that is used in some indirect techniques; Type B (formerly Type I), used for direct techniques; and Type C (formerly Type II), used for indirect techniques in the production of inlays and crowns.

PROPERTIES AND DIRECTIONS FOR USE: Ohashi and Paffenbarger[3] reported average coefficients of thermal expansion over the range of 25 to 37°C as low as 240 x 10^{-6}/°C for a Type B inlay wax and as high as 530 x 10^{-6}/°C for a Type C inlay wax.

A high coefficient of thermal expansion is one of the disadvantages that is inherent in waxes. Unless the dimensional change of a wax pattern going from mouth to room temperature is controlled or compensated for, a shrinkage error of from 0.30 to 0.36 percent will occur in modern Type B inlay waxes.

Linear thermal expansion of the direct type wax (Type B) is permitted, as delineated by Specification No. 4, to a maximum of 0.6 percent linear change in dimension when heated from 25.0 to 37.0°C (77.0 to 98.6°F) and 0.2 percent when heated from 25.0 to 30.0°C (77.0 to 86.0°F). It is not possible to have the wax pattern at room temperature when it fits the cavity.[4] Therefore, one should compensate for the expected linear shrinkage that occurs when the wax is cooled from mouth to room temperature. One method is to hold the pattern at mouth temperature while the investment is setting. This can be accomplished by placing the casting ring with its pattern into a water bath slightly above mouth temperature, 37.8°C (100°F), immediately after investing.[5] However, the possibility of distortion when the pattern is held at an elevated temperature should not be overlooked. In practice, the particular compensating technique employed must consider the thermal shrinkage of the pattern.

Although no requirement concerning thermal expansion of the indirect types of waxes is given in the specification, some manufacturers provide this information with their waxes as a guide to users of the water immersion or water-added

hygroscopic techniques. Type C waxes give appreciably larger castings than Type B waxes when using the warming bath (complete or partial immersion) because of the appreciably greater flow and generally higher thermal expansion of Type C waxes.[1,6]

Two other important properties controlled by the specification are amount of flow and residue after burnout. Each of these may contribute to inaccuracies in restorations if not controlled. The specification prescribes a wax having a maximum nonvolatile residue of 0.10 percent. Incomplete burnout, caused by excessive residue, may prevent the casting of sharp margins or may cause back pressure to impede the flow of gold into the mold which will result in an incomplete casting.

The flow of dental waxes is influenced by the presence of solid-solid and melting transformations that occur in the component waxes. The transformation temperatures can be related to flow indirectly by studying the resistance of the wax to penetration as a function of temperature.[7] At a high stress level, the temperature of the solid-solid transformation associated with the hydrocarbon component of the wax determines the resistance to penetration of a dental inlay wax.

If an inlay wax, used in the direct technique, is too soft, i.e., has too high a flow at mouth temperature, distortion of the pattern may occur upon removal from the tooth. Chilling a soft wax in an attempt to harden it to prevent distortion during removal causes the surface to shrink and sets up stresses which, on partial release at room temperature, may result in distortion. It is best to use a wax that is hard at mouth temperature (maximum of 1.0 percent flow) so that the possibility of distortion is lessened. The same reasoning holds true for the maximum of 1.0 percent flow permitted at 30.0°C (86.0°F) for an indirect inlay wax removed from a die at or near room temperature. The minimum and maximum flow requirements for the three types of waxes at elevated temperatures insure that the waxes will have sufficient flow for forming the wax pattern yet safeguard against a wax which might melt at too low a temperature. The flow requirements of the specification are given in Table I.

The melting ranges, cooling curves, flow and thermal expansion curves have been reported for natural, commercial, and dental waxes as well as mixtures of natural waxes.[8-10] Differential thermal analysis has been used to determine the temperature of transitions of waxes between 20 and 200°C.[11]

Calorimetric analysis has been employed to determine heats of transition and fusion of dental and commercial waxes between 0 and 100°C.[12] In addition, the stress-strain properties

Table I.

Flow Requirements of
A.D.A. Specification No. 5
for Dental Inlay Casting Wax

Flow (percent)		Wax Temperature (°C)		
Min.	Max.	Type A	Type B	Type C
–	1	43	37	34
1	15	46	40	37
50	85	49	43	40
70	90	52	46	43

INLAY CASTING WAXES

Do:

1. Soften a wax uniformly by heating at about 50°C (122°F) for at least 15 minutes before manipulation.[14]
2. Add fresh wax periodically to a molten wax pot, since volatile components may evaporate with time.
3. Use warmed carving instruments and a warmed die to minimize the introduction of residual stresses in the wax.
4. Add wax to the die in small increments to minimize dimensional changes caused by solidification and thermal contraction.
5. Have the temperature of the wax at the moment of contact with the cavity or die well above the annealing temperature of 50°C (122°F) for good impressions.
6. Form indirect wax patterns under hydraulic pressure or swaging for improved accuracy.[15]
7. Use a combination of waxes with a low modulus of elasticity in occlusal areas and a high modulus of elasticity in proximal areas to minimize distortion when a hygroscopic expansion

investment technique is used.[6]

8. Invest a wax pattern immediately to prevent distortion from slight reheating or storage at room temperature for longer than 30 minutes before investing.[16]
9. Store the pattern in a refrigerator, if storage cannot be avoided.[16]
10. Allow a refrigerated wax pattern to warm to room temperature before it is invested.
11. Use a solid wax sprue or hollow metal sprue filled with sticky wax to minimize distortion of the pattern during spruing.
12. Readapt margins if the pattern was stored.
13. Leave the pattern on the die if shipping to a dental laboratory.

Don't:

1. Use a heated solid metal sprue for spruing, because the heat could cause localized warming and distortion.
2. Repeatedly remove and then replace a wax pattern on its die, because the margins are likely to distort.
3. Store at elevated temperatures or for an extended period of time at room temperature.

of natural and dental inlay waxes have been measured.[6] These studies showed that carnauba wax has little and beeswax has no effect on the melting point of paraffin wax; the principal effect of the addition of carnauba wax is to increase the melting range and to reduce the flow. Smaller amounts of carnauba are needed to control the melting range rather than the flow. Addition of beeswax to paraffin wax produces smaller increases in the melting range and decreases in the flow. Increasing the melting range may be accomplished by compounding waxes or by selecting appropriate natural or synthetic waxes with broad melting transitions. The stress-strain properties of waxes have shown that inlay waxes could be prepared with a range of mechanical properties.

EVALUATION PROGRAM: The properties of certain dental waxes are characterized by American Dental Association Specifications.[13] The third revision of Specification No. 4 for Dental Inlay Casting Wax became effective on January 1, 1976.

AVAILABLE PRODUCTS

TYPE B. MEDIUM

Dentsply Biowax, Dentsply International, Inc.
TAGGERT'S BLUE, Mizzy, Inc.
KERR INLAY CASTING WAX: BLUE, GREEN, IVORY, Kerr Mfg. Co., Div. of Sybron Corp.
Inlay Waxes, Regular, Hard; No. 6, Whip-Mix Corp.

BASE PLATE WAX

COMPOSITION: The compositions of the commercial base plate waxes are not published but probably consist of natural and synthetic waxes, resins and hydrocarbon waxes of the paraffin series. A typical composition might include 80 percent ceresin, 12 percent beeswax, 2.5 percent carnauba, 3 percent natural or synthetic resins, and 2.5 percent microcrystalline or synthetic waxes.

PROPERTIES: There is relatively little published information on the properties of base plate wax. Several reports[6-12] provide information on flow and other properties of ingredient waxes which may be used in the formulation of base plate as well as other dental waxes. Ohashi and Paffenbarger[3] list two base plate waxes in a report on the melting, flow and thermal expansion characteristics of some dental and commercial waxes. They report values of 62 and 58°C for melting point and 220×10^{-6} and 390×10^{-6} per °C for the average thermal expansion between 25 and 37°C for the two base plate waxes. These values of thermal expansion and flow at various temperatures are within or near the range of values reported for inlay waxes. As the similarity of properties indicates, base plate waxes have the same disadvantages of high thermal expansion and stress relaxation with associated dimensional changes that are characteristic of inlay waxes. Smyd[17] discussed the effects of the high thermal expansion of base plate wax in causing dimensional changes and called attention particularly to the effect of spot heating of the wax in introducing strains into the wax and subsequent distortion from stress relaxation. He also pointed out that the heat from setting plaster may cause expansion and distortion of the wax pattern. Distortion may be minimized by reducing as much as possible both the temperature to which the pattern is elevated and the time during which it is at an elevated temperature. Smith, Earnshaw and McCrorie[18] determined the flow, brittleness, moldability, carvability and thermal change on solidification of modeling and base plate waxes (on the British market) and concluded that only three of thirty-five tested had the desired combination of low plasticity at mouth temperatures with good ductility.

USES: Waxes which are used in the construction of artificial dentures are classified into three types: Type I, a soft wax for building contours and veneers; Type II, a medium wax; and Type III, a hard wax for use at higher temperatures.

EVALUATION PROGRAM: American Dental Association Specification No. 24, which applies to

Types I, II, and III base plate waxes became effective on December 1, 1971. The three types of waxes are differentiated by requirements which specify different minimum and maximum limits for flow when loads are applied to specimens of the waxes at various test temperatures (Table II). For example, a Type II medium wax must have between 50 and 90 percent flow at 45°C while the flow of Type III hard wax must be between 5 and 50 percent at this temperature. To help minimize dimensional changes and distortion of wax patterns, the thermal expansion of the base plate wax is limited to 0.8 percent between 25 and 40°C.

Requirements relating to working characteristics of the wax specify that softened sheets shall cohere readily, that the wax shall soften without becoming flaky or crumbly and without adhering to the fingers, that it can be trimmed easily and cleanly with a sharp instrument, and that it shall have a smooth glossy surface after gentle flaming. It is also specified that no residue that is visually detectable shall be left after a wax base plate containing plastic or porcelain teeth is flushed from the flask with a boiling water-detergent solution. Other sections of the specification require that the material shall not have an unpleasant odor or flavor, shall not normally irritate oral tissues and that sheets of the wax and separating paper shall separate cleanly after storage.

BASE PLATE WAX

Do:
1. Manipulate the wax at or above its working temperature to minimize incorporation of residual stresses.
2. Flask the waxed denture soon after completion to maintain the greatest accuracy of tooth relations.

Don't:
1. "Pool" the wax with a hot spatula.
2. Overheat areas of wax with an alcohol torch during polishing.

Table II.

Flow Requirements of
A.D.A. Specification No. 24
for Dental Base Plate Wax

Type of Wax	Temperature (°C)	Flow (percent)	
		Min.	Max.
Type I	23	–	1.0
	37	45.0	85.0
	45	–	–
Type II	23	–	0.6
	37	–	2.5
	45	50.0	90.0
Type III	23	–	0.2
	37	–	1.2
	45	5.0	50.0

AVAILABLE PRODUCTS

ALLCEZON BASE PLATE WAX, Mizzy, Inc.
BEAUTY PINK WAX, MEDIUM TYPE II, Moyco Industries, Inc.
Caulk Hi-Heat No. 158; Pink Base Plate, Temproof Wax, L.D. Caulk Co., Div. of Dentsply International, Inc.
Dentsply Neowax Flexible, Dentsply International, Inc.
Dentsply Roll-O-Wax, Dentsply International, Inc.
Dentsply Truwax, Dentsply International, Inc.
HYGIENIC NO. 3 MEDIUM SOFT PINK, Hygienic Dental Mfg. Co.
HYGIENIC EXTRA TOUGH PINK, Hygienic Dental Mfg. Co.
HYGIENIC EXTRA HARD PINK, Hygienic Dental Mfg. Co.
Kerr Set Up Wax #2 Regular, Kerr Mfg. Co., Div. of Sybron Dental Products
Kerr Set Up Wax #5, #10, Kerr Mfg. Co., Div. of Sybron Dental Products
Lab Wax, Modern Materials Mfg. Co.
Mizzy Tuff-Flex, Mizzy, Inc.
Modern Pink No. 3, Modern Materials Mfg. Co.
Red Base Plate Wax, Modern Materials Mfg. Co.
Sure Wax; Sure Wax Extra Hard, Modern Materials Mfg. Co.

MISCELLANEOUS WAXES

Casting Wax

Casting wax is used to fabricate the pattern for the metallic framework of removable partial dentures and other similar structures. These waxes are available in bulk or in the form of sheets or ready-made shapes. Casting waxes probably are formulated from paraffin, ceresin, beeswax, resins, and other waxes. There is no American Dental Association Specification for these waxes, but Federal Specification No. U-W-140[19] includes values for softening temperatures, amount of flow at various temperatures, general working qualities, and other characteristics. The flow characteristics of casting wax show a maximum of 10 percent flow at 35°C and a minimum of 60 percent flow at 38°C. Casting waxes must be pliable, have true gauge dimensions, and vaporize completely at about 500°C with no other residue than carbon.

Sticky Wax

Sticky wax is used on dental stones and plasters and to assemble metallic or resin pieces in a fixed temporary position. Sticky waxes are formulated from yellow beeswax, high or low amounts of rosin and perhaps gum dammar. There is no American Dental Association Specification for these waxes, but Federal Specification No. U-W-00149a (DSA-DM)[19] includes values for flow, residue on burnout, and shrinkage on cooling. At 30°C, sticky wax must have a maximum flow of 5 percent, whereas at 43°C, it must have a minimum of 90 percent. The maximum allowable shrinkage is 0.5 percent at temperatures between 43°C and 28°C. Sticky wax will adhere closely to the surface upon which it is applied when melted, but is somewhat brittle at room temperature. It is desirable for sticky wax to fracture rather than flow if deformed during soldering or repair procedures.

Boxing Wax

Boxing wax is used to form a wax box around an impression of an arch into which freshly mixed plaster or stone can be poured. Usually a narrow stick or strip of wax is adopted around the impression below its peripheral height, followed by a wide strip of wax that produces a form around the entire impression. There is no American Dental Association Specification for boxing wax, but Federal Specification No. U-W-138[19] stipulates that boxing wax should be pliable at 21°C and retain its shape at 35°C. Care should be exercised when application of boxing wax is made to hydrocolloid or rubber base impressions, since these impression materials can distort during the boxing procedure.

Utility Wax

Utility wax is an easily workable, adhesive wax that has numerous applications. For example, utility wax is used to contour trays for use with hydrocolloid impressions or on the lingual portion of a bridge pontic to stabilize it while a labial plaster splint is poured. Utility wax probably is formulated from beeswax, petrolatum and other soft waxes. There is no American Dental Association Specification for utility wax, but Federal Specification No. U-W-156[19] includes requirements for flow, pliability, tackiness, and adhesiveness. The flow of utility wax should not be less than 65 percent nor more than 80 percent at 37.5°C.

Bite Registration Wax

Bite registration wax is used to articulate accurately certain models of opposing quadrants. The wax bite registration for the copper plated die must provide proximal as well as occlusal relations. Bite registrations frequently are made from 28-gauge casting wax sheets or from hard base plate wax, but waxes identified as bite waxes appear to be formulated from beeswax or from hydrocarbon waxes such as paraffin or ceresin.[20] Certain bite waxes contain aluminum or copper particles. There are no American Dental Association or Federal specifications for bite waxes. The flow of several bite waxes as measured by penetration at 37°C range from 2.5 to 22 percent[20] indicating that these waxes are susceptible to distortion upon removal from the mouth.

Corrective Impression Wax

Corrective impression wax is used as a wax veneer over an original impression to contact and register the detail of the soft tissues. It is claimed that this type of impression material records the mucous membrane and underlying tissues in a functional state in which movable tissue is displaced to such a degree that functional contact with the base of the denture is obtained. Corrective waxes appear to be formulated from hydrocarbon waxes such as paraffin and ceresin and may contain metal particles.[20] There are no American Dental Association or Federal specifications for corrective impression waxes. The flow of several corrective waxes as measured by penetration at 37°C is 100 percent. These waxes are subject to distortion during removal from the mouth.

LITERATURE REFERENCES

1. Craig, R.G.; Powers, J.M.; and Peyton, F.A. Thermogravimetric analysis of waxes. J. Dent. Res. 50:450 Mar.-Apr. 1971.
2. Coleman, R.L. Physical properties of dental materials (gold alloys and accessory materials). Res. Paper No. 32. J. Research NBS 1:867 Dec. 1928.
3. Ohashi, M., and Paffenbarger, G.C. Melting, flow, and thermal expansion characteristics of some dental and commercial waxes. JADA 72:1141 May 1966.
4. Taylor, N.O., and Paffenbarger, G.C. A survey of current inlay casting technics. JADA 17:2058 Nov. 1930.
5. Markley, M.R. Compensation by thermal expansion. J. Prosthet. Dent. 3:419 May 1953.
6. Craig, R.G.; Eick, J.D.; and Peyton, F.A. Strength properties of waxes at various temperatures and their application. J. Dent. Res. 46:300 Jan.-Feb. 1967.
7. Powers, J.M., and Craig, R.G. Penetration of commercial and dental waxes. J. Dent. Res. 53:402, 1974.
8. Craig, R.G.; Eick, J.D.: and Peyton, F.A. Properties of natural waxes used in dentistry. J. Dent. Res. 44:1308 Nov.-Dec. 1965.
9. Craig, R.G.; Eick, J.D.; and Peyton, F.A. Flow of binary and tertiary mixtures of waxes. J. Dent. Res. 45:397 Mar.-Apr. 1966.
10. Ohashi, M., and Paffenbarger, G.C. Some flow characteristics at 37°C of ternary wax mixtures that may have some possible dental uses. J. Nihon Univ. Sch. Dent. 11:109 Sept. 1969.
11. Craig, R.G.; Powers, J.M.; and Peyton, F.A. Differential thermal analysis of commercial and dental waxes. J. Dent. Res. 46:1090 Sept.-Oct. 1967.
12. Powers, J.M.: Craig, R.G.; and Peyton, F.A. Calorimetric analysis of commercial and dental waxes. J. Dent. Res. 48:1165 Nov.-Dec. 1970.
13. Guide to dental materials and devices. ed. 7. Chicago, American Dental Association, 1974.
14. Lasaster, R.L. Control of wax distortion. JADA 27:518 Apr. 1940.
15. Mahler, D.B. Casting fit using the water bath technic. I.A.D.R. Program and Abstracts of Papers, p. 80, Abstract 178, 1967.
16. Phillips, R.W., and Biggs, D.D. Distortion of wax patterns as influenced by storage time, storage temperature and temperature of wax manipulation. JADA 41:28 July 1950.
17. Smyd, E.S. Wax, refractory investments and related subjects in dental technology. J. Prosthet. Dent. 5:514 July 1955.
18. Smith, D.C.; Earnshaw, R.; and McCrorie, J.W. Some properties of modelling and baseplate waxes. Br. Dent. J. 118:437 May 1965.
19. U.S. General Services Administration, Federal Supply Service, Federal Specifications No. U-W-138, May 12, 1947, Wax, boxing, dental; No. U-W-140, March 16, 1953, Wax, casting, dental; No. U-W-00149a (DSA-DM), Sept. 9, 1966, Wax, sticky, dental; No. U-W-156, Aug. 17, 1948, Wax, utility, dental.
20. Powers, J.M., and Craig, R.G. Thermal analysis of dental impression waxes. J. Dent. Res. 57:37 Jan. 1978.

GYPSUM PRODUCTS AND INVESTMENTS

Gypsum derived materials serve a wide spectrum of uses in dentistry; as impression plaster, dental plaster for study and reference models, improved dental stones for casts, molds to form complete dentures, and as a binder in soldering and low-temperature casting and investments. The high-temperature casting investments contain phosphate, phosphate and colloidal silica in combination, and organic orthosilicates as binders of quartz and cristobalite grain.

Utilization of gypsum alabaster by man for artistic purposes is ancient. The plaster products of gypsum were investigated by alchemists of the Middle Ages. Phosphate and silicate binders originated in the refractory brick and foundry trades of the later 19th and early 20th centuries.

Gypsum products used in dentistry are produced by heat treatment of mineral gypsum, which chemically is calcium sulfate dihydrate, $CaSO_4 \cdot 2H_2O$. In this heat treatment the dihydrate is converted to the hemihydrate, $CaSO_4 \cdot \frac{1}{2}H_2O$, commonly known as plaster of Paris.

All of the gypsum products of dentistry are chemically the hemihydrates; however, they differ in their physical properties because of differences in the hemihydrate crystal size and arrangement.

PLASTER AND STONE

COMPOSITION: Dental plaster which resembles ordinary building plaster is produced by heating mineral gypsum in an open kettle at temperatures of 110 to 120° C. This produces slender crystals which are porous and relatively soft.

USES: Impression plasters are designated as Type I and are discussed elsewhere in the *Dentist's Desk Reference* (page 182). Type II model plasters are suitable for study, repair and reference casts, interarch registration assemblies, and for flasking dentures.[1]

Unimproved dental stone known as Type III (Hydrocal) is produced by driving off water of crystallization under an elevated steam pressure at about 125° C. The product produced has a lower surface area per unit of mass than dental plaster.[2] Type III stones are particularly suitable for casts used to construct dentures.

Improved dental stone (Type IV Densite) commonly is produced by dehydration in an autoclave in the presence of sodium succinate or in a kettle with a 30 percent calcium chloride solution.[2] Improved stones are recommended because of their accuracy and strength where metal parts are to be fitted over teeth. They function particularly well as crown-and-bridge casts.

DIRECTIONS FOR USE: To mix dental model (Type II), stone (Type III), and improved stone (Type IV) approximately 40 to 50, 30 to 40, and 22 to 24 ml of water are required, respectively, per 100 grams of gypsum product. When the powder is mixed with water, it should be spatulated to obtain a smooth mix, first slightly by hand spatulation and then, under vacuum, by motor-mechanical spatulation. Good mixing yields a dense gypsum product with a minimum of large bubbles.

An increase in the amount of spatulation decreases the initial setting time and increases the setting expansion. The greater the water-to-powder ratio, i.e., the cubic centimeters of water to a gram of powder, the greater the initial setting time and the lower the setting expansion. Within limits, the lower the water-to-powder ratio, the greater the compressive strength. Also, set gypsum products are weaker when wet than dry.

Besides being affected by manipulation and mixing conditions, addition of chemicals may change the setting time and setting expansion. For example, very small amounts of certain chemicals such as K_2SO_4, ground up set plaster, and stone accelerate setting while others such as borax ($Na_2B_4O_7 \cdot 10H_2O$) and sodium citrate retard setting.

Immersion of the gypsum casts in water after mixing and pouring maximizes the setting expansion. The increased expansion so obtained is called hygroscopic or wet-setting expansion. In general, for gypsum products increasing the temperature of water used for mixing from 20 to

---

PLASTER AND STONE

Do:

1. Use the proper ratio of water to powder; if difficulty in volume measurements is encountered, use weight measurements.
2. Use only uncontaminated powder, and avoid any that has crystallized lumps.
3. Place water in a mixing bowl (rubber or soft plastic) first, and slowly sift powder into the water, thereby avoiding the introduction of air bubbles.
4. Pour immediately after mixing.
5. Use a saturated plaster-water solution when casts are soaked for duplication or are placed in boiling water to remove wax in order to prevent loss of the surface.
6. Wait approximately 24 hours to develop the full strength of a cast.

Don't:

1. Store gypsum products in unsealed containers for prolonged periods.
2. Whip or fold the powder mix with water. To do so increases the chance of incorporating air.
3. Scrape or chip casts with a steel instrument while waxing.
4. Use the casts within 45 to 60 minutes after pouring.

37° shortens the initial setting time; above 37° C the initial setting time is lengthened.[2]

EVALUATION PROGRAM: American Dental Association Specification No. 25 for dental gypsum products specifies that all materials must be uniform and free of lumps and when tested according to specifications shall be capable of reproducing a 0.050 mm-wide groove.[3] A setting time of 10 ± 3 minutes is required for all products except impression plaster, which requires 4 ± 1.5 minutes. No plasters are acceptable in Specification No. 25 which when wet sieved have more than 2 weight percent retained on a 100 mesh or more than 10 weight percent on a 200 mesh sieve.

Maximum permitted linear setting expansions, which correspond to the accuracy required for typical uses of the various gypsum products are: for Type II, 0.30 percent; Type III, 0.20 percent; and Type IV, 0.10 percent. The consistency of Types II, III, and IV gypsum products required in Specification No. 25 is the same. Minimum compressive strengths required also reflect differences in use of these products and are for Types II, III, and IV, 8.8, 20.6, and 34.3 MN/m² respectively.[1] Increase in stone hardness appears to be associated with increase in compressive strength.

AVAILABLE PRODUCTS

TYPE I, PLASTER IMPRESSION

Cloverleaf XX Quickset, J. E. Healy Co.
Impression Plaster, Modern Materials Mfg. Co.
Impressotex, Whip-Mix Corp.
Microtrue, Whip-Mix Corp.
R&R Orthodontic Plaster, Ransom and Randolph Company
Snow White Plaster #2, Kerr Mfg. Co., Div. of Sybron Corp.
Solutex, Whip-Mix Corp.

TYPE II, PLASTER, MODEL

CLOVERLEAF LABORATORY PLASTER, J. E. Healy Co.
Easycut Plaster, Modern Materials Mfg. Co.
KERR SNOW WHITE PLASTER NO. 1, Kerr Mfg. Co., Div. of Sybron Corp.
Lab Plaster, Modern Material Mfg. Co.
LABORATORY PLASTER, Whip-Mix Corp.
MODEL PLASTER, GRADE A, Whip-Mix Corp.
Orthodontic Plaster, White, Whip-Mix Corp.
Orthodontic Plaster, Modern Materials Mfg. Co.
Plaster, Pre-Vest, Inc.

R&R MODEL PLASTER, Ransom and Randolph Company

TYPE III, DENTAL STONE

Bitestone-White, Whip-Mix Corp.
CASTONE, Ransom and Randolph Company
COECAL BUFF, WHITE, Coe Laboratories, Inc.
Denstone, Modern Materials Mfg. Co.
Die-Keen, Modern Materials Mfg. Co.
Die Stone, Modern Materials Mfg.Co.
Flasking Stone, Whip-Mix Corp.
Flasking Stone, Modern Materials Mfg. Co.
Hydrotex Dental Stone, Whip-Mix Corp.
India Die Stone, Lactona Corp., Div. Warner-Lambert Corp.
Laboratory Stone, Whip-Mix Corp.
Labstone, Modern Materials Mfg. Co.
MICROSTONE, Whip-Mix Corp.
Mounting Stone, White, Whip-Mix Corp.
Orthodontic Stone, Super White, Whip-Mix Corp.
O-67 Snow White Stone, Modern Materials Mfg. Co.
Pre-Vest Stone, Pre-Vest Inc.
QUICKSTONE, Whip-Mix Corp.
RAPID STONE, Kerr Mfg. Div. of Sybron Dental Products
Surgident Functional Bite Stone, Sterndent Corp.

TYPE IV, DENTAL STONE HIGH STRENGTH

DIE ROCK, Whip-Mix Corp.
DUROC, Ransom and Randolph Company
Master Model Stone, Pre-Vest, Inc.
R&R Laboratory Stone, Ransom and Randolph Company
SILKY ROCK, Whip-Mix Corp.
Super-Die (vivid yellow), Whip-Mix Corp.
True-Stone, True Stone Fast-Set, Modern Materials Mfg. Co.
UTK Blue die stone, Unitek Corp.
VELMIX STONE, Kerr Mfg. Co., Div. of Sybron Corp.

GYPSUM-BONDED INVESTMENTS

COMPOSITION: Gypsum-bonded investment powders contain cristobalite or a mixture of quartz and cristobalite mixed with calcium-sulfate hemihydrate which forms the set bond.

Quartz and cristobalite refractory grain provide most of the thermal expansion on burnout. One investment, Investic (Ticonium Inc., Albany, New York), used for casting partial dentures from a low-melting base-metal alloy, has only quartz as the refractory grain. Other chemicals, e.g., sodium chloride, boric oxide, potassium sulfate, graphite, copper powder, and calcined magnesia, are added in small quantities to modify atmosphere, strength, setting, and thermal expansion properties.[4]

USES: Gypsum-bonded investments usually are used for the casting of gold alloys and should not be heated to temperatures greater than 700°C. The types of gypsum-bonded investments are defined in Specification No. 2 on the basis of their use and method of expansion to compensate for casting shrinkage. Types I and II investments are both used for casting gold alloy inlays and crowns; however, expansion in Type I is effected thermally with some additional expansion resulting from setting in air. Expansion in Type II investments is produced primarily by hygroscopic means with limited expansion produced thermally. Type III investments are used for casting partial dentures of gold alloy and low-melting chromium-base alloys; i.e., those that melt about 1,300°C. The majority of expansion of these investments is obtained thermally while final expansion occurs during air setting.

DIRECTIONS FOR USE: Hygroscopic expansion in Type II investments is accomplished usually by total immersion of the invested wax pattern in water. Ordinarily, the wax pattern is invested inside a steel ring lined with a wet or moistened asbestos liner. Most often, the investment casing is immersed in the water bath immediately after pouring of the investing slurry.

To expand the wax pattern and to lessen its resilience to hygroscopic expansion, the water bath temperature is commonly set at an elevated temperature, most frequently at 37° to 38°C. In the handling of investments in which air or dry setting expansion is desired, either a dry or slightly moist asbestos-lined steel ring may be used to hold the investment casing. A

GYPSUM-BONDED INVESTMENTS

Do:
1. Keep investment well mixed by turning container over and up repeatedly before use, and then let settle for a few minutes.
2. Use only fresh investment; especially avoid investments which have been stored for a prolonged period in a humid atmosphere.
3. Keep investment containers closed.
4. Be particularly careful in controlling times of mixing, pouring, and adding or immersing in water.

Don't:
1. Store investment at elevated temperatures.
2. Heat gypsum-bonded investments to burnout temperatures higher than 700°C.
3. Prolong standing of investment before adding of or immersing in water.
4. Mix in dirty bowls, or bowls in which phosphate-bonded investment has been used.

limited hygroscopic expansion will result if the asbestos liner is wet. Mixing is usually done in a moistened bowl.

If restrictive effects of the wax or plastic pattern are to be encountered, thermal rather than hygroscopic expansion techniques are recommended. It is more likely that hygroscopic expansion will be affected by the restrictive effects of the pattern, particularly in the construction of full crowns.

In general, the investment manufacturer's instructions should be followed carefully. However, difficulty can be encountered, depending upon the melting temperature and fluidity of the particular alloy to be cast.

It is a general rule that for a given investment the lower the fluid-to-powder ratio, the greater the setting and thermal expansions. The more thoroughly the investment is mixed, the greater the setting expansion; therefore, motor-mechanical mixing, commonly 30 seconds or more, is preferable to hand mixing.

EVALUATION PROGRAM: American Dental Association Specification No. 2 for casting investment for dental gold alloy of April, 1961 is applicable to gypsum-bonded investments.[5]

AVAILABLE PRODUCTS

TYPE I, INLAY THERMAL

ACCU-CAST INLAY INVESTMENT, Den-Tal-Ez Mfg. Co.
BEAUTY CAST, Whip-Mix Corp.
KERR CRISTOBALITE INLAY, Kerr Mfg. Co., Div. of Sybron Corp.
LUSTER CAST, Kerr Mfg. Co., Div. of Sybron Corp.
NOVOCAST, Whip-Mix Corp.
SHINY-BRITE CRISTOBALITE, Whip-Mix Corp.
WHIP-MIX CRISTOBALITE INLAY, Whip-Mix Corp.

TYPE II, INLAY HYGROSCOPIC

BEAUTY CAST, Whip-Mix Corp.
RANSOM & RANDOLPH HYGROSCOPIC INVESTMENT, Ransom and Randolph Company, Div. of Dentsply International, Inc.

TYPE III, PARTIAL DENTURE THERMAL

ACCU-CAST GRAY INVESTMENT, Den-Tal-Ez Mfg. Co.
KERR CRISTOBALITE MODEL, Kerr Mfg. Co., Div. of Sybron Corp.
R&R GRAY INVESTMENT, Ransom and Randolph Company, Div. of Dentsply International, Inc.
R&R HFG; R&R #1 Investment, Ransom and Randolph Company
SUPER MOLD, Whip-Mix Corp.

WHIP-MIX CRISTOBALITE MODEL, Whip-Mix Corp.

PHOSPHATE-BONDED INVESTMENTS

COMPOSITION AND PROPERTIES: Phosphate-bonded investments are used to cast high-melting gold alloys and base-metal alloys which melt above 1,300°C. These investments usually have a mixture of quartz and cristobalite refractory grain to give most of the thermal expansion. However, some very high temperature investments used for casting partial dentures have only quartz as the refractory grain.

Magnesium oxide in the form of calcined magnesia is incorporated in the investment powder as a setting agent. Upon addition of alkaline colloidal-silica-containing investment fluid, part of the magnesia is converted to magnesium hydroxide. Solubilized magnesium hydroxide induces precipitation of the colloidal silica and reacts with solubilized phosphate to form the early investment bond.

One of the most common water-soluble phosphates used in dental investment powders is monoammonium phosphate. If only distilled water is added, magnesium phosphates are the sole constituents of the early bond. However, most commonly a mixture of crystalline phosphate and co-precipitated colloidal silica constitute the early bond.

Upon drying at 100°C or higher, and if ammonium phosphates are solubilized to form the green bond, both ammonia and water are evolved. For a given investment brand, early strength and hardness are greater when increased amounts of colloidal silica are added. Upon burnout, a sinter bond is formed.

DIRECTIONS FOR USE: Unlike gypsum-bonded investments, the initial set of phosphate-bonded investments is accompanied by the emanation of heat, which attains in 2 in.-diameter rings, temperatures of at least 40 to 50°C. These temperatures are sufficient to fully expand and greatly soften a wax pattern.

Therefore, pouring of investment into the ring must be done before heat develops in the mix.

Spatulation should act constantly in all parts of the investing slurry so as to keep it cool. This prevents hot spots from forming in the investing slurry, which might catalyze the setting reaction and generate even more heat. The greater the amount of setting investment handled, the greater the build-up of heat.

Mixing is carried out in a moist plastic container. Manufacturers usually recommend fluid-to-powder ratios ranging from 0.14 to 0.18 ml per gm of investment powder. For any given fluid-to-powder ratio of a given investment, the less the investment liquid dilution; i.e. the higher the colloidal silica concentration, the greater the wet or dry setting expansion, and to a small extent the thermal expansion.

Fluid should either be added at once to the powder or, as may be more commonly done, the powder added to a premeasured amount of fluid. Gentle hand spatulation (about 15 seconds), to mix the added fluid, should be followed by rapid motor-mechanical mixing under vacuum (20 to 45 seconds) and then brief vacuum degassing (often 15 seconds) of the investment mix. When only hand spatulation is to be used without a vacuum, mixing should be done on a vibrator for at least 45 seconds. The working times with these investments seldom exceed four or five minutes. One can spatulate the mix at a low speed (to delay fast setting) and then vibrate the mix for 15 to 20 seconds before filling the ring to reduce trapping of bubbles.

One or two layers of asbestos are used to line the steel ring, depending upon the manufacturer's instructions. Nonasbestos ring liner materials have recently become available, which can be substituted for the asbestos liners. If partial hygroscopic expansion is desired, the liners should be wet and never pressed hard after being placed as this will reduce expansion. To obtain total hygroscopic or wet-setting expansion and inhibit overheating the wax pattern, the invested ring is immersed in water after pouring at temperatures ranging from 23 to 39°C.

Air bench setting of the invested ring after hygroscopic expansion is 45 minutes to one hour before transferring to a cold furnace for burnout. There is a high risk that putting wet investment into a furnace at high temperatures (greater than 200°C) will result in explosion or cracking of the investment. It is common practice to scrape off the top end of the investment in the ring to remove accumulated fine particles that are thought to reduce investment permeability.

In order to avoid the formation of cracks in burnout, the investments should be moist but not wet. It is often recommended, especially if the invested ring has dried out for three hours or more, that it be soaked in water 4 or 5 minutes before putting into a cold furnace. This is unnecessary if the ring is placed in a water-saturated atmosphere in a dessicator above a pool of water within one hour after pouring or after hygroscopic expansion.

In the burnout of phosphate-bonded investments, the manufacturer's recommendations should be adhered to carefully. Burnout temperatures must be suitably adjusted to obtain best castability for the particular alloy used. Too low a burnout temperature will cause incomplete filling of the mold and incomplete castings.

The maximum burnout temperatures used to cast precious and semiprecious alloys are 750 to 775°C. A common burnout temperature is 704°C. For achieving the cleanest precious-metal castings, burnout conditions should be adjusted to retain black coloration of the investment, i.e., retention of some of the graphite carbon in the investment formulations, but not that from residual ungraphitized wax which may have penetrated the investment.

For base-metal (nonprecious) alloys, the burnout temperatures used for some investments are as high as 1,000°C and are usually not lower than 844°C. Especially for the higher-melting base-metal alloys, burnout temperatures should be adjusted to achieve thin casting plates so that casting margins will be adequately developed.

Because of the high vapor pressure of base-metal alloys, super-heating to achieve adequate fluidity in an inadequately heated investment casting can result in a build-up of back pressure in the mold. Also, loss of oxygen gatherers, e.g., vaporized manganese and loss of other vaporized elements which may affect the fluidity, can cause poor castings. Attainment of peak burnout temperature usually takes at least one hour. Heat soaks at burnout generally range from 30 to 60 minutes.

EVALUATION PROGRAM: No specification has been developed for phosphate-bonded investments. American Dental Association Specification No. 2 for Casting Investment for Dental Gold Alloy for gypsum-bonded investments may be partly applicable.

PHOSPHATE-BONDED INVESTMENTS

Do:

1. Increase the colloidal silica concentration in the investment fluid to increase compensation for casting shrinkage.
2. Set the invested ring in air from 45 to 60 minutes before burnout.
3. Keep investment liquids refrigerated, but do not freeze; discard if silica precipitate forms at bottom of the container.

Don't:

1. Allow the spatulated mix to heat up before investing so as to avoid deformation of the wax pattern.
2. Cast into investment molds that are too cold to give adequate castability for the particular alloy used.

AVAILABLE PRODUCTS

Biovest, Dentsply International, Inc.
Ceramigold, Whip-Mix Corp.
Complete, J. F. Jelenko & Co., Pennwalt Corp.
Multivest, Ransom and Randolph Company
Seravest, Niranium
Vestra High-Heat Investment, Unitek Corp.

SILICATE-BONDED INVESTMENTS

COMPOSITION AND PROPERTIES: Silicate-bonded investments are the most refractory investments commonly used in dentistry. They are used for the casting of high-melting base-alloys, e.g., Vitallium (Howmedica, Ltd., Chicago, Illinois). They usually consist of refractory quartz (SiO_2) grain bonded by silica derived from the dehydrolysis of silicic acids.

Calcined magnesia is dispersed in small amounts in the investment powder and acts as a setting agent for the silicic acids. These silicic acids usually are dissolved in alcohol as ethyl orthosilicate. Volatilization of part of the alcohol increases the water concentration, which promotes hydrolysis of ethyl orthosilicate to silicic acid. Partial solution of the magnesia increases the alkalinity and dehydrolysis of the formed silicic acids. This condensation reaction forms the strong glass-like green bond between the quartz grains.

DIRECTIONS FOR USE: Refractory casts made from these investments for partial dentures are very friable and must be thoroughly impregnated with rosin and/or wax for use in the laboratory.

Two and sometimes three liquids are mixed with the investment powder; a common fluid-to-powder ratio is 0.21. Hand mixing is commonly adequate. Burnout temperatures range from 1,100 to 1,150°C. Prolonged heat soaks at peak burnout temperatures of one hour or more are common.

Almost no dimensional change occurs in the setting of silicate-bonded investments, and unlike other investments no heat is given off in setting. Therefore, these investments exhibit no expansion other than thermal, and the linear expansion obtainable with essentially no restricting stress is 1.7 percent.

The coarse-grained character of these investments makes it advantageous to use fine-grained protective coats to obtain smooth cast-

SILICATE-BONDED INVESTMENTS

Do:

1. Use protective coats whenever possible to reduce casting roughness and organic liquid attack in wax and plastic patterns.
2. Handle with extreme caution the very friable refractory casts before they are impregnated with rosin and/or wax.

Don't:

1. Store liquid binders in a hot place or where they might explode the container and flow over a flame, hot plate, oven or furnace to cause a fire.
2. Allow cracks to develop in protective coats, as this will cause fins on castings, and possibly permit attack by binder liquid on wax and plastic patterns.

ings. In the construction of partial dentures, these coats are brushed over "engineered" wax and plastic patterns on the refractory casts. In the construction of bridgework, these coats also act to protect the wax and plastic pattern from any attack by organic solvents in the liquid.

Precautions must be taken in the storage of the liquid binders. They should be stored in a cool place but not frozen. If the liquid binder becomes too hot, especially if the containers are partly empty, an explosive mixture with air may form.

EVALUATION PROGRAM: No dental specifications currently apply to these investments. Usually they are much coarser grained than either phosphate or gypsum-bonded investments.

AVAILABLE PRODUCTS

SM Hardshell Ethyl Silicate Investment, Superior Magna Co.

SOLDER INVESTMENTS

COMPOSITION: Gypsum- and phosphate-bonded investments are used as solder investments. The compositions of these investments are similar to casting investments.[6] Solder investments containing only quartz as the refractory grain are preferable to those containing cristobalite.[7] However, phosphate-bonded casting investments containing both quartz and cristobalite have been used successfully for soldering high-fusing-gold and base-metal alloys.

DIRECTIONS FOR USE: Solder investments are poured, after mixing, to encapsulate the parts to be soldered. The "sticky wax" patterns, depending upon the investment, are boiled, poured, or burned out, and the solder is melted with a flame and directed to flow into the joint.

To avoid shifting of parts to be soldered, a low setting and a low thermal expansion are desirable. Solder investments after burnout should be able to withstand heat from the soldering operation without cracking. Also, solder investments should have both a high green and burnout strength. When phosphate-bonded casting investments are used as solder investments, thermal and setting expansion is minimized by mixing only with distilled water and not with the colloidal-silica containing investment fluids.

The bridgework assembly must be firmly fixed. At least one-half to one hour for phosphate-bonded and up to two hours for gypsum-bonded investments should elapse before the set investment is trimmed. No added water must contact the solder investments, as any hygroscopic expansion is considered undesirable.

Furnace burnout, beginning from a cold furnace, rather than burnout over a flame, is recommended. At least a one-half hour soak at the peak burnout temperature is necessary. Furnace burnouts produce a uniform temperature throughout the assembly and make it possible to avoid curvature in the assembly alignment.

For the soldering of some gold alloys, gypsum-bonded solder investment commonly is used. With these investments it has been recommended that they be boiled and the wax pattern poured out. The recommended peak burnout temperature of gypsum-bonded soldering investment is 430°C. When phosphate-bonded investments are used for the higher-fusing gold and base-metal alloys, 650°C burnouts are permissible and the wax may be eliminated by volatilization and oxidation.[8]

Pre-Vest Soldering Investment, Pre-Vest, Inc.
R & R HFG Soldering Investment, Ransom and Randolph Company
R & R Multi-Vest, Ransom and Randolph Company
R & R Soldering Investment, Ransom and Randolph Company
Speed-E Soldering Investment, Whip-Mix Corp.
Whip-Mix Soldering Investment, Whip-Mix Corp.

SOLDER INVESTMENTS

Do:
1. Keep investments free of added water to avoid hygroscopic setting expansion.
2. Wait until the investment is fully set before trimming it, at least 30 minutes.
3. Eliminate all water by heating the investment to at least 400°C, for this water will inhibit soldering.

Don't:
1. Allow porcelain constructions to contact a set investment as it will discolor the porcelain; use wax overlays to prevent this.
2. Heat gypsum-bonded investments above 700°C, otherwise they will decompose.

AVAILABLE PRODUCTS

Aluminum Investment, Whip-Mix Corp.
Crown and Bridge Soldering Investment, Modern Materials Mfg. Co.
Dentsply Biovest Soldering Investment, Dentsply International Inc.
Hi-Heat Soldering Investment, Whip-Mix Corp.
Hi-Temp Liquid, Whip-Mix Corp.
Model Casting Investment, Modern Materials Mfg. Co.

AUXILIARY MATERIALS

The common auxiliaries for the handling of gypsum products and investments are:
1. *Rubber spatulas* both steel and hard rubber for mixing dental plaster and stone.
2. *Rubber and plastic bowls* that are flexible for mixing plaster and stone and sometimes investments by hand or with hand-driven mechanical devices.
3. *Clear, hard plastic containers,* used with motor-driven stainless steel mixing blades, commonly varying in capacity from 25 to 875 cc, used for mixing all gypsum products and investments.
4. *Stainless steel containers* for the same functions as the larger plastic containers.
5. *Vacuum mixers* with 425 to 1,750 RPM, with the higher speed commonly used for small mixes.
6. *Casting rings* of a steel alloy and sometimes plastic of a suitable size.
7. *Asbestos liners* with a width ¼ in. less than the height of the casting ring. Both thick and thin varieties are used, ranging from 0.4 to 0.6 mm.
8. *Sprue and crucible formers,* steel, rubber and plastic.
9. *Constant-temperature baths* for hygroscopic expansions commonly set at the factory at 37.8°C.
10. *Burnout furnaces,* low temperature and high temperature, electric- and gas-fired, respectively.

AVAILABLE PRODUCTS

Alcote Improved Tinfoil Replacement, L. D. Caulk Co.

Caulk Shellac Base Plates, L. D. Caulk Co.

Die Locaters, Pentron Corp.

Divestment, Whip-Mix Corp.

E-Z Part, Whip-Mix Corp.

Gypsum Hardener, Whip-Mix Corp.

Hygrotrol, Whip-Mix Corp.

Ney Die Lube, J. M. Ney Co.

Ney Silk Release Spray, J. M. Ney Co.

Ney Spruing System, J. M. Ney Co.

Ney 24k Gold Plate, J. M. Ney Co.

Ney 22k Light Color Plate, J. M. Ney Co.

Paper Rings, Williams Gold Refining Co., Inc.

Por Sep Release, Ceramco, Inc.

Pre-Vest Chrome Investment, Pre-Vest, Inc.

Pre-Vest Inlay Investment, Pre-Vest, Inc.

Pre-Vest Univest Investment, Pre-Vest, Inc.

R & R Colorguard Tin Foil Substitute, Ransom and Randolph Company

Stone Die & Plaster Hardener, George Taub Products Inc.

T-60 Chrome Investment, Modern Materials Mfg. Co.

Unitek Debubblizer and Wax Pattern Cleaner, Unitek Corp.

Unitek Die Lubricant, Unitek Corp.

LITERATURE REFERENCES

1. Dental gypsum products and investments. In Guide to dental materials and devices, ed. 8, Chicago, American Dental Association, Ch. 10, pp. 104-114, 1976.

2. Gypsum compounds. In Craig, R. G., and Peyton, F. A. (eds.), Restorative dental materials. St. Louis, C. V. Mosby Co., Ch. 9, pp. 252-275, 1975.

3. American Dental Association specification no. 25 for dental gypsum products. Council on Dental Materials and Devices. JADA 84:640, 1972.

4. Phillips, R. W. Skinner's science of dental materials. ed.7, Philadelphia, W. B. Saunders Co., Ch. 26, p. 412, 1973.

5. American Dental Association specification no. 2 for casting investment for dental gold alloy. In Guide to dental materials and devices. ed. 2, Chicago, American Dental Association, 1964.

6. Dental Technician, Prosthetic, Bureau of Naval Personnel NAVPERS 10685-C, 1965 Revision, p. 45.

7. Phillips, R. W. Skinner's science of dental materials. ed. 7, Philadelphia, W. B. Saunders Co., Ch. 33, pp. 563-583, 1973.

8. Friedman, M. Post-soldering ceramic alloys, quintessence of dental technology. J. Dent. Technicians 2:31 Sept. 1978.

SOLDERS AND FLUXES

Soldering is a process dating back to antiquity. Although it cannot be stated with absolute certainty, the first solders were probably lead-tin alloys, as the basic ingredients of lead and tin were readily recovered by the smelting of their ores in open pit fires or furnaces. Pliny, the Roman historian, recorded the use of lead-tin solders over 2,000 years ago. The low melting points of these alloys rendered them particularly suitable for joining sections of lead pipe that were used to supply water to ancient Rome.

Solders which are used in modern dentistry bear little resemblance in composition to those of ancient solders. Dental solders may be described as alloys which are biologically compatible in the oral environment and are specifically designed and/or employed for the purpose of fusing two pieces of dental alloy through the use of an intermediate low temperature molten filler metal. The joining process which uses solder is called soldering.

Joining processes other than soldering include brazing and welding. All can involve the use of molten filler metal; some welding processes however are conducted without filler metal. Solders have the lowest melting points with liquidus temperatures less than 800°F, brazing alloys have liquidus temperatures greater than 800°F, and welding alloys have temperatures close to those of the metal pieces to be joined (by definition of the American Welding Society). Soldering, brazing, and welding all involve the use of molten metal and owe their primary distinctions to the temperatures employed to perform the joining operations and the proximity of those temperatures to the melting points of the pieces joined. Numerous processes which are conventionally called soldering in dentistry actually utilize brazing or welding alloys; the processes are all similar in the application of heat for the purpose of fusing two pieces of metal together.

COMPOSITION AND PROPERTIES: The soldering process involves the use of solders, materials which fuse two dental alloys together, and fluxes, materials which coat the surfaces of alloys to be joined in order to produce clean metal surfaces at the temperatures of joining so that molten solder will fuse with those surfaces.

Solders: Current dental solders are fabricated from primarily corrosion resistant, nontoxic metals, often with additions of limited quantities of tin and minimal quanitites of other elements, some of which could produce toxic effects in the unalloyed state. Table I presents some typical compositions and properties of solders used in dentistry. Each solder is used for specific applications.[1-9] The inherent resistance of the primary ingredients to corrosive attack lends resistance to the overall composition, thereby rendering it safe to use in fabricating appliances to be placed in the oral environment. The precious metals, gold, platinum, palladium, and silver, are the major components of many of the solders used for joining both precious and nonprecious alloys. Some special nonprecious alloy solders also contain nickel, chromium and cobalt as primary ingredients. The variety of compositions available for the soldering of nonprecious alloys (Table I) serves to emphasize the need to use only the solder specifically designed for the alloy to be joined.

Fluxes: Fluxes are predominantly composed of salts and/or oxides of metals. Vehicles such as petroleum jelly or alcohol are often employed to facilitate handling during application.

Table I.
Representative Dental Solder Compositions and Applications

Solder	Major Elemental Composition Weight Percent												Application and Temperature Ranges
	Au	Ag	Cu	Zn	Cd	Pd	Ni	Fe	Al	Cr	Co	Sn	
Low Karat Solder	45	30-35	15-20										Orthodontic Appliances 691-816°C (1275-1500°F)
General Purpose Solder	60	12-22	12-22										Joining of gold alloy prostheses Fastening of wire clasps to partial dentures 724-835°C (1335-1535°F)
High Karat Solder	80	3-8	8-12										Joining of yellow gold alloy prostheses 746-871°C (1374-1600°F)
Nonprecious Alloy Solders	30-40					30-40	25-40			0-20			Nonprecious porcelain alloy pre-porcelain soldering
							70-85	5-10	0-3	10-15			T ≥ 1150°C (2100°F)
							60-90		0-3	3-30	3-30		
Silver Solder	42-67	15-31		15-20	0-24	0-3							Stainless steel orthodontic wires-brackets. Temporary Appliances T ~ 607-688°C (1125-1270°F)
Porcelain-Gold Solders	60-90	10-30	5-20	1-3		5-10	0-1					1-2	Joining of gold alloys prior to porcelain application T ≥ 1065°C (1950°F)

These vehicles burn or evaporate at elevated temperatures before the soldering temperature is attained, leaving behind a uniform coating of flux. Fluxes become molten before the joining temperature is reached and the molten flux flows or spreads to form a continuous coating over the surfaces to which they have been applied. Molten flux protects the underlying metal from the air, thereby preventing formation of surface oxides which would impede fusion and the formation of a strong solder joint. Fluxes may also act to dissolve surface impurities or to leach selectively elements from the surface of the underlying metal. These actions result in a surface free of obstacles to fusion and of a composition which is readily "wet" by the solder.

Antifluxes: Antifluxes are materials used to coat certain surfaces of the parts to be joined to *prevent* solder from flowing to those regions. Antifluxes are not "wet" by the solder and should be removed at the time that flux is removed.

USES: Dental solders and fluxes constitute systems used to assist in the fabrication of dental appliances by joining orthodontic wires, fastening attachments to partial dentures and crown and bridge units, joining crown and bridge units before and after the application of porcelain, and repairing fixed and removable (cast and wrought) dental appliances; for example, reattaching broken parts, "filling" voids and/or breaks in cast appliances and adding and/or improving contours of cast restorations.

DIRECTIONS FOR USE: A solder and its flux are designed to function as a system for joining specific alloys. The first step in any soldering operation is to ascertain that the flux and solder which are to be used are those which are recommended for the alloy to be joined. Once this has been done, the physical operations in preparation for soldering can commence. First, the pieces to be joined must be thoroughly cleaned; abrasive blasting or grinding with a sandpaper disc are two common techniques which are useful. Once the mating surfaces have been cleaned, they should be aligned using an ac-

ceptable procedure such as occlusal index, and stabilized for the soldering operation with an approved investment material. The adjoining parts should be contoured so as to provide only a small gap between the mating surfaces. A space of approximately 0.1 mm is desirable. Alignment of the parts on dies, or with clamps, followed by stabilization with soldering investment is an appropriate procedure. Flux then should be applied liberally to the mating surfaces. In some cases, (those involving deep or inaccessible joints) a thin coating of flux should be applied before placing the parts in a fixture. The flux thusly placed ensures protection of those surfaces against oxidation at elevated temperatures. Frequently, fluxing agents tend to flow beyond the areas intended for joining, thereby allowing the solder to fill or obliterate carefully developed contours in cast restorations. The use of an "antiflux" such as graphite from a soft lead pencil of jewelers rouge mixed with chloroform can be helpful in confining the flow of flux and solder. These materials are coated on the areas for which no solder is desired *before* the fluxing agent is applied.

After the proper surfaces of the appliance have been coated with flux, heat is applied, either with a torch or by placing the appliance into a furnace. In either case it is important to heat the parts slowly and uniformly to prevent possible warpage or inaccuracy in the alignment of the parts. If a torch is used, a slightly reducing or neutral brush flame is usually employed and applied to bulky regions near the surfaces to be joined, but *not* directly to them. The flames should consist of a sharply defined blue inner cone and a long diffuse outer region. Heat is gently applied, to prevent excessive bubbling of the flux while water and vehicles are being eliminated. As the temperature increases, the flux becomes molten and flows over the entire surface to be joined. The temperature should be raised until the solder flows when it is touched to the mating surfaces at the thicker or more bulky section. The solder should flow freely to thinner areas and wet both surfaces throughout the joint. After the solder has been applied, the flame is removed and the soldered appliance is allowed to cool under ambient conditions well below the solidification temperature; it may then be cooled more rapidly to near room temperature. The cooling rate should be chosen according to a predetermined plan to develop either a softened or hardened appliance. The appliance is then removed from the fixture and thoroughly cleaned by any of a combination of abrasive blasting, soaking in hot water or mild acidic solution, wire brushing, and sandpaper discing; manufacturers' directions should be followed. Care must be taken to completely remove old flux as most fluxes contain toxic chemicals or some compounds which could interfere with subsequent operations, such as veneering with porcelain. For example, flux which remains on bridgework which is yet to receive porcelain can cause bubbles and discoloration in the porcelain as well as negatively affect the porcelain-to-metal bond and/or promote corrosion at the joint.

In the case of soldering in a furnace, the same general procedures of heating and cooling are followed, except that a piece of solder can be laid on the junction prior to insertion into the furnace. This melts and flows if the upper furnace temperature is properly set. This temperature should be 25 to 50°F (13.9 to 27.8°C) above the liquidus temperature of the solder or be set at the solder manufacturer's recommended soldering temperature.

Do:

1. Follow the manufacturer's instructions and recommendations.
2. Use only solder and flux which are recommended as a system for joining specific alloys.
3. Clean surfaces completely of oxides, dirt, oil, or any combination in order to obtain sound joints.
4. Coat the surfaces to be soldered with a liberal, uniform application of flux.
5. Use of a gap of 0.125 to 0.250 mm (0.005 to 0.010 in.) is recommended as a guide; many use the width of a calling card for a 0.250 mm gauge.
6. Keep flux away from porcelain veneered surfaces. Coating of porcelain with wax before applying the flux is recommended.
7. Wear safety goggles and protective laboratory clothing. Molten flux can cause corrosive as well as heat burns.
8. Conduct all soldering in a well ventilated area. Fumes are given off by some fluxes and solders which may be hazardous to health.
9. Use only the correctly sized torch tip so that the flame is large enough and hot enough to raise the piece to the soldering temperature as well as supply enough heat so that the solder will melt and flow.
10. Use a neutral to slightly reducing flame. In all cases, follow the alloy and solder-flux manufacturer's suggestions.
11. Use a fine, needle-like flame for soldering orthodontic appliances; heat quickly, solder, and then cool.
12. For soldering inside of a furnace, set the temperature of the furnace at the solder-flux manufacturer's recommended temperature or 25 to 50°F (13.9 to 27.8°C) above the liquidus temperature of the solder.

13. Use solder which melts at a higher temperature than that to be encountered by subsequent soldering or porcelain applications.

14. Cool the appliance after soldering to room temperature under ambient conditions unless this is not recommended by the manufacturer or if this results in an appliance which is too soft. (See #11)

15. Remove the flux thoroughly after the soldering operation. Soaking in hot water and vigorous brushing or other abrasive cleansing is beneficial. The use of an ultrasonic cleaner with hot water or a mild acid indicated by the flux manufacturer is recommended for removing flux from inaccessible areas.

Don't:

1. Substitute for either the recommended solder or flux as they are designed to work together.

2. Rely on flux to clean surfaces. Fluxes may have cleaning capabilities but these should be reserved for cleaning away what cannot be removed by other techniques.

3. Apply flux so thickly that it is difficult to keep it from flowing to areas which should not be in contact with flux.

4. Attempt to cleanse surfaces by the use of rubber wheels or similar abrasive devices which contain organic compounds. These can leave deposits which will interfere with fluxing and soldering operations.

5. Use a flame so large that it is impossible to control the application of heat to desired areas.

6. Overheat orthodontic appliances, heat the surrounding regions, or heat longer than required.

7. Force cooling by quenching the appliance into water or other media.

8. Allow any flux to remain. All fluxing compounds can be toxic to varying degrees. Corrosive flux, allowed to remain, may also cause corrosion and weakening of the soldered joint with time.

AVAILABLE PRODUCTS

490 Fine Solder, J. M. Ney Company
490 Solder, Williams Gold Refining Co., Inc.
500 Fine, Sterngold, Div. of Sterndent
585 Fine Solder, Rx Jeneric Gold Co.
585 Fine, Sterngold, Div. of Sterndent
585 Solder, Williams Gold Refining Co., Inc.
615 Fine Solder, J. M. Ney Company
615 Fine Solder, Rx Jeneric Gold Co.
615 Fine, Sterngold, Div. of Sterndent
615 Solder, Williams Gold Refining Co., Inc.
650 Fine Solder, J. M. Ney Company
650 Fine Solder, Rx Jeneric Gold Co.
650 Fine, Sterngold, Div. of Sterndent
650 Solder, Williams Gold Refining Co., Inc.

660 RS, Rx Jeneric Gold Co.
700 Fine, Sterngold, Div. of Sterndent
729 Fine Solder, J. M. Ney Company
730 Solder, Williams Gold Refining Co., Inc.
750 Fine, Sterngold, Div. of Sterndent
#7 Flux, Williams Gold Refining Co., Inc.
809 Fine Solder, J. M. Ney Company
2225W, Sterngold, Div. of Sterndent
Auramic 1100 (White), Sterngold, Div. of Sterndent
Bak-On Yellow Solder, Ceramco, Inc.
Biobond C & B Solder, Dentsply International, Inc.
Biobond C & M Solder Flux, Dentsply International, Inc.
Ceramalloy Solder, Ceramco, Inc.

Ceramalloy Soldering Flux, Ceramco, Inc.
C. G. Solder, Rx Jeneric Gold Co.
Chrome, Sterngold, Div. of Sterndent
ECS Solder, Rx Jeneric Gold Co.
Gnatho Ceram G Solder, Rx Jeneric Gold Co.
High Fusing White Ceramic Solder, Williams
  Gold Refining Co., Inc.
High Fusing Yellow Ceramic Solder, Williams
  Gold Refining Co., Inc.
High-Temp PNP Flux, Rx Jeneric Gold Co.
Lite White Hard, Sterngold, Div. of Sterndent
Lo-Temp Flux, Rx Jeneric Gold Co.
Low Fusing Solder, Rx Jeneric Gold Co.
Mastercast 615 Solder, Ceramco, Inc.
Mastercast 650 Solder, Ceramco, Inc.
Mastercast White Solder, Ceramco, Inc.
MF-Y (Yellow), Sterngold, Div. of Sterndent
Ney Anti-Flux, J. M. Ney Company
Ney Balanced Line High Fusing Solder, J. M.
  Ney Company
Ney Balanced Line Regular Solder, J. M. Ney
  Company
Neycast Solder, J.M. Ney Company
Ney Casting Flux, J. M. Ney Company
Neydium N. P. Solder, J. M. Ney Company
Neydium N. P. Solder Flux, J. M. Ney Company
Ney Soldering Flux, J. M. Ney Company
NP Flux, Rx Jeneric Gold Co.
NP Solder, Rx Jeneric Gold Co.
Palinay Medium Fusing Solder, J. M. Ney Co.
Palinay #4 Welding Rod, Rx Jeneric Gold Co.
PNP Solder, Rx Jeneric Gold Co.
Protected Electro (White), Sterngold, Div. of
  Sterndent
Protected Electro (Yellow), Sterngold, Div. of
  Sterndent
Rx Low Fusing Flux, Rx Jeneric Gold Co.
Rx NP Flux, Rx Jeneric Gold Co.
Rx PNP Flux, Rx Jeneric Gold Co.
Satin Cast Solder, Rx Jeneric Gold Co.
Silgo Solder, Rx Jeneric Gold Co.
SMG-2 Solder, J. M. Ney Company
SMG-3 Solder, J. M. Ney Company
SMG-YW Solder, J. M. Ney Company
Special CG Solder (SpCG), Rx Jeneric Gold Co.
Steele's Spot-flux, Columbus Dental Co.
Unitek Orthodontic Silver Solder, Unitek Corp.
Unitek Orthodontic Silver Solder/Flux Paste,
  Unitek Corp.

UTK High-Fusing Gold, Unitek Corp.
UTK Low-Fusing Gold, Unitek Corp.
UTK Unibond High-Fusing Solder/Flux Paste,
  Unitek Corp.
UTK Unibond Low-Fusing Gold, Unitek Corp.
White Ceramic Solder, Rx Jeneric Gold Co.
White CG Solder (WCG), Rx Jeneric Gold Co.
White Gold High Fusing Solder, Williams Gold
  Refining Co., Inc.
White Gold Low Fusing Solder, Williams Gold
  Refining Co., Inc.
Wironit Solder, Williams Gold Refining Co., Inc.
Wironium Solder Flux, Williams Gold Refining
  Co., Inc.
Wironium Solder Rod, Williams Gold Refining
  Co., Inc.
Wiron-S Flux, Williams Gold Refining Co., Inc.
Wiron-S Solder Rod, Williams Gold Refining Co.,
  Inc.
Zephyr Foil, Williams Gold Refining Co., Inc.

LITERATURE REFERENCES

1. Brazing manual. American Welding Society, United Engineering Center, New York, 1955.

2. Johnston, J. F.; Mumford, G.; and Dykema, R. W. Modern practice in dental ceramics. Philadelphia, W. B. Saunders Co., 1967.

3. Specification B 32-60aT, ASTM Standards.

4. Soldering manual. American Welding Society, United Engineering Center, New York, 1959.

5. Metals handbook. ed. 8. American Society for Metals, pp. 1188-1189, 1961.

6. Phillips, R. W. Skinner's science of dental materials. ed. 7. Philadelphia, W. B. Saunders Co., Ch. 31-33, 1973.

7. Wise, E. M. Gold: recovery, properties and applications. Princeton, D. Van Nostrand Co., Inc., 1964.

8. Valega, T. M. (ed.) Alternatives to gold alloys in dentistry. Conference proceedings, DHEW Publication # NIH 77-1227, 1977.

9. Stade, E. H.; Reisbick, M. H.; and Preston, J. D. Preceramic and postceramic solder joints. J. Prosthet. Dent. 34:527 Nov. 1975.

RADIOGRAPHIC MATERIALS

RADIOGRAPHIC FILMS

COMPOSITION: Radiographic films consist of emulsions on flat sheetlike bases. The emulsions are capable of interacting with photons of radiation to form a latent image from which a visible image can be created. Typical emulsions consist predominantly of silver halides. Creation of an image on radiographic film involves reduction of silver ions to elemental silver in the regions where photons of radiation were absorbed. Typical film bases consist of transparent polyesters.

Film images are usually viewed by transmitted light. In general, regions of low exposure have high transmissions of light and therefore low optical densities. Regions of high exposure have low transmissions of light and therefore high optical densities. For example, radiolucent structures are characterized by high optical densities and appear as dark regions; radiopaque structures are characterized by low optical densities and appear as light regions.

TYPES: The basic types of radiographic films are those primarily sensitive to x-radiation and those primarily sensitive to visible light. The light sensitive films are intended for use in combination with fluorescent intensifying screens. Intensifying screens give off multiple photons of visible light for each photon of incident x-radiation, and therefore, increase the efficiency of the radiographic process. The light sensitive films can be further subdivided into blue light sensitive films and green light sensitive films. Most intensifying screens have their peak emissions in either the blue or the green regions.

Radiographic films have some sensitivity to both x-radiation and visible light; all films should be protected from inadvertent exposure by either source.

The x-ray sensitive films are usually used for procedures in which films are positioned intraorally. The intraoral film is of necessity packaged individually in moisture resistant packets. Some packets contain two films so that two original images are created.

Light sensitive films are usually used for procedures in which the film is positioned extra-orally. The film is generally supplied in bulk packages and loaded manually into a cassette in combination with intensifying screens.

Screen-film combinations are not ordinarily used intraorally although some research is being directed toward that application.[1,2]

It also should be pointed out that there are non-film types of image receptors. For example, xeroradiography makes use of an electrically charged selenium plate for the formation of the latent image. The image may be transferred to opaque paper or to transparent film.[3]

PROPERTIES: There are many technical factors that collectively influence the performance of radiographic film. Sensitometric curves are one of the fundamental methods for describing the performance of a radiographic film or film-screen combination.[4-8] These curves are a graph of response, usually in terms of optical density, with respect to exposure. Exposure is usually scaled logarithmically. From sensitometric curves a measure of efficiency usually expressed as speed, contrast, exposure latitude, and dynamic range can be obtained.

Speed is usually considered to be the reciprocal of the exposure required to create an optical density of 1.0 above gross fog. Gross fog is base optical density plus net fog. Base optical density is the inherent optical density of the film base. Net fog is the spontaneously caused non-radiographic optical density of the emulsion. Speed is an indication of the amount of exposure required to produce an image. Speed may be categorized by speed groups. Table I gives the speed groups designated in ANSI/ADA Specification No. 22.

Contrast[4-8] is related to the increment of optical density caused by an increment of exposure and is the basic phenomenon that permits differences in the subject to be recorded in an image. Contrast varies as a function of exposure. A sensitometric curve enables one to determine the exposure at which maximum contrast occurs.

Exposure latitude[4-8] is the range of exposure over which useful contrast can be obtained.

Table I.

Speed groups.

Speed group*	Speed Range (in reciprocal roentgens)
C	6.0-12.0
D	12.0-24.0
E	24.0-48.0
F	48.0-96.0

The upper limit of each speed range shall be excluded from that range.

*Speed groups A and B, the two slowest speed groups given in American National Standard Speed Classifications for Intraoral Dental Radiographic Film: Diagnostic Grade, PH6.1-1961, are not covered by this specification because of radiological health considerations associated with excessive radiation exposure.

Latitude is a factor of the variation of tissue types, densities, and thicknesses that can be imaged on a particular film.

Dynamic range[4-8] refers to the optical density range corresponding to the exposure latitude. The optical density range determines the total number of discernibly different gray levels that can contribute to image formation.

Sensitometric curves are generated at constant exposure intensities because time and intensity are not interchangeable for some films and screen-film combinations. This lack of interchangeability is known as reciprocity failure. Due to reciprocity failure, some receptors exhibit an optimum efficiency at a particular time and intensity.[5,6] The optimum is usually skewed toward short times and high intensities.[5,6] Sensitometric curves are also affected by the beam quality of the x-ray generator and by the film processing conditions. Accordingly, a particular radiographic facility should generate sensitometric curves with the radiographic technique factors and processing conditions used at that facility.

Sensitometric curves can be used as a means of film processing quality control. In essence, the procedure is to give a film a series of standard exposures and to make a sensitometric curve when the processing conditions are known to be ideal. The procedure is repeated with film from the same batch at various intervals in the future. If the subsequent curves exhibit poorer responses than the original curve, then an apparent degeneration in the quality of the processing has been detected.

Other important properties of radiographic films that are not derived from sensitometric curves are noise and resolution. Noise in an image is small-scale fluctuations in optical density that are not present in the subject being imaged, but rather, are introduced by the radiographic system. Inherent sources of noise in films and screen-film combinations are the grain structure of the fluorescing agents in the intensifying screens. Resolution is the dependence of contrast upon spatial frequency. Spatial frequency is a measure of the dimensional scale of the subject to be imaged. Both noise and resolution relate to the imaging and perception of small-scale detail.[5,6,9]

The properties of radiographic films are generally interdependent. For example, resolution is usually inversely related to speed, and, exposure latitude is frequently inversely related to contrast.[10]

USES: Radiographic films are used in conjunction with x-ray generators to create radiographic images. The images are used in virtually all aspects of dentistry where radiographic information is desired for diagnosis, treatment planning, and carrying out treatment procedures.

DIRECTIONS FOR USE: A clinician should attempt to select a film or film-screen combination and radiographic technique factors that best perform the visual tasks for which the image is being made. In case of screen-film combinations, it is important to properly match the properties of the screen and the films. The highest speed receptor available that will provide the desired information should be used. This practice helps to minimize the radiational dose to the patient, tends to reduce motion blur, and probably helps to prolong the lifetime of the x-ray generator.[11]

Once a particular film has been selected for a specific task, it is imperative to employ proper exposure and optimum processing conditions to use the radiographic process efficiently and to minimize the radiational dose to the patient. The recommendations are generally included in the manufacturer's instructions.

The instructions for proper darkroom "safelighting" should also be carefully observed. The safelights that are suitable for one type of film are not necessarily appropriate for another type of film. A sensible approach is to use darkroom safelights that are suitable for x-ray sensitive film and both blue and green light sensitive films. It is advisable to test the suitability of darkroom safelighting for all of the films to be used in a particular darkroom.[12] This can be accomplished by covering part of a film with a coin and exposing the remainder to the safelights for the maximum time that film might be unprotected during handling and processing. After the film is processed, if the portion of the film not covered by the coin can be distinguished as darker than the portion covered by the coin, then the darkroom lighting is not "safe" for that film.

Another important consideration is to observe instructions regarding film storage and expiration dates. Time, radiation and heat cause spontaneous conversion of the emulsion such that the optical density of a film is increased without exposure to radiation. The expiration date of film can be prolonged by refrigeration; however, prior to refrigeration one should ascertain that the packaging will protect the film from moisture condensation. Refrigerated film should not be unpackaged until it has returned to room temperature to avoid moisture condensation.

EVALUATION PROGRAM: The Council on Dental Materials, Instruments and Equipment of the American Dental Association has a Specification No. 22 which delineates important features of intraoral dental x-ray film.

AVAILABLE PRODUCTS

Fuji X-Ray Film, Dental Corp. of America
Kodak Blue Brand Film (alternate interleaved), Eastman-Kodak Company

RADIOGRAPHIC FILMS

Do:

1. Match properties of intensifying screens and films for screen-film combinations.
2. Make sensitometric curves for all types of films and screen-film combinations used.
3. Coordinate receptor properties and radiographic technique factors to obtain needed information with the lowest practical radiational dose to the patient.
4. Observe the manufacturer's instructions regarding safelighting, processing, storage, and expiration.

Don't:

1. Overexpose and underprocess films.

Kodak Blue Brand Panoramic (not interleaved), Eastman-Kodak Company
Kodak No Screen Film (interleaved), Eastman-Kodak Company
Kodak No Screen Film-Ready Pack, Eastman-Kodak Company
Kodak Occlusal Ultra-Speed Dental X-Ray Film, Eastman-Kodak Company
Kodak Periapical Ultra-Speed Dental X-Ray Film, Eastman-Kodak Company
Kodak SB Film (interleaved), Eastman-Kodak Company
Kodak SB Panoramic (single coated; blue sensitive; interleaved), Eastman-Kodak Company
KODAK ULTRA-SPEED DENTAL X-RAY FILM, Eastman-Kodak Company
Kodak X-Omat RP Panoramic (not interleaved), Eastman-Kodak Company
Kodak X-Omat RP Film (alternate interleaved), Eastman-Kodak Company
Kodak X-Omat R Panoramic (not interleaved), Eastman-Kodak Company
Kodak X-Omat R Film (alternate interleaved), Eastman-Kodak Company
Kodak X-Omat L Film (alternate interleaved), Eastman-Kodak Company

Kodak X-Omatic G Panoramic (not interleaved), Eastman-Kodak Company
Kodak X-Omatic G Film (not interleaved), Eastman-Kodak Company
RINN "AUTO" SERIES INTRAORAL DENTAL X-RAY FILM, Rinn Corp.

RADIOGRAPHIC FILM PROCESSING CHEMICALS

Radiographic film processing chemicals are solutions used to transform a latent image into a clinically useful visible image on radiographic film. Processing chemicals generally consist of a developer and a fixer solution. An intermediate stop bath may also be used.

TYPES: Processing chemicals may be classified as those for automatic processing and those for manual processing. Manual processing chemicals may be further classified on the basis of processing time as rapid or standard. Some solutions are provided ready to use, others must be made up from powder or liquid components.

DIRECTIONS FOR USE: To obtain good results, it is important to use the processing chemicals recommended for the specific type of radiographic film being processed. Chemicals for processing films should be used with the recommended combination of time and temperature and with adequate agitation during processing.

Proper washing of films between or after use of processing chemicals is important for archival quality films. Momentary washing or a stop bath solution should be used between the developer and fixer solution. Care should be taken to avoid contamination of solutions. It is particularly important that the developer not be contaminated by fixer or stop bath solutions.

Processing solutions may degenerate with use and time. A processing quality control procedure should be conducted routinely to monitor the status of the solutions and to replenish and replace solutions as required.[13,14] The lifetime of processing solutions may be prolonged by storage at reduced temperatures when not being used and by avoiding contact with air. Exposure to air can be minimized by the use of floating tops on processing tanks and by storage in a stoppered container with no air space at the top.

Recovery of silver from processing materials is possible; however, the economics of silver recovery are probably dependent upon the overall number, size and type of films processed.

Care should be taken to avoid skin contact or eye contamination with processing chemicals. See Chapter 1 for further information regarding safe handling of processing chemicals.

RADIOGRAPHIC FILM PROCESSING CHEMICALS

Do:
1. Use processing chemicals recommended for the type of film being processed.
2. Use processing chemicals at recommended times and temperatures and with adequate agitation.
3. Monitor the condition of processing solutions by a processing quality assurance procedure.
4. Replenish and replace processing solutions as indicated.
5. Maintain and store processing solutions in a manner to prolong their lifetime.

Don't:
1. Contaminate the developer with fixer or stop bath solutions.

AVAILABLE PRODUCTS

Formula 1090 Monobath X-ray Solution, J. R. Rand Specialty Co., Inc.

Kodak Anti-Static Solution, Eastman-Kodak Company

Kodak Dental X-ray Developer, Eastman-Kodak Company

Kodak Dental X-ray Developer and Fixer, Eastman-Kodak Company

Kodak Dental X-ray Fixer, Eastman-Kodak Company

Kodak Developer Systems Cleaner, Eastman-Kodak Company

Kodak Farmer's Reducer, Eastman-Kodak Company

Kodak Fixer System Cleaner, Eastman-Kodak Company

Liquid X-ray Developer & Replenisher, Eastman-Kodak Company

Kodak Rapid Fixer, Eastman-Kodak Company

Kodak RP X-Omat Developer Starter, Eastman-Kodak Company

Kodak RP X-Omat Developer Replenisher, Eastman-Kodak Company

Kodak RP X-Omat Fixer and Replenisher, Eastman-Kodak Company

Kodak X-Omatic Intensifying Screen Cleaner, Eastman-Kodak Company

Premier Quik-check, Premier Dental Products Co.

Sta-Kleen, Premier Dental Products Co.

Ten & Twenty X-ray Developer-Fixer Solution Kit, J. R. Rand Specialty Co., Inc.

X-Ray Automatic Processor Fixer, Healthco, Inc.

DUPLICATING FILMS

USES: Duplicating films are specifically formulated for making copies of original radiographs.

DIRECTIONS FOR USE: Copies of radiographs are made by a process similar to that for making contact prints in photography.[15] It is important that good contact is established between the emulsion side of the original film and the emulsion side of the duplicating film to achieve good resolution. If the original is a double emulsion type of film, then either side can be in contact with the emulsion side of the duplicating film. For a single emulsion film the emulsion side can be identified by its dull appearance when viewed obliquely. The non-emulsion side appears shiny when viewed obliquely.

An ultraviolet light source should be used with duplicating films to obtain contrast in the copies that is similar to the original.[15]

Duplicating film is a reversal type of film; namely, the greater the exposure the lower the optical density.

The manufacturer's instructions for processing, safelighting, storage and expiration should be followed carefully to obtain good results.

Do:

1. Use good contact between the emulsion of the original and the duplicating film.
2. Use an ultraviolet light source.
3. Follow instructions for processing, safelighting, storage, and expiration.

AVAILABLE PRODUCTS

DCA X-Ray Film Duplicator, Dental Corp. of America

Kodak X-Omat Duplicating Film (not interleaved), Eastman-Kodak Company

LITERATURE REFERENCES

1. Schoenfeld, C. M.; Moore, B. K.; and Lin, P.J. Measurements of resolution and image noise for dental radiography. J. Dent. Res. 55:B242 Feb. 1976.

2. Dawood, F. F., and Manson-Hing, L. R. Evaluation of new radiographic screens for intraoral radiography. Oral Surg., Oral Med., Oral Path. 48:178 Aug. 1979.

3. White, S. C., and Gratt, B. M. Clinical trials of intraoral dental xeroradiography. JADA 99:810 Nov. 1979.

4. Sensitometric properties of x-ray films. Eastman-Kodak Co. Rochester, New York.

5. Johns. H. E., and Cunningham, J. R. The physics of radiology. Springfield, Illinois, Charles C. Thomas, 1974.

6. Ter-Pogossion, M. M. The physical aspects of diagnostic radiography. New York, Hoeber, 1976.

7. Seeman, H. E. Physical and photographic principles of medical radiography. New York, John Wiley and Sons, 1968.

8. Webber, R. L., and Ryge, G. R. The significance of exposure parameters in dental radiography. Oral Surg., Oral Med., Oral Path. 27:740 June 1969.

9. Wagner, R. F. Toward a unified view of radiological imaging systems. Part II: noisy images. Medical Physics 4:279 Aug. 1977.

10. Rao, G. U. V.; Fatouros, P. P.; and James, A. E. Physical characteristics of modern radiographic screen—film systems. Invest. Rad. 13:460 Sept.-Oct. 1978.

11. Reiskin, A. E., et al. Rare earth imaging in dental radiology. J. Prev. Dent. 4:7 May-June 1977.

12. X-rays in dentistry. Eastman-Kodak Co. Rochester, New York.

13. Gray, J. E., Photographic quality assurance in diagnostic radiology, nuclear medicine, and radiation therapy. HEW Publication (FDA) 76-8043, U.S. Department of Health, Education, and Welfare, 1976.

14. Film processing (supplement to Radiography in modern industry). Eastman-Kodak Co. Rochester, New York.

15. Allen, M. J., and Silha, R. E. New copiers for dental radiograph duplicating film. Dent. Radiog. Photog. 49:14, 1976.

Instruments

ROTARY CUTTING, FINISHING AND POLISHING INSTRUMENTS

DENTAL HANDPIECES

Dental handpieces are precision devices designed to use various types of rotary instruments such as dental burs and diamond stones. The handpieces are driven by connection to a power source, usually either compressed air or an electric motor.

USES: Handpieces provide the means to hold rotary instruments used to cut cavity or crown restorations in human teeth or to perform finishing and polishing operations. They hold rotary instruments for: removing dental or osseous tissue for a surgical procedure, adjusting the occlusion of teeth, adjusting restorations already in the mouth, adjusting removable prosthetic appliances, and cutting, grinding, or polishing restorations.

TYPES: Dental handpieces are usually classified by the maximum rotational speed of a rotary instrument in place. The currently proposed classification is shown in Table I.

Table I.
Classification of Dental Handpieces

Type I, High Speed	
Class A	Greater than 160,000 rpm
Class B	100,000 to 160,000 rpm
Type II, Mid Speed	20,000 to 100,000 rpm
Type III, Low Speed	Less than 20,000 rpm

Dental handpieces also may be classified according to the driving mechanism, such as air turbine, water turbine, electric motor, belt driven or gear driven. They may also be classified as to the use application: a) straight handpiece, b) contra-angle handpiece, and c) prophylaxis angle handpiece.

223

High Speed Dental Handpieces: High speed air turbine dental handpieces are currently available with free-running speeds in excess of 400,000 rpm. The speed depends on the type of turbine, the air pressure and the volume of air used, and the friction in the bearings. The free-running speed may be reduced up to 40 percent during a cutting operation because of the low torque characteristics of Type I handpieces.[1] This low torque feature is, in effect, a safety feature because the handpiece will stall if the operator applies too much force. However, Type I high speed handpieces are by far the most efficient for the removal of tooth structures.

Engineering design features of these handpieces are all similar. Control of the air flow to the handpiece is by a foot controlled valve. Air passing through the handpiece turns the turbine which drives the rotary instrument held concentrically in the shaft of the turbine. Some of the air escapes through the head of the handpiece but most of the air is exhausted through the back end of the handpiece. These handpieces are all of a contra-angle design for convenience and efficiency of use in the mouth.

Air bearing high speed turbine handpieces have been developed in which air suspends the turbine by a thin layer of air between bearing surfaces. These air-bearing handpieces require dry, clean, and pure air for operation. They also require greater operating air pressures than the miniature ball bearing type; pressure between 50 psi to as much as 70 psi is not uncommon,[2,3] while the ball bearing types operate with 30 psi to 50 psi pressure.

Mid Speed Handpieces: Handpieces in this speed range, Type II, are also used for cavity preparation, but they do not remove tooth structures as fast as high speed handpieces. However, Type II handpieces are useful for selected procedures if visibility is difficult or if a better tactile sense is desired by the operator. Handpieces in this group may be air-driven ball bearing type, belt driven, or powered by a miniature electric motor attached to the rear of the handpiece. Both contra-angle handpieces and straight handpieces with contra-angle and pro-phylaxis angles are available. Handpieces designed especially for use in dental laboratories are also available in the mid speed range.

Low Speed Handpieces: Low speed or conventional dental handpieces operating at a free running speed of less than 20,000 rpm are classified as Type III in a forthcoming proposal for a Standard for Dental Handpieces. This handpiece classification includes the motor-operated, belt-driven, conventional dental handpiece, as well as air-driven handpieces designed to be operated at less than 20,000 rpm. Typically these are straight handpieces with right and contra-angle attachments to be used with either latch type or friction grip rotary instruments. Traditionally, these are sleeve bearing handpieces and are suitable for slow speed, high torque applications. They are not very effective for the removal of hard tissue, but are very well suited for finishing and polishing procedures, dental prophylaxis, and laboratory procedures.

PROPERTIES: The evolution of rotary equipment for dental use is summarized in Table II.[4] The dates indicate the approximate year in which the instruments became commercially available to the dental profession and the increase in rotational speed illustrates dentistry's continued efforts and advancements toward the most practical and effective method of removing tooth tissue with the least discomfort and inconvenience for the patient and dentist.

Vibration and Head Dimensions: It was demonstrated very early that rotary instruments operating in the high-speed range caused less vibration perception by the patient than those operating at conventional speeds[5] since the high speed vibration, which carries low force, is of high frequency and above the patient's ability to perceive. This characteristic, combined with the high precision of the bearing and chucking mechanism of the high-speed instruments, makes them relatively free from the sensation of vibration, which is a convenience to the dentist and a comfort to the patient. The low vibration characteristics are a favorable quality of most high-speed handpieces.[2]

Table II.

Historical Background of Rotary
Dental Equipment

Date	Instrument	Speed (rpm)
1728	Hand driven rotary instruments	300
1871	Foot driven engine	700
1874	Electric engine	1,000
1914	Dental unit	4,000
1942	Diamond cutting instruments	5,000
1946	Conversion of old units to increase speed	10,000
1947	Tungsten carbide burs	12,000
1953	Ball bearing handpieces	25,000
1955	Water driven turbine handpiece	50,000
1955	Belt driven angle handpiece	180,000
1957	Air driven turbine angle handpiece with ball bearings	250,000
1961	Air driven turbine straight handpiece	25,000
1962	Air driven turbine angle handpiece with air bearings	800,000

Specially designed rotary instruments with extra length are available. If more length lies beyond the chucking mechanism than is held within the chuck, minor eccentricities may be amplified at ultraspeeds to produce a force sufficient to bend the instrument. Therefore, it is recommended that such instruments be limited to the low- or intermediate-speed range.

The head dimensions of the high-speed, contra-angle handpiece have been reduced in recent years, with the introduction of a miniature head by some manufacturers and a smaller standard head by others.

The smaller heads appear to be serviceable and acceptable to the profession for many operations; this indicates a trend and improvement in design. However, handpieces using standard length rotary instruments have about the same overall length from tip of cutting instrument to back of handpiece. The miniature head design can accommodate the miniature friction-grip bur or diamond instrument, which is about 3 mm shorter in overall length than the regular friction-grip diamond or bur. This total reduction in dimension of the rotary instrument and handpiece head is a definite convenience for certain operations.[2]

Water and Air Coolants: Most dental handpieces are designed to include an air-water spray or a stream of water or air, directed on the rotating instrument in the area of cutting, with some providing adjustment in direction. When the tooth is being cut, these auxiliary facilities are desirable to assist in dissipating the frictional heat of cutting and trauma to pulp tissue. The air-water spray is the most widely used coolant system.[6] Air alone, directed into the area of operation is claimed by some clinicians to be adequate protection, on the basis of clinical response and specific conditions of operation. The ability of the handpiece to direct the air or water stream or spray is critical, and it can vary with the handpiece design and operation to be performed. Under optimum operating conditions, the rotary instrument in the ultra-high speed handpiece causes a minimum of pulp tissue reaction and trauma. Patient apprehension and discomfort is less with instruments in the high speed handpiece provided with coolants, than with handpieces running at conventional operating speeds.[2]

Fiber Optics Illumination: A fiber optics illumination system in high speed handpieces is considered to be a desirable feature by many operators. However, some of these systems transmit a light beam of yellow color which is undesirable to some operators. The fiber optics systems are an aid to improved vision during the shaping of cavity and crown preparations.

Handpiece Sounds and Noise: All dental handpieces have individual noise characteristics related to the design and use. The sound and noise levels produced by dental handpieces should be less than 75 decibels to cause no concern for damage to the hearing of either operator, patient, or dental auxiliary. Permanent hearing loss due to sound from present day dental handpieces is not expected. However, precautions should be used if damage is suspected.

DIRECTIONS FOR USE: There are hazards along with advantages of improved handpieces and rotary cutting instruments operating at high speeds. There is a certain amount of trauma involved with any restorative dental procedure, and numerous pulp studies have been published. The greatest amount of trauma to the pulp occurs during cavity preparations. The heat which is caused by the friction of rotary cutting instruments during the removal of enamel and dentin has been considered to be the greatest cause of injury to the pulp. The amount of heat generated is proportional to 1) an increase in rpm of the instrument, 2) the pressure applied against the tooth, 3) the area of contact of the instrument, and 4) the amount of uninterrupted cutting time. Reducing any of these factors together with the use of a cooling water spray decreases the heating effects.

The operator should be aware of possible pulp damage by excessive heat. The most effective way to minimize the generation of heat when using rotary cutting instruments is by the use of coolants. Air, water, and the air-water spray are commonly used. The air-water spray is the most convenient method of cooling; less water is used but the amount of cooling is comparable to air or water alone.[4-6]

Protection of Soft Tissue: Rotary instruments operated in the mouth are a potential for damage to soft tissue regardless of the operating speed. Tongue, gingiva, lips, and cheeks are very susceptible to injury. Cotton roll holders, rubber dams, tongue depressors, and other devices should be used to assist in protecting the soft tissues from injury. Burs and other rotary instruments should be stopped completely before being placed into or removed from the mouth during a procedure.

Air Contamination: Contamination of air occurs in the area of operation when using either air or an air-water spray. Microorganisms and saliva may combine with an air-water spray to make a potentially hazardous source of cross infection to those in the operating area. Surgical masks worn by the operator are very effective and their use is encouraged. High velocity

---

DENTAL HANDPIECES

Do:

1. Select the appropriate type of handpiece for the procedure to be accomplished.
2. Remember that Type I high speed handpieces should be used at optimum pressure for maximum efficiency.
3. Remember that Types II and III handpieces are operable at much lower speeds but with much greater torque and tactile sense.
4. Recognize that adequate cooling is necessary with higher operating speeds, and that an air-water spray is most efficient.
5. Follow the manufacturer's instructions for routine care and maintenance of handpieces.

Don't:

1. Use high speed handpieces in poorly ventilated areas.
2. Use handpieces which are not capable of being sterilized.
3. Use handpieces which produce a noise level greater than 75 decibels.

---

evacuation equipment helps significantly in the reduction of air contamination.[2].

Lubrication and Sterilization of Dental Handpieces: As the design has been changed along with increased speeds, the proper lubrication of the bearings has become critical to maintain serviceability. Oil, grease or aerosol lubricants are often used. Whatever the lubricant of choice, careful adherence to the manufacturer's directions enhances the reliability of handpieces.

The sterilization of dental handpieces is a necessary routine procedure. This is mandatory to reduce the transmission of infectious diseases between patients. Sterilization may be accomplished by use of an autoclave, dry heat or ethylene oxide.[2] New models of sterilizable high speed handpieces are available and manufacturer's directions must be followed carefully to maintain serviceability.

AVAILABLE PRODUCTS

A-dec Handpiece 5000, A-dec, Inc.

Air Turbine Handpiece, Great Lakes Orthodontic Products

Bur Removing Wrench, J.R. Rand Specialty Co., Inc.

Contra Angle, J. R. Rand Specialty Co., Inc.

Contra Angle, Young Dental Mfg.

Dental Hand Instruments, Healthco, Inc.

Dentsply Airator "GW" Handpiece, Dentsply International, Inc.

Dentsply Borden Airator I, Dentsply International, Inc.

Dentsply Borden Airator II, Dentsply International, Inc.

Dentsply Triad Handpiece, Dentsply International, Inc.

Handpiece Control Unit Components, Zirc Dental Products

Handpiece, Doriot, J.R. Rand Specialty Co., Inc.

Healthco Contra Angle Friction Grip; Contra Angle Latch Type; Contra Angle "U" Type, Healthco, Inc.

Healthco High Speed Air Turbine Miniature Handpiece; Standard Handpiece, Healthco, Inc.

High Speed Ball Bearing Air Turbine, Miltex Instrument Co.

Model 220Z Air Turbine Handpiece System, Shofu Dental Corp.

Premier H-dent Angles & Hand Pieces, Premier Dental Products Co.

Prophy Angle, J.R. Rand Specialty Co., Inc.

Prophy-Solv, Young Dental Mfg.

Slow Speed Doriot, Miltex Instrument Co.

Unitek High Speed Air Turbine Handpiece, Unitek Corp.

Unitek High Speed Straight Handpiece, Unitek Corp.

Unitek Prophy Angles and Contra-Angles, Unitek Corp.

EXCAVATING BURS

The term "bur" applies to all rotary instruments which have cutting blades as part of the head. Dental burs are rotary cutting instruments designed for use in the removal of tooth structure and bone. Prior to the 1940's these burs were made of carbon steel. The availability of tungsten carbide burs about 1947 contributed significantly to the development of high speed handpieces which would not have been practical with carbon steel burs.

PROPERTIES: With the increased use of high speed handpieces, steel burs are rarely used except for a few low speed operations. Larger size burs have been eliminated by some manufacturers. Longer fissure burs are now produced, as well as smaller diameter round burs. The greatest change in bur design may be the slight rounding of sharp corners of inverted cone and fissure burs.[4] Newer burs having 12, 20, and 40 blades have been designed for smoother preparations and finishing procedures. Recently newer crosscut fissure burs have been designed for the rapid removal of old restorations. A summary of the bur shapes and sizes currently available is depicted in Table III.

A comparison of the cutting efficiency of fissure burs at high speed was done by Eames and Nale[7] in 1973. Their study concluded that crosscut fissure burs are more efficient than plain fissure burs. They also found that there was a great variation in the cutting efficiency of burs of nine manufacturers.

USES: Dental burs are mainly used to remove tooth structure in the excavation of caries and the shaping of cavity preparations to receive restorative materials. In addition, they are used in the preparation of teeth to be restored with partial or full veneer crowns.

Dental burs are also used for the adjustment of the occlusal surfaces of natural teeth, the removal of bone during surgery, the shaping and finishing of dental restorations, and the adjustment of prosthetic appliances.

EVALUATION PROGRAM: The sizes, shapes, and dimensions of both steel and carbide burs are given in the revised American Dental Association Specification No. 23. Dental manufacturers continue to produce an even larger vari-

Table III.

Bur Shapes and USA Sizes

Shapes	Sizes
Round (plain and crosscut)	#½-11
Wheel	11½-16
Inverted cone	33½-40
Straight fissure (plain, crosscut, rounded)	55½-563
Tapered fissure (plain, crosscut and rounded end, normal length and long length)	169-702L
Pear shape (normal and long length)	330-333L
End cutting (including end and side cutting)	901-959

ety of burs to meet the dentist's needs; therefore, some newer bur designs are not covered in the specification. Burs are classified according to the type of handpiece with which they are used, either straight or angle handpieces. Angle handpiece burs are categorized as to the type of shank, either latch, taper shank, or friction grip.

Specification No. 23, in addition to standardizing the nomenclature of dental burs, includes test and evaluations for the factors which affect the durability of the burs. The total evaluation of all rotary cutting instruments must include the following: 1) shape and dimensions, 2) strength, and 3) performance characteristics.[8]

AVAILABLE PRODUCTS

Autoclavable Bur Blocks, North Pacific Dental, Inc.
BRASSELER BURS, Brasseler USA, Inc.
Carbide Burs, Healthco. Inc.
Carbide Burs, Pentron Corp., Rx Jeneric Gold Co.
Carbide Excavating Burs, Miltex Instrument Co.
Dica Burs, Mizzy, Inc.
MILTEX MEISINGER BURS, Miltex Instrument Co.
MIDWEST AMERICAN BURS, Midwest American, Div. of American Hospital Supply Corp.

EXCAVATING BURS

Do:
1. Use a bur of appropriate size and shape for the operation being performed.
2. Consider using burs of newer designs for their intended purposes.
3. Take precautions to prevent damage to soft tissues.

Don't:
1. Use burs which are too large for the procedure.
2. Use damaged or worn out burs.

Mini Carbide Burs, Healthco, Inc.
Premier ELA Carbide Burs, Premier Dental Products Co.
Premier ELA Finishing & Burnishing Burs, Premier Dental Products Co.
Premier ELA Steel Burs–Latch Type or Hand Piece, Premier Dental Products Co.
Premier ELA Steel Surgical Burs—Right Angle and Handpiece, Premier Dental Products Co.
R & R Cutwell Carbide Friction Grip Burs, Ransom and Randolph Co.
R & R Cutwell Carbide RA & HP Burs, Ransom and Randolph Co.
R & R Cutwell Steel Burs, Ransom and Randolph Co.
Steel Excavating Burs, Miltex Instrument Co.
Surgical Carbide Burs, Healthco, Inc.
T & F Carbide Burs, Healthco, Inc.

DIAMOND ROTARY INSTRUMENTS

Rotary diamond instruments are cutting instruments consisting of one to three layers of diamond particles bonded to an instrument blank. The mesh size of the diamond grit determines the fineness or coarseness of the diamond instrument.

TYPES: Diamond rotary cutting instruments are available in almost 400 sizes and shapes to fit conventional straight handpieces, latch type and friction grip contra-angle handpieces. All manufacturers use one piece bur blanks; the diamond grit is electro-plated onto the blank using a nickel or chromium bonding material. Some manufacturers use only natural diamond grits but some also use synthetic diamond grits. There is a difference of opinion among manufacturers as to the uniformity of the surface relative to cutting characteristics and durability. The manner in which these instruments are used, particularly at high speed, may be more important than the construction. Reder and Eames[9] found that cutting efficiency varied from lot to lot, and found that the use of water was very important to reduce clogging of the instrument. An evaluation of diamond points was conducted by Janota[10] using scanning electron microscopy. He concluded that there was considerable difference in the quality of the diamond points, and that the best instruments appeared to be those with even spacing of the abrasive diamond grit. He noted also that diamonds are used under arduous conditions, various methods and techniques are used, and the skill and clinical technique of the operator must be considered in trying to evaluate rotary diamond instruments. Many dentists use diamond rotary cutting instruments without a water spray, thereby reducing the effectiveness and the durability of the instrument.

USES: Rotary diamond instruments are used mainly to prepare teeth to be restored with some type of casting, although they may also be used for the removal of old restorations and for making routine cavity preparations.

Rotary diamond instruments are used to a limited extent for the occlusal adjustment of teeth, and for contouring bone during surgery. Extremely fine diamonds may also be used for finishing procedures on selected restorative materials.

DIRECTIONS FOR USE: Diamond rotary cutting instruments should be selected based on the operation to be accomplished. Extra coarse grit instruments are to be used for the removal of bone and fibrous tissue during surgery. Coarse grit instruments are to be used for the bulk removal of tooth structure. Regular or medium grit instruments are designed for routine preparations involving enamel and dentin. Fine grit instruments may be used to finish the walls and margins of preparations. Extra fine, very fine, or super fine grit diamonds are intended for finishing the surfaces of composite restorations.

For maximum efficiency, an adequate volume of water in a spray should be used in the removal of tooth structure, and for the routine preparation of teeth for restorative materials. However, the intermittent use of fine diamonds without water may be desirable for the placement of finish lines on preparations.

DIAMOND ROTARY INSTRUMENTS

Do:

1. Select an instrument of appropriate size, shape and grit for the procedure.
2. Maintain adequate cooling when using high speeds to make preparations.
3. Use precautions to prevent damage to soft tissues.

Don't:

1. Use instruments which are excessively large for a given procedure.
2. Use instruments which are damaged, which do not run true, or which do not cut efficiently.

AVAILABLE PRODUCTS

CFI Precision Tooth Contouring Diamonds, APM-Sterngold, Div. of Sterndent Corp.
Diamond Rotary Instruments-FG, Miltex Instruments Co.
Gingi Curettage Point, Shofu Dental Corp.

Hi-Di Diamonds, Diamond Precision Tools, Ltd.
High Precision FG Diamond & Majestic Diamonds, J.R. Rand Specialty Co., Inc.
Lee Diamond Bur, Lee Pharmaceuticals
New Generation Diamond Instruments, Unitek Corp.
PDP Diamond Points, Rx Jeneric Gold Co.
Red Dot Diamonds & Green Dot Diamonds, Premier Dental Products Co.
R & R Cutwell Diamond Instruments, Ransom and Randolph Co.
Sintered Diamond Instruments, Ceramco, Inc.
SummaPoint & TPE Point, Shofu Dental Corp.
Superfine Finishing Diamonds, Den-Mat, Inc.

FINISHING AND POLISHING INSTRUMENTS

Rotary finishing and polishing instruments are designed to smooth and produce a high lustre on teeth, restorations and appliances.

Rotary instruments for finishing and polishing are available in a wide variety of sizes, shapes, and materials. In addition to finishing burs of 12, 20 or 40 blades, and very fine grit finishing diamonds, numerous wheels and stones are available for finishing purposes.

Finishing and polishing instruments, other than burs and diamonds, may contain the following, or similar, ingredients: emery (alumina), garnet, sand, cuttle, crocus, aluminum oxide, zirconium silicate and silicon carbide. These abrasives are available on discs or strips made of cloth, polyester, or very thin metal. At least some of these abrasive materials are also available as points, wheels, or stones of various sizes and shapes.

More recently manufacturers have produced kits designed specifically for one type of restorative material. These finishing instruments are usually of a rubber material impregnated with a very fine grit abrasive material. The kit usually includes bullet, knife, wheel, and round shaped instruments. Separate finishing and polishing kits are available for amalgams, gold alloys, composite resins, porcelain, chromium-cobalt alloys, and precious and non-precious alloys for use with porcelain.

For use in dental prophylaxis, rubber polishing cups, plain and webbed, and polishing brushes, either of natural or nylon bristle are available. These are used with an appropriate polishing paste, containing a mild abrasive, to polish natural teeth after all plaque and calculus have been removed. The polishing pastes used usually contain pumice or other silicate minerals of very fine mesh size.

FINISHING AND POLISHING INSTRUMENTS

Do:
1. Use instruments appropriate for the procedure.
2. Remember that polishing is merely reducing surface scratches by the use of instruments with increasingly finer grit.

AVAILABLE PRODUCTS

Abrasive Points-Right Angle Latch, Sterngold, Div. of Sterndent Corp.
Abrasive Points-Straight Handpieces, Sterngold, Div. of Sterndent Corp.
Alston TC Ultrafine FG Finishing System, Ransom and Randolph Co.
Arkansas White Stones-FG, Miltex Instruments Co.
Brownie, Greenie and Supergreenie Cups and Mini Points, Shofu Dental Corp.
Ceramalloy Cut-off Disc, Ceramco, Inc.
Ceramiste Mounted Points, Shofu Dental Corp.
Compodent Finishing Kit, Teledyne Dental Products
CompoSite Mounted Points, Shofu Dental Corp.
Cutting Wheels, Sterngold, Div. of Sterndent Corp.
Dental Abrasives, Zirc Dental Products
Dymun-Disc, Ceramco, Inc.
Fine Green Finishing Diamonds, Miltex Instruments Co.
Finishing & Polishing Strips, 3M Company
Grinding Wheels, Sterngold, Div. of Sterndent Corp.

Hand Separator, Mizzy, Inc.

Harperizer, Harper Buffing Machine Co.

Heatless Wheels, Mizzy, Inc.

Identoflex Polishers, Identoflex/Clev-Dent

Interproximal Wheels, Sterngold, Div. of Sterndent Corp.

Laboratory Points, Sterngold, Div. of Sterndent Corp.

Lathe Wheels, Sterngold, Div. of Sterndent Corp.

Mounted Rubber Dentist's Points, Sterngold, Div. of Sterndent Corp.

Mounted Rubber Points, Sterngold, Div. of Sterndent Corp.

Ney-Cheyes Green Abrasive Mounted Points, J.M. Ney Co.

Ney-Cheyes Green Band Stones, J.M. Ney Co.

Ney-Cheyes Green Engine Wheels, J.M. Ney Co.

Ney-Cheyes Green Tooth & Lathe Wheels, J.M. Ney Co.

Ney-Cheyes Red Engine Wheels, J.M. Ney Co.

Ney-Cheyes Red Mounted Points, J.M. Ney Co.

Ney-Cheyes White Acrylic Trimmers and Acrylic Lathe, J.M. Ney Co.

Ney-Cheyes White Polishing Points, J.M. Ney Co.

Pink Corundum Stones, Miltex Instrument Co.

Porcelain Wheels, Sterngold, Div. of Sterndent Corp.

Pumice, Whip-Mix Corp.

Quasite Disk, Shofu Dental Corp.

R & R Faskut Abrasive Points, Ransom and Randolph Co.

R & R Faskut Abrasive Wheel, Ransom and Randolph Co.

R & R Finishing and Trimming Carbide Burs, Ransom and Randolph Co.

Right Angle, Pacemaker Corp.

Rubber Knife-Edge Wheels, Sterngold, Div. of Sterndent Corp.

Rubber Points, Sterngold, Div. of Sterndent Corp.

Rubber Polishing Wheels, Sterngold, Div. of Sterndent Corp.

Sandplastic Disks, Premier Dental Products Co.

Separating Discs, Sterngold, Div. of Sterndent Corp.

Sequential Disc, H.D. Justi Co., Div. of Williams Gold Refining Co.

Sequential Gap Strips, H.D. Justi Co., Div. of

Williams Gold Refining Co.

Sof-lex Brand Finishing and Polishing Disc System, 3M Company

Sof-lex Brand Polishing Strips, 3M Company

3M Brand Hygienist Cleaning and Polishing Strips, 3M Company

Truing Block, Sterngold, Div. of Sterndent Corp.

Twelve Bladed Trimming and Finishing Carbide Burs, Miltex Instrument Co.

UTK Brown Finishing Stones, Unitek Corp.

UTK Green Finishing Stones, Unitek Corp.

LITERATURE REFERENCES

1. Taylor, D. F.; Perkins, R. R.; and Kumpula, J. W. Characteristics of some air-turbine handpieces. JADA 64:794 June 1962.

2. Peyton, F. A. Status report on dental operating handpieces. JADA 89:1162 Nov. 1974.

3. Morrant, G. A.; Powell, J. W.; and Hargreaves, P. Air bearings and their application to dental air turbine handpieces. Br. Dent. J. 116:531 June 1964.

4. Sockwell, C. L. Dental handpieces and rotary cutting instruments. Dent. Clin. N. Am. 15:219 Jan. 1971.

5. Walsh, J. P., and Symmons, H. F. Vibration perception and frequencies. N.Z. Dent. J. 45:106 Apr. 1949.

6. Doer, R. E. Principles associated with the use of high speed rotary instruments. Dent. Clin. N. Am. p. 19, Mar. 1957.

7. Eames, W. B., and Nale, J. L. A comparison of cutting efficiency of air-driven burs. JADA 86:412 Feb. 1973.

8. Council on Dental Materials and Devices. Revised American Dental Association specification no. 23 for dental excavating burs. JADA 90:459 Feb. 1975.

9. Reder, B. S., and Eames, W. B. The cutting rates and durability of diamond stones. J. Dent. Res. 55(B):B186, Abstract 499, 1976.

10. Janota, M. Use of scanning electron microscopy for evaluating diamond points. J. Prosthet. Dent. 29:88, 1973.

INSTRUMENTS AND DEVICES FOR RESTORATIVE DENTISTRY

INSTRUMENTS FOR EXAMINATION

Mouth Mirrors

A variety of sizes and reflecting types of mouth mirrors are available to meet the individual dentist's preferences. Sizes in common use vary from No. 5 (1.0 inch diameter) to No. 2 (0.75 inch diameter). The smaller sizes are valuable in restricted areas of the mouth.

Front and rear surface reflecting types are available as well as plain and magnifying types. Plain, front surface mirrors tend to minimize distortion.

Disposable mouth mirrors are available that are intended for single use. Multiple use mirrors are usually constructed of plated brass that permits moisture sterilization by autoclaving. Cone-socket handles are widely used into which is threaded a mirror of the type required. Such instruments permit continued use of a handle with the insertion of a new mirror following the removal and discarding of a scratched or otherwise unserviceable mirror.

AVAILABLE PRODUCTS

American Dental Mouth Mirrors, A. D. Mfg. Co.
Aqua-Solv Defogger, Teledyne Dental Products
Dental Mirrors, The Lorvic Corp.
Ferrolite Mouth Mirror, J. R. Rand Specialty Co., Inc.
Mirrors, E. A. Beck and Co.
Mirror Handles, Pulpdent Corp. of America
Mouth Mirrors, Kerr Mfg. Co., Div. of Sybron Dental Products
Mirror Defogger, Healthco, Inc.
Mirror Discs, Healthco, Inc.
Mirrors, Miltex Instruments Co.
Mouth Mirror Handles, Healthco, Inc.
Mouth Mirrors #'s 4&5, Healthco, Inc.

Mouth Mirrors, lighted & unlighted, John O. Butler Co.

Parallel Mirrors, Pulpdent Corp. of America

Patient Hand Mirror, Healthco, Inc.

Premier Mirrex Mirrors, Premier Dental Products Co.

Unitek Mouth Mirrors, Unitek Corp.

Explorers

Explorers are delicate pointed instruments used for the digital examination of tooth and restoration surfaces and their margin juncture. A wide variety of explorer designs are used by dental practitioners for the diagnosis of dental caries and assessment of prepared cavity and restoration form. The intended objective should determine the choice of explorer. Three operational factors should be considered when selecting the explorer; 1) sharpness of the point, 2) resilience and stiffness of the tine, and 3) design of the handle, shank and tine (Fig. 1).

AVAILABLE PRODUCTS

American Dental Amflex Explorers, American Dental Mfg. Co.

Explorers, E. A. Beck & Co.

Explorers, Hu-Friedy Mfg. Co., Inc.

Explorers, J. R. Rand Specialty Co., Inc.

Explorers, Miltex Instrument Co.

Explorers, Ivory Eastern Instruments, Inc.

R & R Explorers, Ransom and Randolph Company

R & R Handles for Interchangable Tips, Ransom and Randolph Company

Unitek Explorers, Unitek Corp.

Probes

Probes are similar to explorers in design of all but the tine and its end. Points on probes are rounded, rather than sharp. The length of the tine itself may in cross-section be round or flat, with or without graduations. The instruments are used principally for entering into or measuring the depths of the gingival crevice.

DEVICES FOR "DRY FIELD" OPERATION

Rubber Dam, Frames, Clamps, Forceps, Punch

Isolation of the operative site from oral fluids, lips, cheek and tongue is a major step in the control of the field. Vision, access and patient protection are all enhanced by use of a rubber dam to establish a dry field of operation. This method is considered ideal.

The rubber dam sheet in 5 or 6 inch widths is held open and supported by a metal or plastic frame or clips with an elastic band around the head. Rubber dam clamps are metal devices with jaws that have spring tension in order to secure the clamp to the tooth. The rubber dam that has holes through which the teeth protrude is stabilized by the clamp which is positioned onto the tooth using a clamp forceps. Holes are made in the rubber dam using a punch. Fig. 2 shows the various instruments and devices for rubber dam application.

AVAILABLE PRODUCTS

Premier Mini Dam, Premier Dental Products Co.

Premier Rubber Dam Punch, Premier Dental Products Co.

Premier Rubber Dam Clamp Forcep, Premier Dental Products Co.

Rubber Dam Napkin, Johnson & Johnson Dental Products Co.

Rubber Dam Holder, Brass, Young Dental Mfg.

Rubber Dam Holder, Nylon, Young Dental Mfg.

The Dam Frame, Pulpdent Corp. of America

Saliva Ejectors

Particularly when the rubber dam form of isolation is used, but at other times also, oral fluids and rinse water are required to be removed continuously from the mouth. Saliva ejectors are plastic (disposable) or metal (reusable) devices attached to a suction hose and usually lie in the floor of the mouth. Fluids are withdrawn at a somewhat slow but steady rate to assist in maintaining the dry field and provide

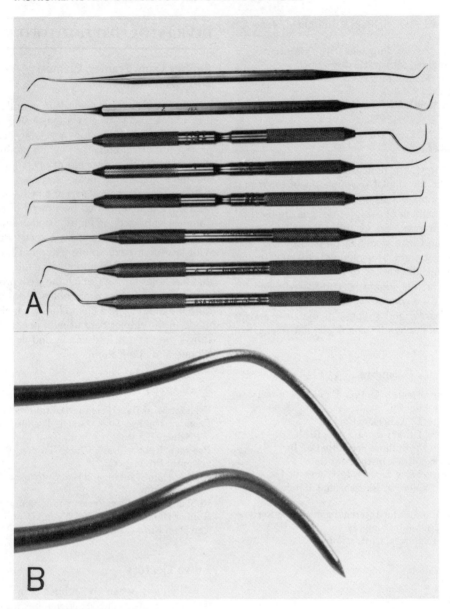

Fig. 1   (A) A variety of explorer designs available for hard tissue examination. (B) Variation between two new identical #3 explorer tips. (Reproduced from Charbeneau, G. T., et al. *Principles and Practice of Operative Dentistry*, Philadelphia, Lea & Febiger, 1975.)

comfort to the patient. Some metal saliva ejectors have rather broad surfaces in addition to the perforated tubes in order to reflect light and/or protect adjacent soft tissues.

Cotton Roll Holders

When the rubber dam is not used for isolation, a less effective means for gaining a dry field may be used. Absorbent cotton rolls can be placed in various areas within the mouth, some of which require holders in order to maintain the position of the cotton roll. These cotton roll holders are hinged devices consisting of an intraoral and an extraoral member and are employed in the mandibular arch. The intra-oral member has a means of grasping the cotton rolls, one on the buccal and one on the lingual side of the arch. These holders are paired, right and left (Fig. 3).

AVAILABLE PRODUCTS

Absorbent Dental Rolls–sterile, Johnson & Johnson Dental Products Co.

Cotton Roll Holders, J. R. Rand Specialty Co., Inc.
Cotton Roll Dispenser, Zirc Dental Products
Cotton Rolls, Healthco, Inc.

Evacuation Equipment

High-velocity evacuation equipment may be used in conjunction with the rubber dam, with cotton rolls or alone to effect the removal of larger volumes of rapidly moving streams of fluids, or the removal of aerosols from the operating site. Evacuating tips made of plastic (disposable) or metal (reusable) are available in a variety of designs for intraoral use.

HAND CUTTING INSTRUMENTS

The intricate and detailed procedures associated with restorative dentistry require a variety of instruments for the shaping of cavities and the placement and finishing of restorative materials. In the preparation of cavities, hand-

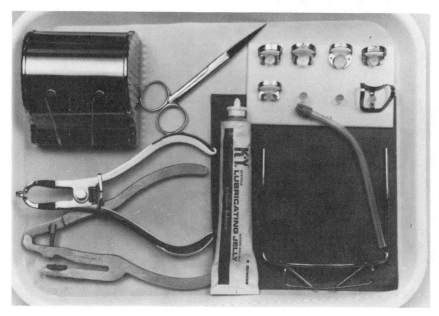

Fig. 2 Instrument tray for application of the rubber dam. (Reproduced from Charbeneau, G. T., et al. *Principles and Practice of Operative Dentistry,* Philadelphia, Lea & Febiger, 1975.)

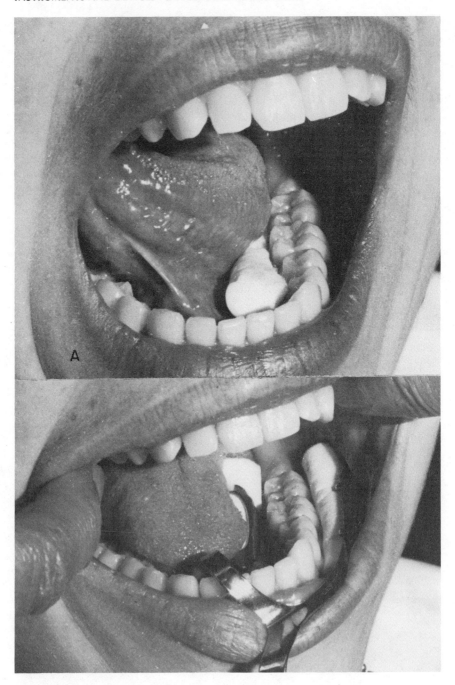

Fig. 3   Cotton roll holder with buccal and lingual rolls. (Reproduced from Charbeneau, G. T., et al. *Principles and Practice of Operative Dentistry*, Philadelphia, Lea & Febiger, 1975.)

cutting instruments are used principally for refining the preparation rather than for bulk cutting of tooth tissue. This change has taken place because of the dramatic transformation in the rotary cutting instruments.

G. V. Black established a formula that describes the dimensions and angulations of the hand cutting instruments. This instrument formula which consists of three of four units is based upon the metric system and is still in current use today by manufacturers.

A hand instrument consists of three parts, the *handle* or *shaft*, the *shank* connecting the handle to the working end, and the *blade* or nib. (Fig. 4) The shank may be straight, single-, double-, or triple-angled. The form or shape of the cutting edge and manner of its use may require an instrument to be "contra-angled." This is the angle of the shank in a manner designed to bring the cutting edge into close proximity to the central axis of the handle and provides improved stability when pressure necessary for cutting is applied.

Hand instruments designed for cutting hard tooth tissue are classified according to the form or shape of the cutting edge as follows:

Chisel. This is an excavator primarily used for planing or cleaving enamel. It is characterized by a blade that terminates in a cutting edge formed by a one-sided bevel (Fig. 5).

Hatchet. In dentistry, a hatchet is a chisel-bladed instrument with the cutting edge in the plane of the handle (Fig. 6). Hatchets are paired "left" and "right" with their blades beveled respectively one opposite to the other.

Hoe. A hoe is a form of chisel in which the angle of the blade more nearly approaches 25 centigrades (90°) to the handle.

Trimmer. Used primarily for beveling gingival margins, a trimmer is a modified hatchet

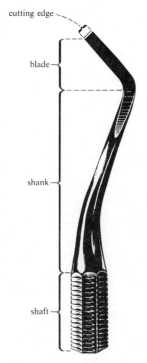

Fig. 4 Essential parts of any hand instrument. (Reproduced from Charbeneau, G. T., et al. *Principles and Practice of Operative Dentistry*, Philadelphia, Lea & Febiger, 1975.)

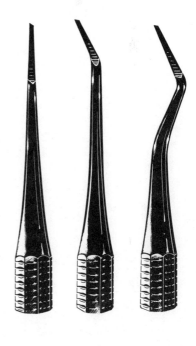

Fig. 5 Chisel. Left to right, straight, monangle and biangle. (Reproduced from Charbeneau, G. T., et al. *Principles and Practice of Operative Dentistry*, Philadelphia, Lea & Febiger, 1975.)

with 1) the cutting edge at other than a right angle to the axis of the blade and 2) a curved blade (double-plane). These are paired "left"

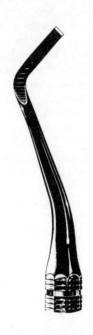

Fig. 6 Biangle hatchet. (Reproduced from Charbeneau, G. T., et al. *Principles and Practice of Operative Dentistry*, Philadelphia, Lea & Febiger, 1975.)

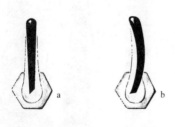

Fig. 7 (a) Single plane enamel hatchet. (b) Double plane, gingival margin trimmer. (Reproduced from Charbeneau, G. T., et al. *Principles and Practice of Operative Dentistry*, Philadelphia, Lea & Febiger, 1975.)

and "right" instruments used with a lateral scraping action (Fig. 7).

Angle former. The cutting edge of the hand instrument classified as an angle former is sharpened at an angle to the axis of the blade (Fig. 8). This blade is beveled on its sides as well as the end to form three distinct cutting edges. It is used especially to form convenience points for gold foil preparations.

Spoon. The spoon-excavator has a curved blade (double-plane) with a rounded cutting edge (Fig. 9). It is used with a lateral scraping action to remove carious dentin.

Carbon steel instruments attain a better cutting edge and maintain their cutting effectiveness for longer periods than do stainless steels. The cutting ends of carbon steels are, however, subject to corrosion because they are not plated for protection. If left unprotected during autoclaving they will deteriorate during repeated sterilization cycles. Several corrosion inhibitors are available for instrument protection during autoclaving, and a chemical vapor sterilizer is also marketed. This system involves limited moisture and is reported as resulting in less corrosion than normal steam under pressure. Dry heat or ethylene oxide sterilization will eliminate the corrosion problem, but such methods require extensive time and may be impractical for the dental office.

Hand cutting instruments must be sharp to be effective. Sharpening of the various instruments with flat cutting edge bevels is done with a soft, very true rotating Arkansas wheel or by free-hand application of a boxed Arkansas stone. The rotary sharpening consists of an oscillating wax-impregnated wheel (2½ inches in diameter) that revolves on a reciprocating shaft. A slotted sharpening guide provides support for the instrument being sharpened. This guide permits the shaping of a flat cutting edge bevel approximately 12.5 centigrades (45°) angulation on the face of the instrument terminating in the cutting edge.

Freehand application of a boxed Arkansas stone is useful once the technique has been mastered. Freehand application of a handpiece mounted small-diameter Arkansas stone can reduce the quality and accuracy of the edge particularly in the hands of an inexperienced operator.

EVALUATION PROGRAM: In 1976, a new American Dental Association Specification No. 29 for hand instruments was approved.[1] This specification is of a general nature and covers requirements and tests for dental instruments. It is intended to be used in conjunction with detailed specifications covering such additional requirements as are applicable to each instrument. The detailed specification for specific designs of hand instruments is now being prepared.

Instruments covered by this specification are of various classes depending upon the material used for construction. Included within this specification are characteristics of material hardness, corrosion resistance, resistance to permanent change in shape, style, design and dimensions, finish, plating identification and workmanship.

AVAILABLE PRODUCTS

EXCAVATORS

American Dental Excavators, American Dental Mfg. Co.
Excavators, E. A. Beck & Co.
Excavators, Hu-Friedy Mfg. Co., Inc.
Excavators, J. R. Rand Specialty Co., Inc.
Excavators, Miltex Instrument Co.
R & R Excavators, Ransom and Randolph Company
Unitek Excavators, Unitek Corp.

CHISELS

American Dental Chisels, American Dental Mfg. Co.
Bone Chisels, J. R. Rand Specialty Co. Inc.
Chisels, E. A. Beck & Co.
Chisels, Miltex Instrument Co.
Chisels, Hu-Friedy Mfg. Co. Inc.
Chisels, J. R. Rand Specialty Co., Inc.
Premier Chisels, Premier Dental Products Co.
R & R Wedelstadt Chisels, Ransom and Randolph Company

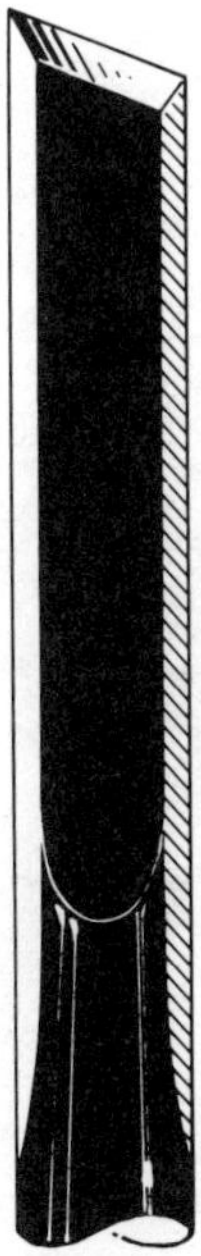

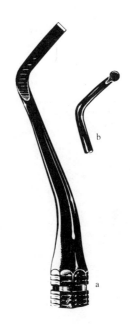

Fig. 8 Angle former, triple-cutting-edge instrument. (Reproduced from Charbeneau, G. T., et al. *Principles and Practice of Operative Dentistry*, Philadelphia, Lea & Febiger, 1975.)

Fig. 9 Spoon excavator (b) is a modified hatchet (a). (Reproduced from Charbeneau, G. T., et al. *Principles and Practice of Operative Dentistry*, Philadelphia, Lea & Febiger, 1975.)

Premier Chisels, Premier Dental Products Co.
R & R Wedelstadt Chisels, Ransom and Randolph
  Company

INSTRUMENTS AND DEVICES FOR AMALGAM

Cavities involving two or more surfaces require a matrix when restoring with amalgam. Matrices help provide the general contour for the restoration and confine the plastic amalgam during its insertion (Fig. 10). The matrix assembly ready to receive the mixed amalgam consists of 1) the *matrix band*, 2) the *matrix retainer* and 3) the *wedge* (Fig. 11). Matrix bands are curved nickel alloy or stainless steel strips 0.0015 or 0.002 inch thick. The band is held in position by a matrix retainer, a mechanical device capable of drawing the band snugly around the tooth. The band should be con-

toured to proper form according to the shape of the tooth being restored, as well as the position of the adjacent teeth. A wedge, usually consisting of wood or a slightly resilient plastic, is forcefully positioned at the cervical area of the teeth to separate the teeth slightly during condensation of the amalgam. This makes up for the thickness of the band material, and minimizes the excess amalgam that might otherwise be condensed beyond the cavity form. High fusing dental compound is often used to enhance the stability of the matrix band.

Since the proportion of dental amalgam alloy to mercury is one factor that determines the mechanical properties and manipulative characteristics of the amalgam, some means of reliable proportioning is required. Consistency can be attained conveniently using preweighed disposable capsules, but all such systems are not necessarily accurate. Many mercury dispensers and other devices for proportioning provide acceptable accuracy when used ac-

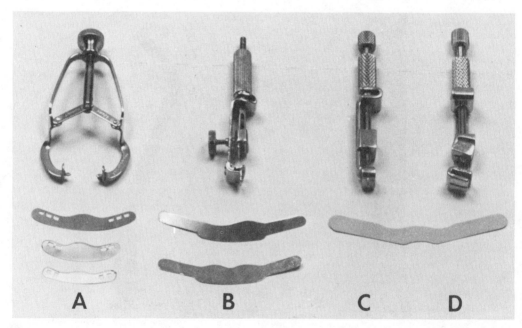

Fig. 10   (A) Ivory No. 1. (B) Ivory No. 9. (C) and (D) Tofflemire [Straight (C) and contra-angle (D)] matrix retainers and bands. (Reproduced from Charbeneau, G. T., et al. *Principles and Practice of Operative Dentistry*, Philadelphia, Lea & Febiger, 1975.)

cording to specific instructions. Human variables can void that accuracy, thus careful attention to manipulative detail is essential. Due to
the potential hazards of mercury vapor, care
should be taken in the handling of any mercury
containing products. Additional information
regarding effects, safe vapor levels and recommendations for hygiene are covered in
Chapter 1.

AVAILABLE PRODUCTS

MATRIX RETAINERS

Automatrix Dental Matrix, L. D. Caulk Co.
Caulk Crown Forms, L. D. Caulk Co.
Cervical Matrix Strip, L. D. Caulk Co.
Caulk Metal Strip, L. D. Caulk Co.
Dead-Soft Metal Matrix, Den-Mat, Inc.
Getz Contour Band, "The Dixi-land Band," Tele-
dyne Dental Products
Incisal Corner Matrix, Premier Dental Products
Co.
Ivory Matrix Retainers, Ivory Co.
Lactona Pre-contoured Matrix Bands, Lactona
Corp.
Matrix Bands, Healthco, Inc.
Matrix Retainers, Healthco, Inc.
Matrix Retainers & Bands, Miltex Instrument
Co.
Matrix Retaining Wedges, Den-Mat, Inc.
Modern Foil, Modern Materials Mfg.

PCA T-Bands, Pulpdent Corp. of America
Premier Anatomically Carved Wedges, Premier
Dental Products Co.
Premier Cervical Matrix Forms, Premier Dental
Products Co.
Rand Matrix Retainers, Matrix Bands for Ivory
and Tofflemire Matrix Retainers, Matrix Rolls,
T-bands, and Myler Rolls, J. R. Rand Specialty
Co., Inc.
Strip-Tite Matrix Retainers, Premier Dental
Products Co.
Strip Holders, Pulpdent Corp. of America
Strip Holder Matrix Clip, Healthco, Inc.
Tofflemire Matrix Bonds, Teledyne Dental Prod-
ucts
T-LCR Retainer, T-LCR Laboratory
Unitek Matrix Bands, Unitek Corp.
Unitek Matrix Retainers, Unitek Corp.

AMALGAM CARRIERS

PCA Amalgam Carriers, Pulpdent Corp. of America
Premier Never-Clog Amalgam Guns, Premier
Dental Products Co.
Rand Amalgam Carriers, J. R. Rand Specialty
Co., Inc.
Unitek Amalgam Carriers, Unitek Corp.

AMALGAM SQUEEZE CLOTHS

Amalgam Squeeze Cloths, J. R. Rand Specialty
Co., Inc.
Caulk Amalgam Squeeze Cloth, L. D. Caulk Co.

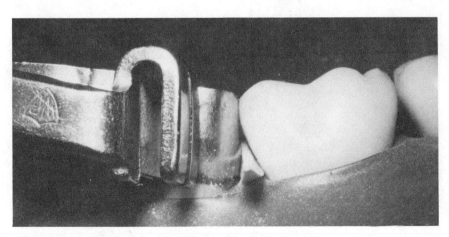

Fig. 11   Clinical application of matrix with wedge to a mandibular bicuspid. (Reproduced from Charbeneau, G. T., et al.
Principles and Practice of Operative Dentistry, Philadelphia, Lea & Febiger, 1975.)

AMALGAM DISPENSERS

Caulk Alloy Pellet Dispenser, L. D. Caulk Co.

Caulk Capsule Holder, L. D. Caulk Co.

Indiloy Powder and Mercury Dispensers, Shofu Dental Corp.

Saf-T-Cote Mercury Dispensers, L. D. Caulk Co.

"Safety-Seal" Amalgam Mixing Capsule, Shofu Dental Corp.

Tab-Mate Hand Held Dispenser, Shofu Dental Corp.

Amalgamators

Amalgamators are mechanical devices used to triturate the amalgam alloy with mercury in order to wet the particles (Fig. 12). Mixing me-

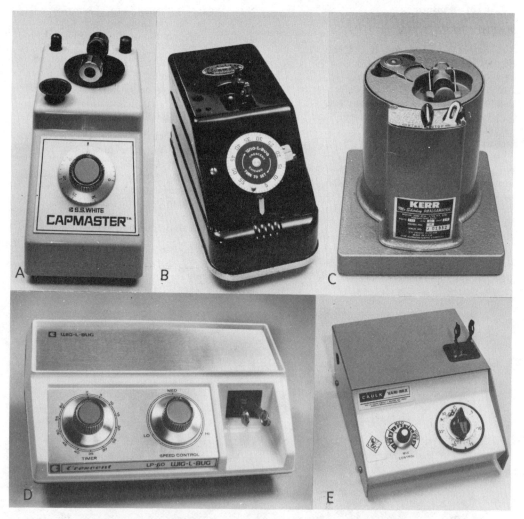

Fig. 12 Mechanical amalgamators. (A) S. S. White Capmaster. (B) Crescent Wig-L-Bug. (C) Kerr McShirley. (D) Crescent Wig-L-Bug LP-60. (E) Caulk Vari-Mix. (Reproduced from Charbeneau, G. T., et al. *Principles and Practice of Operative Dentistry*, Philadelphia, Lea & Febiger, 1975.)

chanically, as opposed to hand trituration, is more efficient and effective because of the work or energy required. The thrust the machine utilizes, its speed and duration of the mixing activity are all interdependent factors that bring about adequate mixing.

The plastic mass of amalgam, after proper trituration, is free of dry alloy particles and is a coherent mass that should not adhere to the mixing container. Suitable carrying instruments are used to transport portions of the mass from the working area to the prepared tooth. Here, condensing instruments are used to adapt the amalgam to the walls and margins of the prepared cavity, to compact the mass into a uniform and as void-free restoration as possible, and to reduce the mercury content to its lowest possible level consistent with the other objectives.

AVAILABLE PRODUCTS

Capmaster, S. S. White Dental Products, Div. of Pennwalt Corp.
Crown, Harry J. Bosworth Co.
Dentomat, Pfingst and Company, Inc.
Hanau, Hanau Engineering Co.
Kerr-McShirley, Kerr Mfg. Co., Div. of Sybron Corp.
Silamat, H. D. Justi Co., Div. American Tooth Co.
Torit, H. D. Justi Co., Div. American Tooth Co.
Wig-L-Bug, Crescent Dental Mfg. Co.
Wig-L-Bug LP 60, Crescent Dental Mfg. Co.

Condensers

Packing instruments are classified as hand or mechanical condensers. Hand condensers vary in face design (smooth or serrated), size, outline shape and face contour (flat or curved). Mechanical condensers are either of "vibratory" or "impact" types, and particular attention must be given to the latter type so as not to fracture enamel margins. Excellent restorations can be placed with either hand or mechanical condensers with no superiority of one demonstrated over the other.

AVAILABLE PRODUCTS

Amal-Pak, J. R. Rand Specialty Co., Inc.
American Dental Amalgam Condensors, American Dental Mfg. Co.
Condensors, E. A. Beck & Co.
Condensors, J. R. Rand Specialty Co., Inc.
Premier Condensors, Premier Dental Products Co.
Unitek Condensers, Unitek Corp.

Carvers and Burnishers

Carvers and burnishers are instruments used to further shape and smoothen the condensed restoration. Carvers are bladed instruments usually used with a knife-like cutting action (Fig. 13), while burnishers are blunted instruments of a variety of sizes and shapes used for rubbing the newly inserted restoration in order to attain a smoother surface finish. Although burnishing

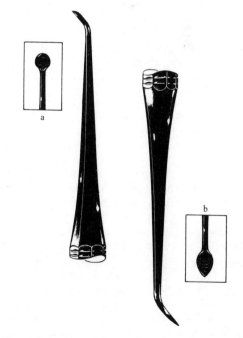

Fig. 13 Cleoid-discoid instruments. Discoid end (a), cleoid end (b). (Reproduced from Charbeneau, G. T., et al. *Principles and Practice of Operative Dentistry*, Philadelphia, Lea & Febiger, 1975.)

the newly placed amalgam surface was at one time looked upon as being detrimental to the physical properties of the amalgam, such a light smoothening action is suggested as routine by many clinicians since this does enhance surface finishing.

Available Products

American Dental Burnishers, American Dental Mfg. Co.

American Dental Carvers, American Dental Mfg. Co.

Carvers & Burnishers, Hu-Friedy Mfg. Co., Inc.

Carvers & Burnishers, Miltex Instruments Co.

Ivory Eastern Carvers and Burnishers, Eastern Instruments, Inc.

Nurlite Carvers & Burnishers, J. R. Rand Specialty Co., Inc.

#3 & #5 Acorn Carver, Shofu Dental Corp.

Premier Carvers and Burnishers, Premier Dental Products Co.

R & R Hollenback Carvers, Ransom & Randolph Company

Unitek Carvers, Unitek Corp.

INSTRUMENTS AND DEVICES FOR CAST RESTORATIONS

Various instruments are used in the placement of chemical tissue packs in order to reflect gingival tissues and reduce seepage of tissue fluid prior to taking impressions with elastic materials or preparations for castings. When reversible agar hydrocolloid is used as the impression material, a device for conditioning and storage is required. Such devices may consist of three water baths maintained at prescribed temperatures to liquify [210 to 212°F (98.9 to 100°C)], store [145 to 150°F (62.8 to 65.6°C)], and temper [115 to 120°F (46.1 to 48.9°C)] the agar for use. Hydrocolloid syringes capable of withstanding these temperatures and the moisture environment and having removable tips in sizes ranging from 19-gauge to 23-gauge are used to deliver the semi-fluid material to all areas of the prepared teeth. Syringes of similar design are used for the elastomeric impression materials.

The finally adjusted and polished alloy casting is cemented into the prepared tooth using a variety of instruments for mixing the cement (Fig. 14), inserting the casting, and finishing margins. Cements that require a controlled, cool environment are usually mixed upon a thick glass or plastic slab capable of being cooled. Thin blade mixing spatulas are used to incorporate cement powder into the cement liquid upon the surface of the slab. Paper mixing tablets are sometimes used for certain cements that are not critically affected by the temperatures at which they are mixed. When the alloy casting is ready to place using finger pressure, devices are often used to assure complete seating of the casting with the expression of the maximum amount of unset cement possible from beneath the casting. Such devices merely concentrate forces delivered by the patient's closing the jaws to the casting being cemented. Both hand burnishing instruments as well as rotary abrasive and burnishing instruments are used to smooth or adapt the margin of the casting closely to the tooth.

Inlay and crown removers are available to assist in the removal of the cemented castings from the tooth. They are of two types. One requires the drilling of a slightly undersized hole through the casting and the self-threading of the device into the gold to a depth where the threading stud contacts tooth tissue. The force delivered to the casting then is one that tends to unseat it. The second type of crown removing device merely works on the principle of delivering a sharp blow to some aspect of the casting in a direction that attempts to parallel as much as possible a direction that will unseat the casting. These can be potentially dangerous in that the force direction is less controlled and fracture of the tooth may result.

Available Products

CROWN AND BRIDGE REMOVERS

Crown & Bridge Remover w/ 3 points, Pulpdent Corp. of America

Crown & Removing Adapter Removers, J. R. Rand Specialty Co., Inc.

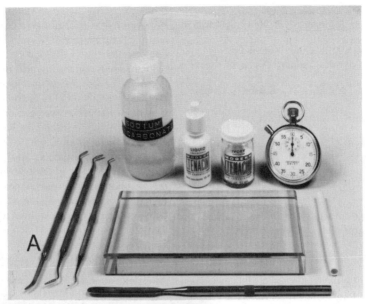

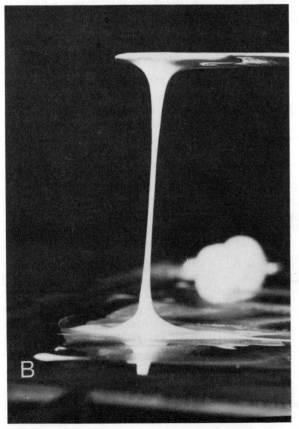

Fig. 14 (A) Materials dispensed for mixing zinc phosphate cement. (B) Consistency approximation. (Reproduced from Charbeneau, G. T., et al. *Principles and Practice of Operative Dentistry*, Philadelphia, Lea & Febiger, 1975.)

Crown Removers, E. A. Beck & Co.

Crown Remover Hammer, J. R. Rand Specialty Co., Inc.

Crown Removers, Miltex Instruments Co.

Crown Setters–Plastic, Pulpdent Corp. of America

Lactona/Medart Pressure Applicator, Lactona/Surgident

Premier Crown Removers, Premier Dental Products Co.

Simcrest Crown & Bridge Remover, Crescent Dental Mfg. Co.

PLIERS AND SPATULAS

American Dental Cotton & Dressing pliers, American Dental Mfg. Co.

American Dental Matrix Pliers, American Dental Mfg. Co.

American Dental Spatulas, American Dental Mfg. Co.

Cement Spatulas, Pulpdent Corp. of America

College Pliers, Pulpdent Corp. of America

College Pliers, Healthco, Inc.

Cotton & Dressing Pliers, J. R. Rand Specialty Co., Inc.

Crimper Cutter Pliers, Pulpdent Corp. of America

Dent-O-Lux Silver Point Plier, Charles B. Schwed Co. Inc.

Dis-Spat, The Marshall Weiner Co.

Impression Paste Spatula, Kerr Mfg. Co., Div. of Sybron Dental Products Corp.

Inserter Pliers, Pulpdent Corp. of America

Pliers & Spatulas, E. A. Beck & Co.

Pliers & Spatulas, Hu-Friedy Mfg. Co., Inc.

Pliers & Spatulas, Miltex Instruments Co.

Premier Pliers & Spatulas, Premier Dental Products Co.

Spatulas—White Plastic, Zirc Dental Products

Tissue Plier, J. R. Rand Specialty Co., Inc.

Unitek Pliers, Unitek Corp.

Wax Spatulas, Pulpdent Corp. of America

INSTRUMENTS AND DEVICES FOR COMPOSITE RESIN

Matrices are used in placing composite resin materials into prepared cavities to assist in establishing general contour and to provide slight compression so as to minimize air voids in the mix. Plastic matrix strips made from Mylar or other materials are most often used. Soft burnishable metal is also used in certain areas for matrices and these can be stabilized with dental compound.

Instruments for mixing and placing composite resins are best made from plastic rather than metal. Materials such as Teflon do not impart a gray color to the composite as do stainless steels and even stellite instruments. The hard inorganic fillers most often used in composite resins abrade the metal spatulas and insertion instruments thus imparting a distinct discoloration to the restoration. The use of metal instruments with microfilled composites should be undertaken only according to manufacturers' instructions.

AVAILABLE PRODUCTS

American Dental Permacoated Instruments, American Dental Mfg.Co.

American Dental Plastic Instruments, American Dental Mfg. Co.

Caulk Celluloid Strips, L. D. Caulk Co.

Caulk Unistrips Matrix, L. D. Caulk Co.

Composite Instruments & Mix Sticks, Zirc Dental Products

Ivory/Eastern Plastic Instruments, Eastern Instruments Inc.

Mylar Matrix Strips, Healthco, Inc.

Nurlite Plastic Instruments, J. R. Rand Specialty Co., Inc.

Plastic Instruments, E. A. Beck & Co.

Plastic Instruments, Miltex Instrument Co.

Poly Instruments, H. D. Justi Co., Div. of Williams Gold Refining Co. Inc.

Premier Composite Strips, Premier Dental Products Co.

Premier Strip-Aids, Premier Dental Products Co.

3-M Brand Composite Placement Instruments, 3M Company

Unitek Mix-N-Ject Syringe Kit, Unitek Corp.

INSTRUMENTS AND DEVICES FOR COHESIVE GOLD

Cohesive golds are rendered cohesive when all surface contaminants are removed. Contaminants, including moisture, are removed by heating the gold during a process called "annealing." Annealing can be accomplished by placing the gold on a tray heated by an electric or gas source, or by passing each piece over an alcohol flame. Devices for delivering proper temperatures to the gold are required.

Carrying instruments for cohesive gold are finely pointed so as not to compress the gold when picking up a piece, nor remove heat because of the bulk of the instrument when annealing by the piece method.

Condensing instruments are of two general types, hand and mechanical. The faces of the condensing points of both types are serrated. Hand condensers are designed to be used either with a sustained force or by the delivery of sharp blows to the end opposite the condensing face. Mechanical condensers are spring loaded (automatic), air driven (pneumatic), or electrically activated (Electromallet).

Hand and rotary finishing instruments are used to alter contours, adapt margins, and smooth and polish as well as cold work the metal surface.

AVAILABLE PRODUCTS

American Dental Gold Foil Annealing Instruments, American Dental Mfg. Co.
Gold Foil Malleting Devices, E. A. Beck & Co.
Gold Matrix Foil, Williams Gold Refining Co., Inc.
Twenty Four k Gold Foil, J. M. Ney Co.

LITERATURE REFERENCES

1. Council on Dental Materials and Devices. New American Dental Association specification no. 29—General specification for hand instruments. JADA 93:818 Oct. 1976.

ENDODONTIC INSTRUMENTS

Endodontic instruments are instruments used within the root canal system of a tooth. The complexity of the endodontic armamentarium has increased significantly in the last two decades paralleling the growth of endodontics as a special area of dental practice as well as the increased emphasis upon endodontics in the general practice of dentistry. Not only would a current listing of endodontic instruments reveal the expected intracanal files, reamers, and broaches but also such diverse items as endodontic handpieces, measurement aids, irrigating needles and syringes, and devices and instruments used in root canal filling.[1,2]

ROOT CANAL FILES AND REAMERS

The principal instruments in endodontic practice are root canal files and reamers designed for hand use only. Root canal files and reamers are used to cleanse and shape the root canal space of the tooth. There is a near universal conviction in dentistry that the cleansing, shaping, and sealing of the root canal system lies at the heart of the successful practice of endodontics.[3-5]

Most members of the dental profession admit the necessity for removal of pulpal tissue or debris from the root canal system, enlargement of the pulp canal space to admit root canal filling materials, and cleansing and smoothing of the dentinal walls to provide for lateral sealing of the root canal filling. Root canal files and reamers are the principal instruments used to achieve these ends. The efficacy of instrumentation has been examined by several authors all of whom admit that results are less than optimum under most clinical circumstances.[6-18] The use of the scanning electron microscope has renewed interest in this problem and focused attention on the efficacy of dentinal surface preparation within the root canal.[19-23] The concurrent use of irrigating solutions with filing and reaming techniques has been emphasized by many of these investigations.

TYPES: The major types of root canal files and reamers include: Type K files and reamers and Type H (Hedstrom) files.

Type K Files and Reamers: Root canal instruments of type K are manufactured from steel wires which are prestressed, cut into short straight rods and machined into either three or four sided tapered pyramidal blanks. The terminal tapered portion of the blank is then twisted to introduce a series of spirals which become the operating head of the instrument. A blank twisted to produce from less than one quarter to less than one tenth of a spiral per millimeter of length, dependent upon size, produces an instrument having from 0.80 to 0.28 cutting flutes per millimeter of operating head and is designated as a root canal reamer. A blank twisted to produce from one quarter to over one half of a spiral per millimeter of length dependent upon size, produces an instrument having from 1.97 to 0.88 cutting flutes per millimeter of operating head and is designated as a root canal file. The larger reamers are likely to be twisted from blanks which are three sided. Root canal instruments of type K are size for size stiffer and stronger than comparable types of instruments. This is due in large part to their mode of manufacture wherein the grain structure of the wire blank is preserved and the entire bulk of metal in the working portion of the instrument makes up the blade with its cutting edges. The ductility of the instrument varies according to the work hardening induced during drawing and fabrication. Work hardening is a function of size, shape, tightness of twist, and the variety of steel used. Stainless steel, besides being relatively free from corrosion, is more ductile than carbon steel and has largely replaced carbon steel for endodontic instruments. For a given amount of twist the large instrument, assuming the same shape, is more work hardened than its smaller counterpart due to greater strains at its outer surfaces and edges. Similarly, a four sided instrument with greater bulk at its outer extremities has more work hardening than a three sided instrument. The tighter the twist of a given size and shape blank the more work hardening is introduced. In efforts to provide the profession with flexible root canal instruments with good cutting characteristics many manufacturers alter

the steel, the number of twists, or more particularly the shape of the instrument blank in their root canal files.

The shape of the instrument operating head, whether four sided or three sided can be of importance in clinical practice. An instrument with a three sided blade gives a deeper cut with thicker cutting chips than does an instrument with a four sided blade which has a smaller contact angle with the root canal wall. The three sided instrument is not only significantly more effective in cutting but having less volume of steel is also significantly more fragile. Some manufacturers of root canal files change from four sided to three sided instruments as the size progression increases in order to gain flexibility and cutting efficacy. The clinician who is not aware of this change in shape is likely to experience an increase in instrument breakage if he assumes a naturally increasing progression of applied forces based upon size alone in his instrumentation technique.[24]

This characteristic is shown graphically in Figure 1 wherein the flexibility curves for type K files and reamers show a lateral displacement to the right corresponding to only slight increases in stiffness as the blade shape is changed from four to three sides. The dotted lines show the increasing stiffness of root canal files had not this change in blade shape occurred. Table I compares the clinical usefulness of type K reamers and files.[1] Root canal reamers with low helical angles to the cutting edges are used primarily with a rotary cutting action. The looseness of the spiral of a reamer does not permit very effective cutting action in linear motion or removal of debris by the blades while being withdrawn from the root canal (carrier effect). Root canal files with larger helical angles to their cutting edges (45° or more) are used with either a rotary or linear cutting action. The tightness of the spiral of a file determines its effectiveness in linear motion and the extent of its carrier effect. In current endodontic practice the root canal file has largely replaced the root canal reamer as it can perform a dual role in root canal preparation.

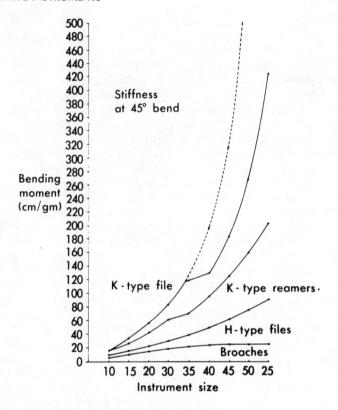

Fig. 1   Flexibility of root canal instruments

Table I.   Clinical Usefulness of Type K Root Canal Files and Reamers

Feature	Reamers	Files
Helical angle of edge	Small	Large
Carrier effect	Poor	Good
Ratio of spiral numbers	Few	Many
Tactile sense inside canal	Rough	Smooth
Cutting mode	Clockwise turn only	Clockwise turn with pull, or pull only

Type H (Hedstrom) Files: Root canal files are also available in the Hedstrom (type H) design. This design is manufactured by machining a spiral groove into a metal blank to produce a tapering and pointed instrument. The grooves are shaped to produce the gross appearance of a series of interstacking cones along a central core of metal. The design of the type H file is such that the bulk of metal in the working blade that supports the outer cutting edges of the instrument occurs as a central unmachined core. The helical angle of this instrument is large (90° or less) contributing to the extreme effectiveness of the instrument when withdrawn from a tooth along a dentinal surface. The instrument is not effective when used with a rotary motion. The relationship between the overall size of the instrument and its inherent strength can be deceptive as the instrument is only as strong or as flexible as the central core of steel from which the cutting edges project. A comparison of type K and type H files is shown in Table II.

USES: For maximal effectiveness, type K files should be used for preparation of the cylindrical apical retention form and type H files for the shaping of the occlusal or incisal flare.[25]

DIRECTIONS FOR USE: The filing sequence adopted today by increasing numbers of clinicians is to cleanse and shape the root canal(s) by serial filing using type K files with rotary clockwise twists of a quarter turn or more followed by withdrawal strokes thereby creating a conical preparation in the apical portion of the root. Type H files are then used to create a flaring of the preparation for accessibility from the apical third of root to the occlusal or incisal orifice.[26] Type K files produce clean, smooth surfaces whereas the surfaces produced by type H files are clean but not as smooth.[27]

As indicated, the resistance to fracture exhibited by root canal files varies according to design, the type H being much more susceptible to fracture than the type K. Type K files are not as susceptible to fracture when subjected to torsional force applied in a clockwise manner (Fig. 2) but are extremely susceptible to fracture when torsional force is applied in a counter clockwise movement.[28] Few type K files (or reamers) can survive a counter clockwise rotation of 180° or less if their tips are bound firmly and will fracture suddenly, and cleanly, in a brittle fashion.[29] This is distinguished from the slow tearing fractures encountered with clockwise rotation. Type H files fracture both by twisting and withdrawing when used with excessive force.

Table II. A Comparison of Type K and Type H Root Canal Files

Feature	*K*	*H*
Mode of use	Clockwise turn with pull, or pull only	Pull only
Rake angle of edge	45°	90°
Cutting efficiency	Average to good	Excellent
Carrier effect	Good	Good
Shaping of nonround canal	Average	Good
Resistance to fracture	Average to good	Poor
Cross section of prepared canal	Circular	Variable

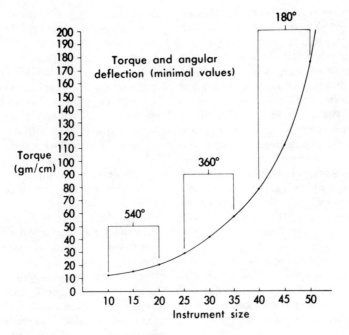

Fig. 2   Type K root canal files and reamers torqued in a clockwise manner

EVALUATION PROGRAM: Until very recently, endodontic instruments had not been scientifically evaluated although they had been used with significant clinical success in a wide variety of root canal techniques for over fifty years. The principal investigations of root canal instrument designs and physical characteristics were initiated in the 1950's concurrent with increased concern in the profession for standardization of the instruments and materials used in endodontics.[30-34] These were culminated in the adoption of American Dental Association Specification No. 28 for Root Canal Files and Reamers in 1975 and the work of the Technical Committee 106–Dentistry of the International Standards Organization in the development of world standards of instrument design and performance.[24,35-39]

American Dental Association Specification No. 28 encompasses root canal files and reamers of type K only and does not cover root canal files of type H (Hedstrom) or root canal broaches or rasps. These latter instruments will be covered under a separate specification currently under development. At present, there are no acceptance programs for other types of root canal instruments or devices.

The files and reamers of Specification No. 28 are divided into two Classes: (A) carbon steel and (B) stainless steel. The specification calls for detailed dimensions and tolerances for the diameters, taper, and tip of the instrument as well as the length of the spiral cutting section. Specific procedures for the measurement of these dimensions are noted. The specification includes physical tests of the instruments detailing the equipment and procedures to be used to record acceptable limits of resistance to fracture by twisting, stiffness to bending, and corrosion resistance. Requirements for the packaging and labeling of instruments as well as color coding are also included in the specification. Figure 3 shows the dimensional features of the specification which are contained in Table III.[39]

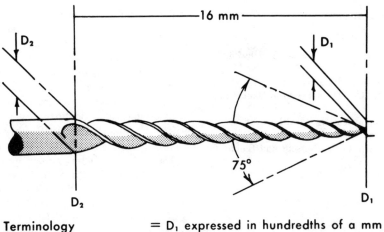

Terminology   = D_1 expressed in hundredths of a mm
Diameters D_2 = D_1 plus 0.32 mm
Taper   = 0.02 mm per mm
Tip angle   = 75° ± 15° included angle
Tolerance   = ± 0.02 mm
Length blade (D_1 to D_2) = 16.0 mm

Fig. 3   Standardized root canal instruments: American Dental Association Specification No. 28

Table III.   Terminology and Color Coding of Standardized Root Canal Instruments

Size	Diameter of instrument		Color	Abbreviation
	D_1 (mm)	D_2 (mm)		
10	0.10	0.42	Purple	Pur
15	0.15	0.47	White	Wh
20	0.20	0.52	Yellow	Yel
25	0.25	0.57	Red	Red
30	0.30	0.62	Blue	Blu
35	0.35	0.67	Green	Grn
40	0.40	0.72	Black	Blk
45	0.45	0.77	White	Wh
50	0.50	0.82	Yellow	Yel
55	0.55	0.87	Red	Red
60	0.60	0.92	Blue	Blu
70	0.70	1.02	Green	Grn
80	0.80	1.12	Black	Blk
90	0.90	1.22	White	Wh
100	1.00	1.32	Yellow	Yel
110	1.10	1.42	Red	Red
120	1.20	1.52	Blue	Blu
130	1.30	1.62	Green	Grn
140	1.40	1.72	Black	Blk
150	1.50	1.82	White	Wh

AVAILABLE PRODUCTS

ROOT CANAL FILES

Antaeus-Hedstrom Files, Charles B. Schwed Co. Inc.
Endodontic Files, Healthco, Inc.
Files, Kerr Mfg. Co., Div. of Sybron Dental Products
Hedstrom Endodontic Files, Healthco, Inc.
K-Files, Midwest American
R & R Endodontic Files, Ransom and Randolph Company
R & R Hedstrom Files, Ransom and Randolph Company
Unitek Endodontic Files, Unitek Corp.

ROOT CANAL REAMERS

Antaeus Reamers, Charles B. Schwed Co., Inc.
Dent-O-Lux Peeso Reamers, Charles B. Schwed Co., Inc.
Dent-O-Lux Modified Peeso Reamers, Charles B. Schwed Co., Inc.
Endodontic Reamers, Healthco, Inc.
Hand Reamers, Midwest American
Peeso Reamers, Pulpdent Corp. of America
Reamers, Kerr Mfg. Co., Div. of Sybron Dental Products Corp.
Root Canal Reamers, E. A. Beck & Co.
R & R Endodontic Reamers, Ransom and Randolph Company
Unitek Endodontic Reamers, Unitek Corp.

ROOT CANAL BROACHES AND RASPS

Historically root canal broaches, rasps, applicators, and probes are the oldest forms of endodontic instruments, dating prior to the early 19th century. Probes are usually light, slender, fairly flexible, smooth or edged, pointed and tapered soft iron wires used for exploring root canals. Broaches, rasps, and applicators are similar soft iron wires manufactured with a series of incisions along the shaft of the wire; the edge of the incision is elevated to create either a pointed barb, semicircular cutting edge, or roughened surface. The depth and angle of the incision cut into the shaft is the principal determinant of the instrument type.

Barbed broaches are the only instruments of this generic type which have retained any popularity of use in current clinical practice. They are used primarily for the removal of intact masses of pulp tissue or the retrieval of medicated dressings from the pulp chamber or root canal. The instrument is introduced slowly until wall contact with dentin is first encountered, rotated to entangle the pulp tissue or dressing in its protruding barbs, and then withdrawn.

The barbed broach is a fragile instrument and should be used with caution. The incisions creating the barbs in the soft and flexible iron wire extend for some distance into the metal and increase the potential for fracture. If the instrument is forced apically into a tapering and confined root canal, the tips of the barbs are compressed against the metal shaft giving a false sense of security. When attempts are made to withdraw an instrument forced into a narrow root canal the barbs engage the surrounding tooth structure and the more force that is used to pull the broach from the tooth the deeper they penetrate. If enough force is applied the barbs of the instrument (1) bend back on themselves allowing withdrawal (rare), (2) fracture in the walls of the root canal (not common), or (3) tear at the base of the incision resulting in fracture of the instrument itself (the most likely occurrence). A fine tactile sense is required for the safe use of barbed broaches; therefore, the use of a heavy "broach holder" is not recommended. Rather, barbed broaches without handles or with short light handles are to be preferred.

AVAILABLE PRODUCTS

Antaeos Broaches, Charles B. Schwed Co., Inc.
Barbed Broaches, Midwest American
Barbed Broaches, Kerr Mfg. Co., Div. of Sybron Dental Products Corp.
Endodontic Barbed Broaches, Healthco, Inc.
Premier Beutelrock Broaches, Premier Dental Products Co.
R & R Nerve Broaches, Ransom and Randolph Company
Unitek Endodontic Broaches, Unitek Corp.

ENGINE DRIVEN ROOT CANAL INSTRUMENTS

Although, historically, engine driven root canal instruments have not been extensively advocated in the United States, due principally to the hazards of root perforation and/or instrument breakage associated with their use, a number of types have been developed for dental contra-angles and handpieces. Introduction of contra-angles designed specifically for endodontics have rekindled long smoldering interest in engine driven root canal instrumentation. Two types of endodontic contra-angles are available. The first, and most popular type at present, operates by a rotary reciprocal movement of the instrument through a 90° arc. The second type produces a vertical oscillation of the instrument as well as the rotary reciprocal motion. Neither type of endodontic contra-angle rotates a root canal instrument 360° as would the typical dental contra-angle. Several varieties of root canal instruments are available for endodontic contra-angles, including type K files and reamers, type H files, barbed broaches and rasps, and special quarter-turn reamers which are not unlike the blanks of metal from which type K files and reamers are twisted.

The mechanical principle of reciprocating rotary motion with or without an accompanying vertical oscillation and its application to the use of endodontic instruments is not new. Ingle refers to it as 'vaiven' motion which he interprets from the Spanish as a "rolling-rotating" motion and advocates its use in pathfinding.[40] Use of the endodontic contra-angle for root canal exploration is not without merit due, no doubt, to sustained mechanical application of this principle. The ease of root canal negotiation with these devices coupled with significant losses of tactile sensation create the principal hazards accompanying their use, these being inadvertent penetration and laceration of the apical tissue and/or lack of accurate control over the working length of the root canal instrument.[41,42] Those endodontic contra-angles which provide vertical oscillation of the root canal instrument present the problem of length control as well as the additional hazards of impacting debris in the root canal or forcing it beyond the apical foramen. No engine driven root canal instruments have been demonstrated to be as effective as hand manipulated types K and H root canal files in cleansing or shaping root canal systems.[31, 34, 43-48] Nor have claims of shortened operating time and decreased incidence of instrument fracture when compared to hand instrumentation been documented at this time.[46]

Most endodontic instruments designed for use with either a straight or contra-angle dental handpiece are manufactured with the shaft and operating head as one piece much as are dental burs. The two types most familiar to dentists in the United States are the Gates-Glidden drill (Type G) and the Pease reamer (Type P) although other special types are included in developing international specifications. Both the Type G and Type P instruments have a long and checkered history in endodontics but currently are enjoying a revival for finishing and enlarging the orifice and cervical third of a root canal following serial filing and flaring with root canal files. The use of either of these instruments to enlarge an uninstrumented root canal or to prepare the root for a post core retainer carries the dangers of perforation and/or excessive loss of tooth structure.

To register or control the working length of a root canal instrument during use several varieties of instrument markers or stops made from multicolored nylon, rubber, or soft plastics are available commercially.[49] These are in the form of small circular discs or in the shape of a tear drop. The point of the tear drop indicates the direction of the curvature of the root canal instrument (or root canal) to the clinician when the instrument is placed in the tooth. These types of markers are placed on the shaft of the root canal instrument and adjusted for proper length. Also available are instrument stops made of colored plastic which are tubular in form encircling the shaft and clipping onto the base of the instrument handle.[50] One type uses a fine tubular extension which sheaths the instrument shaft, thus providing a stop at the floor of the pulp chamber.

A more sophisticated system is the unigauge test handle and instruments. The root canal instruments, which come in a variety of types, are unmounted with a short portion of the terminal end of the shaft bent at a right angle to fit a specially designed adjustable handle. A knurled locking nut on the forward portion of the handle in combination with a slotted posterior portion adjusts the length of the working blade from 20 to 28 mm. The system is available with accessory gauges, wrenches, and special instrument stands. Rather than use commercially available stops or instrument markers many practitioners prefer to use short segments of rubber bands or punchings from rubber dams which they can make themselves.

Available Products

Dent-O-Lux Gates Glidden Drills, Charles B. Schwed Co., Inc.
Engine Reamers, Midwest American
Engine Reamers, Pulpdent Corp. of America
Gates Glidden Drills, Midwest American
Gates Glidden Drills, Pulpdent Corp. of America
Orifice Opener (Pesso Drill), Midwest American
Paste Fillers, Midwest American
Unitek Endodontic Engine Reamers, Unitek Corp.

DEVICES FOR INTRACANAL IRRIGATION

Irrigation during endodontic instrumentation is not only desirable but usually necessary. While sodium hypochlorite solutions with or without the intermittent use of hydrogen peroxide are conceded to be the irrigant of choice in endodontic practice, ethylene diaminetetraacetic acid (EDTA) solutions, lubricating gels, or pastes are often recommended due to their chelation effects on calcified tissues. Evidence obtained through scanning electron microscope investigations reveals that solutions of sodium hypochlorite are particularly effective in removing organic debris whereas EDTA solutions, not gels or pastes, are effective in removing calcific debris.[20-23] The usage of both solutions appears to result in the cleanest and most debris free dentinal surfaces. The removal of debris appears to be a function of the quantity of the irrigant used as well as its particular biochemical properties.[51, 52] Several technical problems are associated with endodontic irrigation; these are supplying sufficient volumes of irrigant to the working area particularly in fine or tortuous root canal systems, aspirating the expended fluid and debris from the root canal and operating field and preventing extrusion of either irrigant or debris beyond the apex of the tooth.

Two types of irrigating needles for use within the root canal system have been developed; one has a blunted tip and a slit along one side extending from the tip for four or five millimeters toward the hub, and the other has a sealed tip with lateral perforations into the needle lumen from the tip toward the hub.[53] Both needles are designed to provide an escape for irrigating fluids laterally and occlusally or incisally out of the tooth should the needle bind in the root canal. Without this feature the root canal would in effect become an extension of the irrigating needle should the needle be forced into place. The perforated needle provides for greater lateral lavage of the root canal system.

Several types of syringes have been developed for use with endodontic irrigating needles.[54-57] Some are simple disposable injection syringes while others provide for aspiration of solution from the tooth as well as irrigation of the root canal system. The aspirating/irrigating types vary in degree of sophistication from simple adoptions of injection syringes to specially designed devices. Some of the more sophisticated devices have raised questions as to their sterilizability and operating safety and none has as yet received acceptance by the Council.

Several severe injuries have been caused by the inadvertent injection of irrigating solutions into apical tissues during endodontic procedures.[58-61] The severity of the reaction is dependent upon the volume of irrigant injected, the toxicity of the solution, and the location of the insult. Air embolisms have been reported as a fatal consequence of blowing compressed air into the open root canals of teeth.[62] Instrumentation with large size instruments (45 and larger) has been shown to increase the potential for extruding debris and irrigant beyond the root canal in experimental situations. Selection of the type of irrigating solution to use, the proper device for using it, and the safest method of use for a particular clinical procedure should be made with these potential hazards firmly in mind.

AVAILABLE PRODUCTS

503ED Endodontic Syringe, Monoject

EndoLock Endodontic Root Canal Irrigation Needle w/Syringe, NPD Dental Systems, Inc.

PERC Perforated Endodontic Root Canal Irrigation Needle, NPD Dental Systems, Inc.

INSTRUMENTS AND DEVICES FOR ROOT CANAL FILLING

The instruments used in endodontic filling procedures differ little from those used in restorative dentistry. A general listing of an endodontic armamentarium includes such items as mirrors, explorers, excavators, cotton forceps, and plastic instruments. Several of these basic types of instruments have been redesigned specifically for endodontic use. Endodontic explorers such as the DG16, DG16-17 and DG16-23 in which the exploring tines are twice as long as those of their restorative counterparts to permit examination of the depths of a pulp chamber have been found useful by many dentists. Root canal excavators, which are spoon excavators with extra long shanks, are a necessity. Cotton forceps can be obtained in several patterns such as college pliers, lock forceps, and back action forceps with either serrated, grooved, or smooth beaks. The plastic instruments most useful for manipulation of temporary filling materials and bases encountered

in endodontic practice are the Woodson #2 (small plugger-hatchet beaver tail blade); Woodson #3 (larger plugger-hoe beaver tail blade); Mortonson (truncated cones of two sizes); or the Ladmore (dome ended cylinders of two sizes). Several variations of these basic patterns have been proposed by individual practitioners.

Most of the specialized endodontic instruments in the dental armamentarium are used in root canal filling procedures. These include pluggers, spreaders, special forceps, and paste filling instruments and devices.

Root canal filling spreaders are smooth, pointed and tapered, metal instruments used to compact filling materials laterally in a root canal. When inserted into the root canal along with the root canal filling material they act much as a wedge, forcing the material laterally against the surrounding dentinal walls. Spreaders have long handles of stainless steel or chromium-plated brass similar to instruments used in restorative dentistry. The working portion of the instrument is usually biangular in design with varying degrees of angulation between the axis of the handle and the axis of the working portion of the instrument dependent upon the particular design. Short handled root canal spreaders, the so-called finger spreaders, which are not unlike root canal files in size and shape are also available for use in posterior teeth. Spreaders are available in a variety of working point sizes.

Root canal filling pluggers (condensers) are smooth, flat ended and slightly tapered, metal instruments used to compact filling materials vertically in a root canal. As with root canal filling spreaders they are available in a variety of sizes and patterns, the most common of which are biangular in design. A uniangular design (Luks) is also available as are the finger, or short handled, pluggers for use in posterior teeth. Some designs, particularly those adopted for use with vertical condensation techniques, have serrations designating five millimeter sections of the working portion for quick assessments of depth of penetration.

For use with silver cone root canal filling

ENDODONTIC INSTRUMENTS

Do:

1. Use standardized and certified stainless steel root canal files and reamers.
2. Purchase instruments from a single manufacturer and familiarize yourself with the cutting and tactile characteristics of that brand.
3. Wipe the instruments with 2x2 gauze moistened with alcohol after removing from the package and prior to use.
4. Sterilize root canal instruments with autoclaving (stainless steel) or dry heat (carbon steel) prior to use.
5. Adopt a technique for determination of tooth length prior to and during endodontic treatment. Develop consistency and skill in the technique you adopt.
6. Place instrument markers or stops on all root canal instruments when you are using them in a tooth.
7. Use root canal files type K to prepare the bulk of the root canal and for serial filing or recapitulation.
8. Use barbed broaches for the removal of intact pulp tissue or medications from the root canal.
9. Rotate type K instruments in a clockwise manner when using as well as in a linear motion out from the canal. If the instrument binds, rotate clockwise while withdrawing from the root canal.
10. Use a sufficient quantity of a suitable irrigant during instrumentation, allowing for debris removal and avoiding apical irritation.
11. Use the natural progression of instrument sizes with the next size in progression only when the size being used can be worked freely in the root canal.
12. Use type H files for the occlusal or incisal flaring of the root canal after apical preparation by type K files.
13. Dry the root canal system with sterile cotton and/or paper points.
14. Use engine driven root canal instruments in endodontic contraangles as pathfinders only with adequate length control. Use hand manipulated files to finish root canal preparations.
15. Prepare a definite seat (apical collar/retention form) in the apical third of the root canal when using solid core filling materials such as silver points.
16. Prepare a sufficiently flaring root canal to permit root canal spreaders or pluggers to reach the apical third of the root when using semi-solid filling materials such as gutta percha.
17. Use root canal spreaders to compact root canal filling materials laterally.
18. Use root canal pluggers to compact root canal filling materials vertically.
19. Use a suitable device for the proper placement of paste root canal fillings.
20. Use suitable amalgam carriers and condensers when placing retrograde root canal fillings in conjunction with apicoectomies.

Don't

1. Use non-standardized or non-certified instruments. Avoid the use of carbon steel instruments whenever possible.
2. Mix brands of instruments in your armamentarium.
3. Use root canal files and reamers directly from the package.
4. Flame root canal files or reamers or use cold disinfectants for sterilization. Use bead sterilizers with caution for accessory sterilization only.

5. Attempt endodontic treatment without approximation of tooth length prior to treatment and a definite determination during treatment. Avoid changing techniques from case to case.

6. Attempt to instrument teeth without adequate indication of the length of instrumentation.

7. Use reamers or broaches for the preparation of the full length of a root canal.

8. Attempt to prepare root canals with barbed broaches or force these instruments into narrow root canals.

9. Rotate type K instruments in a counterclockwise manner when using. Do not attempt to remove a bound instrument by 'unscrewing' it from the root canal.

10. Work on the root canal without irrigation. Do not use potentially irritating irrigants. Do not extrude apically.

11. Deviate from the size progression sequence when using instruments. Avoid using larger sizes too soon or when the smaller sizes continue to bind or do not reach working length.

12. Use type H files for preparation of narrow or fine root canals.

13. Blow air into an open root canal.

14. Use engine driven root canal instruments in endodontic contra-angles without knowing the precise length of the tooth. Do not use these instruments exclusively for root canal preparation.

15. Attempt to seat root canals with solid core filling materials if you do not have an apical preparation for the proper retention of these.

16. Attempt to seal root canals with semi-solid filling materials if the shape of the canal after cleansing and shaping will not allow compaction of the material in the apical third of the root.

17. Use root canal pluggers to compact root canal filling materials laterally.

18. Use root canal spreaders to compact root canal filling materials vertically.

19. Attempt to seal root canals with paste root canal fillings using paper points or root canal files or reamers.

20. Attempt to use amalgam in the periapical region without suitable means of controlling excess material and/or fragments.

techniques, two types of special forceps are available: the Steiglitz Ring-type forceps which has locking handles not unlike a small splinter forceps or hemostat and the grooved beak point forceps which is similar to a fine plier in design with angled and grooved beaks to hold the silver cone during insertion.

When inserting a root canal filling consisting entirely of a paste material or placing sealer cement deep within a root canal special instruments are often used. A paper point or a root canal file or reamer may be used to coat root canal walls with sealer cement in many cases but for a complete seal of the system with a paste filler this will not suffice. Lentulo paste fillers can be used in a contra-angle handpiece to spread paste evenly throughout a root canal, but are not very satisfactory if the paste mixes are of the high viscosity or stiffness consistent with maximum dimensional stability and low tissue toxicity. For use with heavy bodied paste systems, modified disposable tuberculin syringes have been recommended and specially designed devices have been developed.[63] Most notable of these is the Pulpdent Pressure Syringe of Greenberg and Katz which is capable of placing controlled amounts of very heavy pastes into all sizes of root canals.[64] This particular device has been demonstrated to be very effective for the purposes for which it was intended. Pastes as thick as those used for temporary coronal restorations can be used with the device provided the mesh size of the zinc oxide or other base particles permit extrusion through a variety of sizes of injection needles.[65]

Occasionally the endodontist must seal a root canal with zinc-free dental amalgam following apicoectomy. Amalgam carriers with small apertures for the material have been developed for this special purpose. One variety is the Messing root canal gun which is, in effect, a metal syringe available with three sizes of stainless steel needles and styluses which act as pluggers. A second type of carrier resembles a straight tweezer with a cylinder attached to the tip of the lower portion. These are available in large and small sizes. Several amalgam condensers of the angled back action variety are available for retrograde root canal filling.

AVAILABLE PRODUCTS

Endodontic Instruments, Dentool Co. Inc.

Endodontic Instruments, Hu-Friedy Mfg. Co., Inc.

Luks Pluggers-Single End, Pulpdent Corp. of America

PCA Root Canal Discs and Measuring Stand, Pulpdent Corp. of America

PCA Root Canal Stops, Pulpdent Corp. of America

Premier Beutelrock Endodontic Instruments, Premier Dental Products

Premier Dual Pin Pliers, Premier Dental Products Co.

Premier Endodontic Hand Instruments, Premier Dental Products Co.

Premier Endodontic Locking Pliers w/Grooves, Premier Dental Products Co.

Premier Endodontic Plier, Premier Dental Products Co.

Premier Endo Magazine #104 & #106, Premier Dental Products Co.

R & R Endodontic Rubber Stops, Ransom and Randolph Company

R & R Schilder Endodontic Pluggers and Heat Carriers, Ransom and Randolph Company

R & R Spiral Fillers, Ransom and Randolph Company

Root Canal Pluggers-double end, Pulpdent Corp. of America

Root Canal Spreader Dryers, Pulpdent Corp. of America

Rubber Dam Punch & Clamp Forcep, J.R. Rand Specialty Co., Inc.

Unitek Endodontic Condenser, Unitek Corp.

Unitek Endodontic Finger Pluggers, Unitek Corp.

Unitek Endodontic Hand Instruments, Unitek Corp.

Unitek Endodontic Root Canal Fillers, Unitek Corp.

LITERATURE REFERENCES

1. Heuer, M.A. Instruments and materials. In Cohen, S. and Burns, R. (eds.) Pathways of the pulp. ed. 1, St. Louis, C.V. Mosby Co., 1976.

2. Heuer, M.A. Endodontic materials. In Craig, R.G. (ed.) Dental materials: A problem oriented approach. ed. 1, St. Louis, C.V. Mosby Co., 1978.

3. Heuer, M.A. The biomechanics of endodontic therapy. Dent. Clin. N. Am. p. 341, July 1963.

4. Sampeck, A.J. Instruments of endodontics: Their manufacture, use and abuse. Dent. Clin. N. Am. p. 579, Nov. 1967.

5. Schilder, H. Cleansing and shaping the root canal. Dent. Clin. N. Am. p. 269, Apr. 1974.

6. Nicholls, E. The efficacy of cleansing root canals. Br. Dent. J. 112:167 Feb. 1962.

7. Shoji, Y. Studies on the mechanism of the mechanical enlargement of root canals. Nihon Univ. Sch. Dent. J. 70:71 June 1965.

8. Haga, C. Microscopic measurements of root canal preparations following instrumentation. Northwestern Univ. Dent. Sch. Dent. Res. Grad. Study Bull. 57:11, 1967.

9. Gutierrez, J.H., and Garcia, J. Microscopic and macroscopic investigations on results of mechanical preparations of root canals. Oral Surg., Oral Med., Oral Path. 25:108 Jan. 1968.

10. Vessey, R.A. The effect of filing versus reaming on the shape of the prepared root canal. Oral Surg., Oral Med., Oral Path. 27:543 Apr. 1969.

11. Schneider, S.W. A comparison of canal preparations in straight and curved root canals. Oral Surg., Oral Med., Oral Path. 32:271 Aug.

1971.

12. Davis, S.R.; Brayton, S.M.; and Goldman, M. The morphology of the prepared root canal: A study utilizing injectable silicone. Oral Surg., Oral Med., Oral Path. 34:642 Oct. 1972.

13. Oliet, S., and Sorin, S.M. Cutting efficiency of endodontic reamers. Oral Surg., Oral Med., Oral Path. 36:243 Aug. 1973.

14. Jungman, C.L.; Uchin, R.A.; and Bucher, J.F. Effect of instrumentation on the shape of the root canal. J. Endod. 1:66 Feb. 1975.

15. Coffae, K.P., and Brilliant, J.D. The effect of serial preparation versus nonserial preparation on tissue removal in the root canals of extracted mandibular human molars. J. Endod. 1:211 June 1975.

16. Weine, F.S.; Kelly, R.F.; and Lio, P.J. The effect of preparation procedures on original canal shape and on apical foramen shape. J. Endod. 1:255 Aug. 1975.

17. Walton, R.E. Histologic evaluation of different methods of enlarging the pulp canal space. J. Endod. 2:304 Oct. 1976.

18. Littman, S.H. Evaluation of root canal debridement by use of a radiopaque medium. J. Endod. 3:135 Apr. 1977.

19. Mizrahi, S.J.; Tucker, J.W.; and Seltzer, S. A scanning electron microscope study of the efficacy of various endodontic instruments. J. Endod. 1:324 Oct. 1975.

20. McComb, D., and Smith, D.C. A preliminary scanning electron microscope study of root canals after endodontic procedures. J. Endod. 1:238 July 1975.

21. McComb, D.; Smith, D.C.; and Beagrie, G.S. The results of in vivo endodontic chemomechanical instrumentation—a scanning electron microscope study. Br. Endod. Soc. J. 9:11 Jan. 1976.

22. Moodnik, R.M., et al. Efficacy of biomechanical instrumentation: A scanning electron microscopic study. J. Endod. 2:261 Sept. 1976.

23. Dupont, A.A.; Brady, J.M.; and del Rio, C.E. Scanning microscope evaluation of canal debridement as compared to present methods. Oral Surg., Oral Med., Oral Path. 44:113 July 1977.

24. Lilley, J.D., and Smith, D.C. An investigation of the fracture of root canal reamers. Br. Dent. J. 120:364 Apr. 1966.

25. Shoji, Y. Systematic endodontics. Buchenid Zeitschriften-Verlag, "Kie Quintessenz" Berlin—Chicago, 1973.

26. Serene, T.P., et al. Principles of preclinical endodontics. ed. 2, Dubuque, Kendall/Hunt, 1975.

27. Fromme, H.G., and Reidel, H. Treatment of dental root canals and the marginal contact between filling material and tooth, studied by SEM. Br. Endod. Soc. J. 6:17, 1972.

28. Chernick, L.B., et al. Torsional failure of endodontic files. J. Endod. 2:94 Apr. 1976.

29. Lautenschlager, E.P., et al. Brittle and ductile torsional failures of endodontic instruments. J. Endod. 3:175 May 1977.

30. Sommer, R.F.; Ostrander, F.D.; and Crowley, M.C. Clinical endodontics: A manual of scientific endodontics. ed. 3, Philadelphia, W.B. Saunders Co., 1966.

31. Ingle, J.I. The need for endodontic instrument standardization. Oral Surg., Oral Med., Oral Path. 8:1211 Nov. 1955.

32. Green, E.N. Microscopic examination of root canal files and reamers. Oral Surg., Oral Med., Oral Path. 10:532 May 1957.

33. Craig, R.G., and Peyton, F.A. Physical properties of carbon steel root canal files and reamers. Oral Surg., Oral Med., Oral Path. 15:213 Feb. 1962.

34. Craig, R.G., and Peyton, F.A. Physical properties of stainless steel endodontic files and reamers. Oral Surg., Oral Med., Oral Path. 16:206 Feb. 1963.

35. Sargeant, J.E., and Stemler, J. Torsional properties of endodontic instruments. IADR Program and Abstracts of Papers. Abstract M43, 1964.

36. Oliet, S., and Sorin, S.M. Torsional tester for root canal instruments. Oral Surg., Oral Med., Oral Path. 20:654 Nov. 1965.

37. Craig, R.G.; McIlwain, E.D.; and Peyton, F.A. Bending and torsion properties of endodontic instruments. Oral Surg., Oral Med., Oral Path. 25:239 Feb. 1968.

38. Gutierrez, J.H.; Gigoux, C.; and Sanhueza, I. Physical and chemical deterioration of endodontic reamers during mechanical preparation. Oral Surg., Oral Med., Oral Path. 28:394 Sept. 1969.

39. Council on Dental Materials and Devices, American Dental Association new specification no. 28 for endodontic files and reamers. JADA 93:813 Oct. 1976.

40. Ingle, J.E., and Beveridge, E.E. Endodontics. ed. 2, Philadelphia, Lea and Febiger, 1976.

41. Frank, A.L. An evaluation of the giromatic

endodontic handpiece. Oral Surg., Oral Med., Oral Path. 24:419 Sept. 1967.

42. Laws, A.J. Preparation of root canals—an evaluation of mechanical aids. N.Z. Dent. J. 64:156 July 1968.

43. Molven, O. Engine and hand operated root canal exploration. Odont. Tidskr. 76:61, 1968.

44. Molven, O. A comparison of the dentin removing ability of five root canal instruments. Scand. J. Dent. Res. 78:500, 1970.

45. Harty, F.J., and Stock, C.J.R. A comparison of the flexibility of giromatic and hand operated instruments in endodontics. Br. Endod. Soc. J. 7:64 July 1974.

46. Harty, F.J., and Stock, C.J.R. The giromatic system compared with hand instrumentation in endodontics. Br. Dent. J. 137:239 Sept. 1974.

47. O'Connell, D.T., and Brayton, S.M. Evaluation of root canal preparation with two automated endodontic handpieces. Oral Surg., Oral Med., Oral Path. 39:298 Feb. 1975.

48. Weine, F.S.; Kelly, R.F.; and Bray, K.E. Effect of preparation with endodontic handpieces on original canal shape. J. Endod. 2:298 Oct. 1976.

49. Saunders, M. Length control of root canal instruments: An improved system. Br. Dent. J. 129:337 Oct. 1970.

50. Guldenor, P., and Imobersteg, C. New method of measuring the exact length of root canal instruments. Br. Endod. Soc. J. 6:51, 1972.

51. Senia, E.S.; Marshall, F.J.; and Rosen, S. The solvent action of sodium hypochlorite on pulp tissue of extracted teeth. Oral Surg., Oral Med., Oral Path. 31:96 Jan. 1971.

52. Baker, N.A., et al. Scanning electron microscopic study of the efficacy of various irrigating solutions. J. Endod. 1:127 Apr. 1975.

53. Goldman, M., et al. New method of irrigation during endodontic treatment. J. Endod. 2:257 Sept. 1976.

54. Goodlin, I.F. An endodontic suction adaptor kit. Can. Dent. Assoc. J. 39:195 Mar. 1973.

55. Kahn, H., et al. An improved endodontic irrigation technique. Oral Surg., Oral Med., Oral Path. 36:887 Dec. 1973.

56. Malmin, O. Endovage the safer one. Akron, Endovage Co., 1973.

57. Rowe, A.H. An assessment of the 'Aspir' endodontic irrigator/aspirator. Br. Endod. Soc. J. 9:23 Jan. 1976.

58. Harris, W.E. Unusual endodontic complication: Report of a case. JADA 83:358 Aug. 1971.

59. Bhat, K.S. Tissue emphysema caused by hydrogen peroxide. Oral Surg., Oral Med., Oral Path. 38:304 Aug. 1974.

60. Becker, G.L.; Cohen, S.; and Borer, R. The sequellae of accidently injecting sodium hypochlorite beyond the root apex. Oral Surg., Oral Med., Oral Path. 38:633 Oct. 1974.

61. Walker, J.E. Emphysema of soft tissues complicating endodontic treatment using hydrogen peroxide: A case report. Br. J. Oral Surg. 13:98 July 1975.

62. Rickles, N.H., and Joshi, B.A. A death from air embolism during root canal therapy. JADA 67:397 Sept. 1963.

63. Ireland, J.F., and Dolce, J.L. Modification of technique for injection obturation. J. Endod. 1:156 May 1975.

64. Greenberg, M. Filling root canals by an injection technique. Dent. Dig. 69:61 Feb. 1963.

65. Berk, H., and Krakow, A. Efficient endodontic procedures with the use of the pressure syringe. Dent. Clin. N. Am. p. 387, July 1965.

SURGICAL INSTRUMENTS

EXTRACTION FORCEPS

There are many designs and shapes of extraction forceps. The present standard model is the anatomical forcep which is adapted to measurements of average crown width and length. The beak of the instrument is not the only consideration in the anatomical forcep but when the instrument is closed upon the type tooth for which it is designed the beaks make maximum contact with a favorable force distribution to the tooth to provide a firm, nonslipping grasp. In addition, the handles of the forcep remain separated sufficiently for a good handhold without causing strain.

Bayonet and angled shapes allow for clearance over the mandible when extracting maxillary teeth. Forceps with essentially straight handles and beaks angled about 45 to 90 degrees allow good access and visibility when removing mandibular teeth.

There is a practical limit to the number of forceps an office may have available as the instruments are expensive. In general practice,

at least two complete sets of forceps are needed as immediate resterilization is impossible if accidental contamination should occur during surgery. Personnel must understand the use of each instrument. After the practitioner has become familiar with the basic armamentarium, specialized instruments may be added. American firms have furnished an excellent basic line of instruments plus many specialized instruments; some designed by various practitioners are named after the designer. Recently, European instruments with many design variations have been introduced. It is impossible to comment adequately on these instruments and the purported advantages of their designs, since the advantages have to be experienced by the individual user. However these instruments, by and large, are excellent in construction and materials.

The tendency today is toward use of universal anatomical forceps rather than paired anatomical instruments. An example is the 10S maxillary molar forcep which fits the left as well as the right molars. For the practitioner who removes many carious teeth in a robust population, rather than periodontally involved teeth in an aged population, right and left cowhorn type maxillary forceps (88R and 88L) might be more appropriate. These forceps have a buccal prong that slides between the buccal roots. The handle is considerably longer. A disadvantage is that two forceps must be purchased, which increases the cost if many complete sets of instruments are bought, and office personnel must select the instrument for the proper side.

Stainless steel equipment is more costly initially, but it is more durable than plated carbon steel. Proper care and sterilization procedures must include oiling the hinges regularly to assure free and easy movement.

Often overlooked in the general office is the need for periodic refurbishing of the beaks. Normal wear or damage by dropping blunts the beaks or causes indentations which can be corrected at nominal cost by sending the instruments back to the manufacturer.

AVAILABLE PRODUCTS

Extraction Forceps, E. A. Beck and Co.
Extraction Forceps, Miltex Instruments Co.
Forceps, Hu-Friedy Mfg. Co., Inc.
Forceps, J. R. Rand Specialty Co., Inc.
Mosquito Forceps, Lee Pharmaceuticals
Steiglitz Forceps, Pulpdent Corp. of America
Unitek Pedodontic Extraction Forceps, Unitek Corp.

ELEVATORS

There are many techniques for elevator use, and consequently, many elevator designs. Minimal equipment includes paired (right and left) molar root exolevers (Winter type), paired triangular exolevers (Winter type) and a straight exolever. Several sizes of instrument tips are available and the user selects the size best suited for the situation. The Winter elevators are available with straight or cross bar handles. Many operators prefer the cross-bar handle, which is more efficient, but others prefer the smooth round handle because the cross bar handle may deliver unnecessary force. The straight handle elevator is made with a wide as

well as a thin, delicate tip. Smooth or serrated tip elevators are available and both function well if their edges are sharp.

Again, stainless steel is preferred. The tips must be resharpened periodically in the office or returned to the manufacturer for sharpening. A dull elevator is ineffective.

AVAILABLE PRODUCTS

American Dental Periosteal Elevator, American Dental Mfg. Co.
Elevators, E. A. Beck & Co.
Elevators, Hu-Friedy Mfg. Co., Inc.
Elevators, Miltex Instrument Co.
Nurlite Elevators, J. R. Rand Specialty Co., Inc.

RETRACTORS

Surgical retractors range from simple instruments designed to retract normal structures such as the tongue or cheeks, or to hold the surgical flap away from the operative site, to extremely specialized instruments for major jaw surgery.

The retractors designed for minor surgery often have two sides in a right angle bended instrument, one side smooth and the other side with small prongs on the end to hold the surgical flap. Some have one side only, the other side being a rounded handle for a more comfortable grip by the assistant during long procedures.

Newer major surgery retractors are being designed continuously for an efficient approach to difficult areas. Some are designed for intraoral vertical mandibular ramus procedures. Others are designed for extraoral procedures in the vertical ramus, with different designs for different techniques. Some have fiber-optic attachments for better visibility in deep wounds.

AVAILABLE PRODUCTS

Gingi Retractor, Pulpdent Corp. of America
Gingival Retraction Packing Instruments, North Pacific Dental, Inc.
Retractors, E. A. Beck & Co.
Retractors, Hu-Friedy Mfg. Co., Inc.
Retractors, Miltex Instruments Co.

CURETS

Various sizes of curets are available. The original purpose of the instrument was to remove pathologic soft tissue or spongiosa. Although still used for this purpose, curets have been modified into the "feelers" for many oral surgery procedures, such as impaction removal and breaking the free gingival attachments around teeth to be removed. Larger curets may be used as periosteal elevators.

Some designs have several sizes of straight instruments and several sizes of bi-angled instruments. Some curets are provided in a double ended design with right and left on one narrow handle. Handles of single-ended instruments are often more substantial, and a choice is offered of a round handle or a square handle. The advantage of the square handle is the ability to orient the curet tip in an obscure surgical area by the position of the handle.

Available Products

American Dental Curettes, American Dental Mfg. Co.
American Dental Goldmal-Fox Surgical Curette, American Dental Mfg. Co.
Curettes, Miltex Instruments Co.
Curettes, E. A. Beck & Co.
Curettes, Hu-Friedy Mfg. Co., Inc.

SCISSORS, NEEDLE HOLDERS AND HEMOSTATS

Surgical scissors are used in the dental office for cutting tissue and for cutting sutures. In the operating room good surgical scissors are never used for cutting sutures, but rather for two surgical dissection procedures, namely cutting tissue and dissecting fascial planes by placing the closed scissors in the tissue and opening them to spread the tissue in order to push aside nerves and vessels. The instruments are precision made and kept extremely sharp.

For occasional surgical use, serrated scissors may be used. They require less sharpening care; however, they are not as effective. A substantial handle length, six inches, is desirable for reaching into the mouth. A combination scissors and needle holder instrument is often used for suturing in minor office surgery.

The needle holder used for oral surgery should not be less than 6 inches long. It should be noted that a suture needle breaks if it is clamped by the needle holder over or close to the eye of the needle. Hemostats should not be used as needle holders.

Hemostats are used primarily to clamp bleeding blood vessels. A secondary role is blunt dissection, used in the same manner as the dissecting scissors. For oral surgery, the mosquito hemostat is commonly used for its delicacy. These instruments should not be used for applications other than those requiring delicacy since they distort if misused. No dental office should be without them, for they could be life saving.

Available Products

Needle holders, Hu-Friedy Mfg. Co., Inc.
Scissors & Hemostats, J. R. Rand Specialty Co., Inc.
Scissors & Hemostats, Miltex Instruments Co.
Scissors & Hemostats, E. A. Beck & Co.
Scissors, Hu-Friedy Mfg. Co., Inc.

SURGICAL HANDPIECES

All modern surgical handpieces are high speed turbines, usually propelled by compressed air or gas. Several of these instruments are needed in an office that performs extensive surgery. These instruments can be autoclaved if the manufacturer's directions are followed carefully by the office staff.

Some of the newest surgical air turbines feature decreased speed in order to increase torque. They revolve at approximately 30,000 to 50,000 rpm in contrast to 300,000 to 400,000 rpm of current handpieces. Straight handpieces are used for most major oral surgery as well as for intraoral bone surgery, as for example, the removal of unerupted teeth. However, a contra-angle handpiece is available for better access to the third molar area, but the bur can be too short for vertical cutting of the lowest portion of the impacted tooth when the horizontal portion of the 90° instrument lies on the occlusal plane of the second molar. New instruments offer a compromise between the two, such as a 45° handpiece that makes access better for the third molar impaction area. Many of the surgical handpieces have a water coolant stream built in. The advantage of the high speed handpiece is fast cutting of bone with very light pressure. The advantage of the slower speed handpiece with torque is better tactile sense with the instrument.

Other instruments in this field include reciprocating bone cutting instruments that have various attachments for specific applications. Improvements are offered continually. For example, several instruments have been designed for use in intraoral vertical osteotomies in the ascending ramus of the mandible. The reciprocating (oscillating) saws are noted for their lack of injury to adjacent soft tissues in the depth of the wound beneath the bone that is being sectioned.

Surgical burs are available in various lengths, sizes, and shapes for different surgical uses. In unerupted tooth removal a round bur is used often for bone removal as well as for tooth division. Manufacturers suggest the use of bone burs made for their surgical handpieces; however, some practitioners use ordinary carbide dental burs. Larger bone burs are made for special uses such as torus removal and alveoloplasty, but again, many operators prefer dental burs.

Available Products

Impact-Air 45, Innovators, Inc.
Surgical Instruments, Healthco, Inc.

SUTURES

Much research has been directed toward developing the ideal suture material. New fibers have been tested and improvement is evident; however, no single material has been found to satisfy all needs. Sutures are used for many purposes in different areas of the body and therefore the prime consideration lies in careful selection of the type of suture and the size of the strand for a particular situation.

Basically, sutures are absorbable or nonabsorbable and monofilaments or multifilaments (usually braided). Absorbable sutures are represented by catgut, plain or chromic, which is tanned for slower absorption; polyglactin 910; and polyglycolic acid. Catgut is a monofilament, while the others are braided multifilaments. Nonabsorbable sutures are represented by silk, cotton, nylon, polyester, polypropylene and stainless steel.

The advantage of monofilament sutures is less "wicking" action as compared to the braided materials which allow secretions, fluids and bacteria to follow the suture into the deeper tissues. This is especially likely with silk and cotton which absorb such contaminants. Furthermore, granulocytes and macrophages are too large to work their way between tightly packed suture filaments to act upon the contaminants.[1]

The multifilaments tie more easily, stay tied longer compared to monofilaments, and their knots are not as irritating to nearby surface tissues. A disadvantage of some monofilaments is their low friction combined with "memory," so that knots tend to untie spontaneously and return to the original straight fiber shape.

Tissue reaction to suture material is the subject of extensive research. This factor may be most significant for major oral surgery where sutures are embedded in tissue. For superficial oral surgery in the mucous membranes of the mouth, there is a less critical requirement for tissue compatibility since most oral sutures are removed spontaneously or by the surgeon in several days. In a study of tissue reaction to many types of sutures,[1] responses for each material were noted at 7, 21 and 180 days. Although differences were noted in the longer term sites, all 7-day reactions were noted as minimal for monofilaments and multifilaments, natural and synthetic fibers. Apparently wicking is of minimal importance if sutures are removed within a short time.

Strength is important in such procedures as hernia and tendon repair. It is less important in oral surgery, except possibly in bone sutures where wire is used. Loss of strength with time is equally unimportant in many oral surgery or periodontic procedures.

Handling characteristics are best with braided materials such as silk, cotton and braided nylon. Most oral mucous membrane flaps are sutured with silk because of low cost, ease of handling and ease of visibility. However, catgut or the newer polyglycolic acid sutures are advantageous in areas where they may be difficult to find (a buried silk suture can cause a granulomatous lesion) or in children and some adults where suture removal is mentally and physically traumatic.

The use of the suture with swedged needle in a presterilized package is ideal, although more expensive. The swedged needle precludes the larger tissue hole made by the eye of the reusable needle, and it is used for all fine flap suturing. Although the initial expense is higher, it eliminates the labor of preparing the suture in the office, and it guarantees sterility.

The characteristics and applications of suture materials are summarized in Table I.[2]

SCALPELS

The present structure of scalpels, namely metal handles and disposable blades, is satisfactory, and no major changes are required. The metal handles are available in three sizes, the standard most commonly used #3 handle which is 6 inches long and two longer sizes.

Table I.
Characteristics of Suture Materials

Suture Material	Advantage
Metallic	Strong
Polyester	Good handling properties Prolonged retention
Synthetic Monofilaments	Strong Knot security Lack of deterioration
Cotton and Silk	Superb handling properties Accurate knot placement
Catgut	Absorbable in tissues (Poor handling properties)
Absorbable Synthetics	Strong, inert Flexible Average handling properties

Disposable blades are manufactured in seven designs. Primarily the small straight #11 blade, the sickle #12 blade, and curved #15 blade are used in dentistry.

New designs of scalpels adapted for microsurgery as well as general surgery have been developed. The handles are pencil-shaped and the disposable blades are finer, and available with different angles; some have two cutting edges.

A disposable scalpel has been designed. It has not found general use outside of emergency rooms. It consists of a plastic handle to which a conventional blade is fused. Perhaps one of the reasons for its lack of popularity is the difficulty of disposal so that cleaning and trash crews are not cut by blades which pierce through the plastic trash bags. Special foam fold-over containers are used by operating rooms to dispose of blades. The fused handle-blade disposable scalpel is the most difficult to render harmless.

AVAILABLE PRODUCTS

Scalpels, E. A. Beck & Co.
Scalpels, Hu-friedy Mfg. Co., Inc.
Scalpels, Miltex Instrument Co.

LITERATURE REFERENCES
1. Van Winkle, W., and Salthouse, T. N. Biological response to sutures and principles of suture selection, Ethicon Inc.
2. Herrmann, J. B. Modern surgical sutures: Their characteristics and applications. International Symposium: Sutures in wound repair, Ethicon, 1972, p. 31.

PULP TESTERS

Pulp testers are instruments that attempt to determine whether the pulp of a tooth is vital or nonvital. Usually the instruments supply a stimulus to the tooth and the test for vitality is then based upon the ability of a patient to perceive the stimulus.

USES: Pulp testers are used for any diagnostic or treatment planning situation in which the vitality of tooth pulps needs to be determined. Probably the most common specific use of pulp testers is in helping to determine a need for endodontic treatment.

TYPES: The most common types of pulp testers supply an electrical stimulus to a tooth. These pulp testers are powered either by house current or by batteries. Other types of pulp testers are based upon thermal stimuli.[1,2] Electric resistance heaters or a heated hand instrument have been used to apply a heat stimulus to a tooth. Cold stimuli have been applied by thermoelectric coolers,[3,4] by ice, or by a refrigerated hand instrument. Assessment of tooth vitality has also been performed on an experimental basis by measuring the temperature of the crowns of teeth.[5,6] Measurements have been made with thermistors applied to teeth, by infrared thermography, and by application of liquid crystals to teeth.[1,5] The thermal stimulus and thermal measuring types of pulp testers have been used only on a limited or experimental basis, and accordingly, further discussion will concentrate on the more commonly used electrical stimulus type of pulp testers.

COMPONENTS: Commercially available pulp testers generally consist of a variable voltage output unit, a cathodal electrode to be applied to the crown of a tooth, and a grounded electrode usually incorporated into the portion of the instruments held in the hand of the clinician administering the test. The current path is generally considered to be from the tooth electrode, through the crown and the pulp to the apex of the root, through other tissues of the patient to a point of contact between the patient and the clinician, and through the clinician to the grounded electrode.[7,8] This single tooth electrode situation is known as monopolar stimulation. Limited use, mostly on an experimental basis, has been made of pulp testers which apply both electrodes to the crown of a tooth.[8-10] This is known as bipolar stimulation. For bipolar stimulation the current path is considered to be only through the crown and the pulp between the two electrodes.[8,11]

The currents produced by pulp testers are pulsed, D.C. currents. The duration of the pulses, the frequency, and the wave form vary with different brands of pulp testers.[2,12,13]

In general, the safety of electric stimulus pulp tests has been established by animal experimentation.[6] However, electrical phenomena caused by a pulp tester may interfere with electronic life support devices. Accordingly, electric stimulus pulp testers should not be used if the clinician or the patient has an electronic pacemaker or other electronic life support device unless the safety of use is reliably established. In this situation, pulp tests based upon thermal principles may be the procedure of choice.

DIRECTIONS FOR USE: A pulp test procedure, in essence, consists of: isolating and drying the teeth to be tested, establishing good electrical contact between the tooth electrode and a tooth, and increasing the voltage output of the stimulator from its lowest setting until a response is elicited from the patient. If no response is elicited from the patient, then presumably the tooth pulp being tested is not vital.

The physical stimulus to which the pulp of a tooth responds is the amount of current flow through the pulp or more precisely the current density within the pulp.[7,8,13,14] For a given electrode area of contact and for a particular location of contact on a tooth, the current density in the pulp is undoubtedly proportional to the current through the pulp tester circuit.

The threshold of stimulation typically occurs at currents between 1 and 20 uA;[2,10,15] however, thresholds depend upon the pulse duration, the frequency, the polarity, and the wave form of the stimulating current.[2,10] Tooth resistances and capacitances range from about $1M\Omega$ and over 100 pF to 55 $M\Omega$ and 25 pF.[13,16,17] The electrical resistances of different teeth vary considerably due at least partly to differences in size and shape of the teeth. Voltages greater than 200 V may be required to exceed threshold stimulation. Some pulp testers, for example, deliver 800 V at maximum settings.[13] Care should be taken not to short circuit the two electrodes during handling.

Since the circuit resistance is high, a conductive medium should be used to establish good electrical contact between a tooth and the tooth electrode. A small portion of toothpaste is usually suitable to establish electrical contact. The contact medium should be sufficiently viscous and should be used in a small enough quantity so that the contact area between the electrode and the tooth is not substantially greater than the electrode area itself. Otherwise, the current density may be affected by changes in the effective contact area. Also, the conductive medium should not be allowed to contact the gingiva, thereby forming a low resistance circuit path to bypass the tooth and the pulp. For the same reason, it is essential to dry the crown of a tooth in preparation for a pulp test. In addition, the conventional pulp test cannot be used for a restored tooth if the restoration makes electrical contact with the gingiva or adjacent teeth, since a bypass circuit would be established. Probably, bipolar pulp testers could be used for teeth restored with intracoronal restorations.

The clinician operating a conventional pulp tester must establish good electrical contact with the patient and with the handheld electrode. Undoubtedly factors, such as the amount of moisture in the clinician's hand, affect the resistance of the circuit. Surgical gloves should not be worn by the clinician during a pulp test procedure unless special provisions are made to complete the electrical circuit. Bipolar stimulation would eliminate these types of electrical contact problems.

Since a tooth responds to the amount of electric current, it would be most germane to monitor this property during a pulp test. However, most commercial pulp testers provide only an indication of relative voltage and do not provide an indication of current flow.[13,18] Monitoring voltage in the presence of unknown and highly variable circuit resistances does not provide a measure of current flow. In view of this situation, it is important to test several teeth believed to be normal to calibrate the pulp tester to each patient. The control teeth should be about the same size and shape as the test teeth and a consistent position of contact for the electrode on the teeth should be used.

LIMITATIONS OF USE: A pulp test cannot be regarded as totally reliable. For example, false positive tests for vitality can occur if a patient response is evoked by stimulation of periodontal nerves. Periodontal stimulation can occur with monopolar testing, even if the current path is properly routed through the pulp, because periodontal tissues can be involved in the current path beyond the root apex. False positive tests could result from stimulation of an adjacent vital tooth, due to a low resistance path through contacting restorations. Presumably, false positive tests are minimized by properly administered bipolar stimulation. Also, it should be noted that a vital pulp is not necessarily a normal healthy pulp. In fact, an inflamed or hyperemic pulp may have a lower stimulation threshold than a normal pulp.[2]

False negative tests for vitality can occur if part of the current is diverted around the tooth by poor test techniques, such as moisture contamination on the tooth surface. The electrical resistance of some teeth may be great enough that a pulp tester cannot develop sufficient voltage to create a current above the threshold. Failure to make good electrical contacts at any point in the pulp test circuit could result in a false negative test. Obviously, false negative tests could also occur in the presence of local anesthetics, analgesics and psycholeptic drugs.

The many complicating factors emphasize the need to supplement pulp tests by other information such as: radiographic analysis, tooth percussion, existence of periapical tenderness, evidence of a sinus tract, evidence of trauma, and patient testimonial regarding the onset and nature of a particular situation.

Do:

1. Isolate and dry teeth to be examined.
2. Use an appropriate contact medium, such as toothpaste between the tooth electrode and the tooth.
3. Use a consistent location of electrode contact on the teeth.
4. Stimulate teeth believed to be normal as a control for the test teeth.
5. Supplement a pulp test with other diagnostic information to help eliminate false positive and false negative tests.

Don't:

1. Use an electric stimulus pulp tester if the patient or clinician has a pacemaker or other electronic life support device unless the safety of use is reliably established.
2. Use a pulp tester for anesthetized teeth or in the presence of analgesic or psycholeptic medication.
3. Use conventional pulp testers with surgical gloves unless special means are taken to complete the pulp test circuit.
4. Use conventional pulp testers for teeth with restorations that can establish a bypass circuit around the tooth to be tested.
5. Rely upon pulp testers exclusively for diagnosis of pulpal status.

Literature References

1. Stoops, L.C., and Scott, D., Jr. Measurement of tooth temperature as a means of determining pulp vitality. J. Endod. 2:141 May 1976.

2. Sommer, R.F.; Ostrander, F.D.; and Crowley, M.C. Clinical endodontics. In Clinical evaluation of diagnostic aids. ed. 3, Philadelphia, W.B. Saunders, 1966.

3. Mumford, J.M., and Bowsher, D. Pain and protopothic sensibility. A review with particular reference to the teeth. Pain 2:233, 1976.

4. Reynolds, R.L. The determination of pulp vitality by means of thermal and electrical stimuli. Oral Surg., Oral Med., Oral Path., 22:231 Aug. 1966.

5. Howell, R.M.; Duell, R.C.; and Mullaney, T.P. The determination of pulp vitality by thermographic means using cholesteric liquid crystals. Oral Surg., Oral Med., Oral Path. 29:763 May 1970.

6. McDaniel, K.F.; Rowe, N.H.; and Charbeneau, G.T. Tissue response to an electric pulp tester. J. Prosthet. Dent. 29:84 Jan. 1973.

7. Mumford, J.M. Path of direct current in electric pulptesting using one coronal electrode. Br. Dent. J. 106:243, 1959.

8. Hannan, A.G.; Sui, W.; and Tom, J. A comparison of monopolar and bipolar pulptesting. J. Can. Dent. Assoc. 40:124, 1974.

9. Mitchell, C.L. Central nervous system responses to tooth pulp stimulation and their modification by drugs. Adv. Oral Biol. 4:131, 1970.

10. Matthews, B.; Horinchi, H.; and Greenwood, F. The effects of stimulus polarity and electrode area on the threshold to monopolar stimulation of teeth in human subjects with some preliminary observations on the use of a bipolar pulp tester. Arch. Oral Biol. 19:35, 1974.

11. Mumford, J.M. Path of direct current in electric pulp-testing using two coronal electrodes. Br. Dent. J. 106:243, 1959.

12. Jones, E.H. Battery powered vitality testers. Aust. Dent. J. 12:147 Apr. 1967.

13. Matthews, B., and Searle, B.N. Some observations on pulp testers. Br. Dent. J. 137:307, 1974.

14. Mumford, J.M., and Newton, A.V. Zone of excitation when electrically stimulating human teeth. Arch. Oral Biol. 14:1383, 1969.

15. Matthews, B., et al. Thresholds of vital and non-vital teeth to stimulation with electric pulp testers. Br. Dent. J. 137:352 Nov. 1974.

16. Mumford, J.M. Resistivity of human enamel and dentine. Arch. Oral Biol. 12:925, 1967.

17. Matthews, B., and Searle, B.N. Electrical stimulation of teeth. Pain 2:245, 1976.

18. Hietanen, J., and Rantanen, A.V. Screening some modern pulp vitality testers. Proc. Finnish Dent. Soc. 69:113, 1973.

PROSTHODONTIC INSTRUMENTS AND DEVICES

ARTICULATORS

During the past two centuries, a great variety of articulators have been developed. Changing concepts of occlusion have stimulated a constant search for improved instruments. New materials, new technology, and research in the physiology of occlusion have contributed refinements in structure and function of articulators in recent years. The general practitioner surveying this field today is likely to be confused by the number of articulators and their apparent complexity.

The dentist using the articulator is the critical factor in the successful application of these devices. The dentist's concepts and understanding of occlusion are the deciding elements for success. The articulator, simple or complex, assists the dentist in applying wisdom and skill to a clinical problem.

The articulator attempts to reproduce the movements of the mandible and the various tooth-to-tooth relationships in those movements. It is a rigid device with movement patterns determined by solid guiding pathways. The mandible, however, is guided by muscles, ligaments, and joint surfaces that are not rigid, by the teeth, and by the complex neuromuscular system. The mandible itself is resilient and has been shown to flex under normal biological stresses, and the teeth are suspended in membranes that respond to stress in an elastic manner. It follows that any instrument can give only a mechanical equivalent of the natural movement potential of the mandible and the teeth. No currently available articulator allows for the resilient surfaces of the temporomandibular joint or the periodontal membrane, all of which may affect occlusal registrations and the final biologic acceptance of the restoration. No matter what articulator system is used, the newly established restoration must be observed, interpreted, and adjusted in the mouth with the aid of various occlusal indicators.

In general, the more adjustable the articulator is, the more accuracy there is in reproducing the factors of mandibular movement. It is not within the scope of this survey to outline and discuss the various aspects of mandibular movements, and the reader is referred to the excellent texts in this area.[1,2]

USES: Articulators are used in diagnostic procedures to mount casts and to study the occlusion of a patient as an aid in planning treatment. Articulators also are used in the production of prostheses of all types and, in this context, they serve to stimulate the patient's masticatory system. The closer the mounted casts reproduce the relations and movements of the patient's teeth and jaws, the more accurate the prosthesis will be and fewer adjustments will be required when the prosthesis is delivered.

The significant role of an articulator in clinical dentistry varies with the complexity and extent of the prosthesis in question. The fabrication of a Class II inlay does not require the degree of instrument sophistication that is required for full-mouth reconstruction. Between these two extremes are cases with various degrees of complexity. The dentist learns to select the preferred instrument for each situation and avoids, wherever possible, oversophistication in technique as being time-consuming and expensive.

TYPES: Several classifications of articulators have been reported in the literature. Perhaps the most suitable one is a simple classification that divides articulators into five groups: hinge articulators, fixed condyle articulators, semiadjustable articulators, fully adjustable articulators, and fossa molded articulators.

Hinge articulators: The hinge articulator, well known to all dentists, is a simple hinge and simulates only opening and closing movements of the mandible. No lateral, retrusive, or protrusive movements of the casts are possible. These articulators reproduce only one relation, that of centric occlusion. They reproduce this relation only to the degree of accuracy with which the relation is obtained in the mouth in an interocclusal registration. Simple as they are,

there are hidden sources of error. The relation of the mounted casts to the hinge axis of the articulator is usually incorrect. The hinge axis of the articulator is inferior and anterior to that of the patient. The casts open and close on an arc of lesser radius than the teeth in the mouth, and the angle of approach is different. Errors of horizontal and vertical relations are produced. The greater the thickness of the interocclusal registration, the greater the degree of error. Often with the use of these devices a restoration with correct occlusal relations on the articulator is high when placed in the mouth. Methods of compensation for these errors are described in the literature.[3]

Hinge articulators, when correctly used, are suitable for small intracoronal restorations that do not involve cusps and are limited to the occlusal fossa region of the teeth. They are satisfactory when used with the functionally generated path technique for more complex restorations.

Fixed condyle path articulators: Fixed condyle path articulators (average value settings) allow lateral and protrusive movements at a fixed condylar inclination and at a fixed intercondylar distance. The degree to which these two elements coincide with those of a patient is one of chance. The degree of coincidence can be identified clinically by comparison of the relation of casts mounted on a fixed condyle articulator in protrusive and lateral excursions with the relation of the patient's teeth in similar movements. The patient's occlusion should be examined in both working and balancing relations on the left and the right sides. The accuracy of reproduction of these tooth-to-tooth relations on the mounted casts then can be assessed and, if satisfactory, work may proceed. If the condyle characteristics of the patient and the articulator do not coincide, restorations can be designed only to centric relations. Contouring of the cusps and inclines cannot be made to relate to lateral and protrusive relations of the teeth, nor can the retruded position of the mandible be reproduced. Projection of canine or other tooth guidance onto the anatomy of posterior restorations cannot be made satisfactorily. The balancing relations of the posterior teeth are especially liable to faulty occlusal design with these devices. Functional incisal relations are difficult to develop on these articulators, and the potential incisal relation errors are greater with an increasing vertical overlap. Fixed condyle articulators are subject to the same errors of closure as the hinge articulator in relation to misrepresentation of position of the hinge axis. These latter errors can be reduced considerably by mounting the casts with a mounting jig to locate the maxillary incisor point that will ensure some standardization of the cast relation to the hinge axis of the articulator.

Fixed condyle articulators can be used for individual posterior restorations and short span (three to four units) posterior bridges where a well-developed canine rise is present in the patient or for individual anterior restorations and short span anterior bridges with a minimal vertical and horizontal overlap (1 mm or less). They should not be used for posterior restorations or posterior bridges when the canine rise is minimal and where close balancing relations exist. They are not suitable for the more extensive work involving posterior and anterior units as fixed bridges nor for making complete dentures. It is always wise to compare the relations to the mounted cast with similar relations in the mouth.

Semi-adjustable articulators: In the semi-adjustable articulators, condyle path mechanisms are adjustable in the sagittal plane; they also include adjustable incisal guide tables, an adjustment for lateral mandibular movement (Bennett), occasionally an intercondylar adjustment, and a facebow to relate the casts to the hinge axis. The setting of the condyle path angulation is achieved by a protrusive interocclusal registration or lateral interocclusal registrations. The articulator condyle path is usually a flat surface. The condyle path may be incorporated in the maxillary arm of the articulator—an arcon articulator, or it may be incorporated in the mandibular arm of the articulator—a nonarcon articulator. A cranial reference plane allows remounting of casts to

recorded readings. Some of these articulators have adjustments to adapt to the retruded mandibular position and for the development of a long centric occlusion. The skilled operator can achieve a high degree of accuracy with these articulators, and a satisfactory reproduction of mandibular movements and tooth relations can be developed. Restorations can be built to be in harmony with lateral and protrusive relations, and posterior and anterior restorations of greater complexity can be constructed; when placed in the mouth, these require a minimum of adjustment. Semi-adjustable articulator techniques usually use an approximation of the hinge-axis position and, therefore, changes in the vertical occlusal dimension cannot be routinely made on the mounted casts. Semi-adjustable articulators are not recommended for tripodized occlusal relations built to a point centric position. Examples of semi-adjustable articulators are the Whip-Mix Articulator, the Hanau H2 Articulator, and the Dentatus Articulator. Each of these instruments is very satisfactory in complete denture occlusion.

Fully adjustable articulators (hinge axis): The fully adjustable articulators have a complex condylar mechanism adjustable in three planes. Adjustment of the curvature of the condyle pathway is possible by modification of the standard path or by replacement with paths of differing curvatures. Lateral mandibular movement (Bennett) is adjustable, and the intercondylar distance can be varied. Adjustable and custom incisal guide tables can be used. A cranial reference plane enables remounting to be done to recorded readings. When used with a kinematic hinge-axis bow, modifications to the vertical dimension of occlusion may be made without change of the horizontal relation.

These articulators can be adjusted to trace the recordings made by a pantograph. In so doing, the articulator is adjusted to reproduce the border movements of the mandible, and the assumption is made that the intraborder pathways are included. The fully adjustable articulator gives a more accurate reproduction of mandibular movements and the interarch relations than the three previously described types.

These articulators are valuable in occlusal analysis and treatment planning of complex reconstruction work and in the fabrication of complex restorations. They are especially important in posterior restorations with minimal canine guidance and close tooth-to-tooth interarch relations in the balancing positions.

Examples of fully adjustable articulators are the Denar Articulator, the Stuart Articulator, and the Aderer Simulator.

Fossa molded articulators: Methods for custom molding an articulator condyle to reproduce the patient's pathway have been attempted since the earliest articulators were designed.

Two methods are currently in use. In one, intraoral functional registrations are made on removable templates. The templates then are mounted on the articulator and copied on the condyle mechanism in a cold-curing plastic resin which, on curing, forms two condyle pathways. The advantage claimed for this type of registration is that the functional pathways are used to set the condyle pathways and not tracings of the borders of mandibular movement.

In the other method,[4,5] the condyle pathway of the patient is copied with a facebow, and air-turbine cutting devices are used to carve a duplicate pattern in acrylic blocks placed extraorally alongside the temporomandibular joint. These carvings then are set in an articulator, and the case is mounted in the usual way. Here again, the claim is made that functional pathways are registered.

An example of the first type of instrument is the TMJ Articulator; the second type is represented by the Dento Dynamics System.

AVAILABLE PRODUCTS

Aderer Simulator, J. Aderer, Inc.
Articulators, United Dental Service
Articulators and Base Accessories, Charles Development Co.
Denar Articulators, Denar Corp.
Dentatus Articulators, Almire International Co.
Dento Dynamics System, Dentonamics Corp.
Die Locators
Galletti Articulator, Silvermans

Hanau H2, Teledyne Dental, Hanau Division
Handy II Articulator, Shofu Dental Corp.
Improved New Simplex Articulator, Dentsply International, Inc.
Quick Mount Face-Bow, Whip-Mix Corp.
Stephart Articulators, Crescent Dental Mfg. Corp.
Stuart Articulator, C.E. Stuart
TMJ Articulator, TMJ Instrument Co.
Whip-Mix Articulator, Whip-Mix Corp.

IMPRESSION TRAYS

The trays used to hold impression materials in registering the oral structures may be either manufactured (stock) trays or custom made for a particular case. Stock trays are available in a range of sizes designed for either the maxillary or the mandibular arch and may be made of metal or plastic. They may be intended for use once only or for reuse indefinitely. Section trays for making impressions of a part of the dental arch and trays for edentulous or dentulous mouths are available. Impression trays may be plain or perforated; the perforations are intended to retain the impression material in the tray as the impression is removed from the mouth. Another retention device used in trays is the rim-lock design in which an enlarged rim around the periphery of the tray serves as an undercut to prevent the impression material from detaching from the tray. For use in the agar hydrocolloid impression technique, water cooled trays are manufactured. Tubes run along the edge of the tray and emerge in the tray handle to which hoses can be attached and water circulated around the tray to cool and solidify the agar impression material. Special trays for use in the mouths of children are usually listed by the manufacturer as orthodontic trays as they are mainly used by orthodontists in making impressions for diagnostic casts in the analysis of occlusal irregularities.

Special or custom trays are usually made for a particular case on a study cast which has been made from a preliminary impression made with a stock tray. The custom tray gives a more accurate adaptation of the tray to the oral structures to be registered and facilitates border molding where required, an important contribution where the more expensive impression materials are being used. Tray compound (American Dental Association Specification No. 3) was at one time used extensively for making custom trays but has largely been replaced in recent years by resins. The resin tray materials are available as powder-liquid preparations similar to those used for denture bases or as preformed blanks which are softened by heat and adapted by hand or by the use of a vacuum adaptation device. Usually a spacer is first adapted to the cast to provide room for the impression material; the thickness of the spacer varies with the impression materials and the particular technique to be used. Base plate wax can be used conveniently as a spacer for the powder-liquid resins, but for the thermoplastic materials, an asbestos sheet, softened by immersion in water, is required.

AVAILABLE PRODUCTS

Anterior-Bite Impression Trays, Columbia Dentoform Corporation
Bridge Trays, Teledyne Dental Products
Caulk Trayresin Resin, L.D. Caulk Company
Disposable Die Tray, Dental Plastics and Products Company
Hold, Impression Tray Adhesive, Teledyne Dental Products
Impression Tray 4-in-1 Disposable, Kerr Mfg. Co., Div. of Sybron Dental Products Corp.
Impression Trays, Crescent Dental Mfg. Co.
Justi Tray Material, H.D. Justi Co., Div. of Williams Gold Refining Co., Inc.
Kwik Tray, Kerr Mfg. Co.
Mounting Impression Trays, Whip-Mix Corp.
PCA Dispos-a-trays, Pulpdent Corp. of America
Perforated Impression Trays, Healthco, Inc.
Premier Disposable Bite Trays, Premier Dental Products Co.
Rim-Lock Trays, L.D. Caulk Co.
Rim Lock Impression Trays, Healthco, Inc.
Rim Lock Water Cooled Impression Trays, Healthco, Inc.
Sani-Trays, Teledyne Dental Products
Shur Tray, Modern Materials Mfg.

Surgident Die-Lok Trays, Lactona/Surgident
Surgident Water Cooled Trays, Lactona/Surgident
Tra-tens, Teledyne Dental Products
Unitek Impression Trays, Unitek Corp.

WAXING INSTRUMENTS

A great variety of waxing instruments are available. They are all essentially spatulas, specially designed to be heated and then to melt and pick up waxes for development of a pattern or other wax device. Dental catalogues list wax spatulas of many shapes and sizes that range from the insulated handled Fahnstock to the all metal slender No. 7 spatula. Spatulas have become known by the name of the designer or by a generally accepted catalogue number. In some cases both number and name are used.

AVAILABLE PRODUCTS

Waxing Instruments, Hu-Friedy Mfg. Co., Inc.
Waxing Instruments, Miltex Instrument Co.
Rapid Waxer, J.M. Ney Company

WAX CARVING INSTRUMENTS

Wax carving instruments are available in many designs. The names of dentists have become attached to many instruments; Ward, LeCron, Hollenback, P.K. Thomas, Wall, Roach, Capon, Frahm, Reeves, Vehe, Mortinson, Mave, Evans, Lacey, and Thompson are some of those listed in current catalogues. These instruments are used for carving wax patterns of restorations in the laboratory in the indirect technique or in the mouth in the now less frequently used direct technique.

ARTICULATING PAPER AND TAPE

Articulating paper and tape or ribbon are pressure sensitive materials that transfer coloring to objects against which they are brought into contact. The essential difference between paper and tape is the form in which the paper is supplied. Articulating paper is sold in strips, usually in book form, in sheets or as a roll. The description is further complicated as some of these forms may be sold with thin plastic or silk as the vehicle for the coloring agent. A roll of paper in a dispenser is usually described as tape. Articulating paper in any of its several forms is used clinically to detect and locate occlusal contacts between the maxillary and mandibular teeth or between teeth and restorations that occlude with them. It is used also in the laboratory in a similar manner when adjusting restorations of the working casts. The choice of paper, tape or sheet is a matter of individual preference and the nature of the particular case. Articulating paper is made in several thicknesses (0.20 mm, 0.12 mm, 0.04 mm) and usually in blue or red color. The thinner the paper the smaller the occlusal discrepancy it detects. The colorings used are food dyes.

Available Products

Articulating Paper, Healthco, Inc.

Articulating Paper Forcep, J.R. Rand Specialty Co., Inc.

Articulating Silk-Mark Ribbon, J.R. Rand Specialty Co., Inc.

Bauch Articulating Papers and Silk, Pulpdent Corp. of America

Bauch Articulating Paper Holder, Pulpdent Corp. of America

Lactona Disposal Articulating Paper, Lactona Corp.

Miller Forceps, Articulating Paper Holder Forceps, Pulpdent Corp. of America

Optow High Spot Paste, Teledyne Dental Products

PCA Exact Liner, Pulpdent Corp. of America

Miscellaneous Available Products

Al-Cote, L.D. Caulk Co.

Biolon Processing Unit, L.D. Caulk Co.

Film AC, H.D. Justi Co., Div. of Williams Gold Refining Co., Inc.

412 Single-Use Curved Tip Syringe, Monoject

Plastipin, J.M. Ney Company

Premier Retra Rings, Premier Dental Products

Literature References

1. Posselt, U. The physiology of occlusion and rehabilitation. ed. 2. Philadelphia, F. A. Davis, 1968.

2. Ramfjord, S. P., and Ash, M. M. Occlusion. ed 2. Philadelphia, W. B. Saunders Co., 1971.

3. McPhee, E. R. The simple class II non-adjustable articulator. Mich. State Dent. J. 56:68 Mar. 1974.

4. Lee, R. L. Jaw movement engraved in solid plastic for articulator controls. J. Prosthet. Dent. 22:209 Aug. 1969.

5. Lee, R. L. Jaw movement engraved in solid plastic for articulator controls. II. Transfer apparatus. J. Prosthet. Dent. 22:513 Nov. 1969.

LOCAL ANESTHETIC INSTRUMENTS

Control of pain and anxiety are vital to the contemporary practice of dentistry. The dentist must accept responsibility for management of the pain/anxiety complex. Within the past decade, the dental graduate has become increasingly accustomed to recognizing early signs of anxiety, and preventing dentally induced pain. The dental profession is fortunate in that it has at its disposal a wide variety of techniques and chemical agents which can be utilized in the management of pain and anxiety.

Sedation is the calming of a nervous, apprehensive individual by use of systemic drugs without inducing the loss of consciousness. Consciousness is the capability of the patient to elicit a rational response to a question or command and demonstrate that all protective reflexes are intact, including the ability to clear and maintain his airway in a patent state. Within recent years the phrase "conscious sedation" has been used to describe the techniques of anxiety control which have come to be employed, primarily to distinguish them from various unconscious techniques (general anesthesia). The acceptance of conscious sedation by the dental profession has added immeasurably to

the acceptance of dental therapy by many previously unmanageable patients.

Conscious sedation techniques are frequently described as a part of a spectrum of pain and anxiety control.[1-3] The function of this spectrum is to demonstrate to the dental profession that a wide range of techniques are available for patient management and that no one technique is a panacea.

The four most frequently employed techniques of conscious sedation which utilize drugs to accomplish their goals are: oral premedication, intramuscular premedication, inhalation, and intravenous sedation. Each of these techniques has its own distinct advantages and disadvantages, indications and contraindications, which must be weighed heavily when selection is being made for the ideal technique of conscious sedation for a given patient. Factors which must be considered include the following. Prior to initiating a sedative technique the dentist should note the degree of anxiety present in the patient, the physical status of the patient, and the patient's age, weight and previous drug experience. After evaluating the patient, the dentist must then select a sedative technique which will be effective for the length of the dental procedure and yet impose a minimum degree of stress upon the patient. Dentists are advised to use techniques and drugs with which they are familiar.

Following a thorough evaluation of these factors, the least potent technique and drug which will produce the desired result should be selected. Bennett[1] has listed the objectives to be sought in conscious sedation. They are: 1) the patient's mood must be altered; 2) the patient must remain conscious; 3) the patient must be cooperative; 4) all protective reflexes must remain intact and active; 5) vital signs must remain stable and within normal limits; 6) the patient's pain threshold should be elevated and 7) amnesia may be present. Several other objectives should be added to these: 8) the ultimate goal in the use of drugs for conscious sedation should be to eliminate the need for drugs on the patient; 9) the administrator of the drugs must never sedate a patient beyond the level at which the dentist is comfortable and competent, and 10) the quality of dental care performed under conscious sedation should be at least equal to or better than the same therapy carried out on the same patient without the benefits of conscious sedation.

Inhalation sedation with nitrous oxide and oxygen and intravenous sedation are two techniques which have become quite popular in dentistry. It is estimated that approximately 35 percent of practicing dentists utilize inhalation sedation to some degree.[4] The greatest safety factor in either of these techniques is the operator. It is only through complete and adequate training programs that these techniques can be employed safely. Recent and future graduates have or will receive undergraduate training in these techniques. The untrained dental graduate is strongly urged to enroll in a continuing education course of these techniques which adheres to Part III of the Guidelines for Teaching the Comprehensive Control of Pain and Anxiety in Dentistry.[5] Training programs in these two techniques should include the actual treatment of dental patients.

Of even more far reaching importance than the management of anxiety in dental practice is the management of pain. It may be stated that virtually every dentist in clinical practice administers drugs for the relief of, or prevention of, pain which is associated with dental therapy. Without doubt the drugs of choice for pain control in dentistry are the local anesthetics. Local anesthetics are topical applications or regional injections of drugs to eliminate sensations, especially pain, in one part of the body. Many highly effective local anesthetics are available today for pain control, yet in spite of these excellent drugs, problems and complications still arise. Many of these problems are minor annoyances, such as inadequate anesthesia; however, others can be more serious, such as the inadvertent injection of local anesthetic drugs into the vascular system. Thorough discussion of the various components of the local anesthetic armamentarium will eliminate many of these problems and complications from future occurrence.

Injection of local anesthetics became possible through the invention of the Pravaz syringe, a forerunner of the modern hypodermic needle. Significant changes have occurred since the initial days of local anesthesia. The early glass syringe has been superseded by the modern metal cartridge holding syringe and in recent years by the plastic disposable syringe. Needles which were nondisposable in prior years have given way to the newer stainless steel disposable needles, with their greatly increased safety and comfort. The solutions themselves have changed considerably over the years. No longer must the dentist compound his own local anesthetic solution from tablets, adding quantities of vasoconstrictor for effective anesthesia. The nature of the drugs has changed and the manufacturing process of these agents has advanced steadily to the present time in which prefilled cartridges of high quality solution are readily available. The basic local anesthetic armamentarium includes a needle, syringe and solution containing cartridge. Table I summarizes the recommended procedure for preparing a typical needle-cartridge-syringe unit for use in administering local anesthetics.

Table I.
Recommended Preparation of Local Anesthetic Armamentarium

Preparing the needle-cartridge-syringe unit:

1. Insert the cartridge into the syringe.
2. Holding the syringe as for injection, gently push the piston forward with moderate pressure until the harpoon is firmly embedded. DO NOT TAP OR HIT THE PISTON as this will cause the cartridge to crack.
3. Attach the needle to the threaded portion of the syringe.
4. A few drops of anesthetic solution are expressed to ensure that the unit is ready for use.

Removing a used cartridge from the syringe:

1. Retract the piston, pulling the cartridge away from the needle.
2. The harpoon will disengage the plunger and the cartridge will fall from the syringe.

Loading a second cartridge:

A. Remove the needle and repeat the steps previously described,

   or

B. Use the following procedure:
   1. Retract the plunger fully.
   2. Insert the cartridge into the syringe.
   3. Prevent the needle from penetrating the diaphragm with the fingers of one hand, while the second hand gently embeds the harpoon in the plunger.
   4. Release the cartridge, permitting the needle to penetrate the diaphragm.
   5. Express a few drops of solution to ensure that the unit is ready for use.

NEEDLES

COMPONENTS: Needles for use on dental syringes are usually manufactured of stainless steel, although a variety of other materials may also be used. The needle consists of three sections: the hub, the shank, and the bevel. The *hub* of the needle may be either metal or plastic. It is sealed in a plastic covering and is attached directly to the syringe. The *length* of the shaft of a disposable needle is measured from the hub to the point of the bevel. Disposable dental needles are manufactured in two sizes, long and short. While it is commonly stated that the short needle is 1 in. long, and the long needle is 1⅝ in. long, Aldous[6] reported that in actuality the length of dental needles ranged from 19.4 to 41.5 mm.

The bevel of the needle is of importance. Bevels are defined by manufacturers as micro-sharp, unimpaired sharp, long bevel, medium bevel and short bevel. All needles bend during the penetration of tissue. This factor is of particular importance in those injections which deeply penetrate tissue (especially the inferior alveolar block). Aldous[6] demonstrated that the greater the angle of the bevel with the long axis of the needle, the greater the degree of deflection. Needles with the point centered on the long axis deflected less than beveled, pointed needles.

Another significant feature of needles is the gauge, the internal diameter of the needle lumen. The three most commonly used gauges in dental practice are the 25, 27 and 30 gauge needles, with the 27 gauge the most commonly used.[7] While there are industry standards established for lumenal diameters, Wittrock and Fischer[8] demonstrated that there is significant variation in actual lumenal diameter amongst various manufacturers. The gauge of a needle is of importance for several reasons. Aldous[6] showed that less deflection is produced by larger caliber needles and needles with greater rigidity in their metal. Where accuracy is needed in injection techniques the degree of deflection is important. For this reason larger gauge needles (lower numbers) are recommended for injections which require deeper tissue penetration (i.e., block injections). Also, there is less likelihood of needle breakage and a greater degree of reliability of aspiration with the use of larger gauge needles.

An argument commonly voiced against the use of larger needles is that they are more painful to the patient on insertion. Clinical evidence, however, consistently disproves this statement. Needles of 25, 27 and 30 gauge can be inserted atraumatically into mucous membrane without the patient being aware of the difference in needle gauge. This factor when considered with other positive attributes of larger gauge needles, speaks strongly for the use of the 25 gauge long needle for all block injections.

USES: At no time should a needle be introduced more than one-half to two-thirds of its shaft length into tissue. For this reason it is recommended that long needles be employed for inferior alveolar, posterior superior, and infraorbital nerve blocks. Short needles may be used for injections in which tissue penetration is not as deep, such as palatal nerve blocks, maxillary infiltrations, mental and buccal nerve blocks.

DIRECTIONS FOR USE: The practitioner must always take precautions to prevent contamination of the needle. Contamination of the needle, leading to subacute infection in the injection site, is apparently underestimated in its frequency of occurrence.[9] Clinical observation of dentists over the past five years has shown a decided lack of concern for this complication. Contamination of the needle can occur once the sterile package has been opened. With the lower protective cap removed the portion of the needle that is attached to the syringe should not be permitted to touch any non-sterile substances (i.e., fingers). After the needle is attached to the syringe the needle cap is removed prior to insertion into tissue. Care must be taken to avoid touching the needle tip to any foreign objects. A common cause of needle contamination is the placement of the needle and the syringe on the bracket table between injections. Often times the needle will not be covered at this time, permitting possible contamination to occur. In most cases, subacute tissue infection is manifested clinically as

soreness at the site of the injection, limitation of movement, possible erythema, edema, swelling of local lymph nodes, and elevation of temperature. The clinical picture most frequently is mistaken for trismus; however, trismus is normally a self-limiting process, whereas infection may persist.

Disposal of needles is an important consideration. Never should a needle be unscrewed from the syringe and simply thrown into a trash receptacle; persons cleaning an office can easily be stuck by an uncapped needle, leading to the possible contraction of hepatitis. All disposable dental needles should be destroyed before they are discarded to prevent their possible harm to or reuse by others. Minimally, the needle shaft should be broken off the needle. All remnants of the needle should be stored and then disposed of properly. In many cities the police department collects and disposes of used needles for dentists and physicians.

LIMITATIONS OF USE: Disposable dental needles are supplied in presterilized, sealed packets. In spite of the apparent lack of standardization in the industry, the dental profession has been supplied with sterile, sturdy needles which are quite sharp. Care and handling of the needles is important in minimizing potential complications including dullness, barbs on needles, needle breakage, and contamination of needles. While initially sharp, disposable stainless steel needles dull rapidly when penetrated into tissue. If a needle is penetrated into tissue three or more times a distinct tearing of tissue and increased resistance to the needle can occur. Clinically this relates to increased pain on insertion, and postoperative inflammation at the injection site. It is recommended that needles be changed following every two or three penetrations.

Nondisposable needles are not recommended by the American Dental Association[10] because of significant problems with initial sharpness, resharpening procedures, metal fatigue during resharpening, and sterilization techniques.

Barbs may occur on needle tips during the

manufacturing process or during clinical use if the needle is permitted to impact against bone. Clinically, barbs produce a tearing of tissue as the needle is withdrawn from the injection site, causing discomfort to the patient. Examining new needles for barbs is not difficult; however, care must be taken to prevent contamination of the needle tip during this process. The needle tip is gently pulled back over a sterile, dry gauze. Should any barbs be present, they will catch in the gauze. The needle should then be discarded in the recommended manner.

Bending of needles is not recommended for any intraoral injection. The process of bending a needle weakens it, increasing the possibility of breakage. While the incidence of broken needles is quite low for disposable needles, such unfortunate situations have occurred.[11-14] Bending of needles is most frequently used in inferior alveolar and posterior alveolar blocks. Unfortunately these two injections also require the deepest penetration of tissue. Should a needle break off during injection (especially if the needle is embedded in tissue to its hub) its removal proves quite difficult, as the elastic mucous membrane bounces back, covering the broken segment of the needle. For this reason long needles are recommended for these injections. Average depth of soft tissue penetration for inferior alveolar nerve block is 23.6 mm.[15] Short needles average from 19.4 to 25.5 mm in length. Should bone be impacted firmly, or should the patient make a sudden movement, the needle may bend and possibly break. Since the weakest portion of a needle is at the point where the shank and hub meet, breakage is most likely to occur there.

SYRINGES

COMPONENTS: The most commonly used syringes today are the breech or side loading metal cartridge syringes. The disposable needle is attached to the barrel of the syringe by screwing it onto a threaded hub. Syringes available in

---

NEEDLES

Do:

1. Use only disposable needles for local anesthetic administration.
2. Use long needles for block injections such as inferior alveolar, posterior superior alveolar and infraorbital. Short needles may be used for other injections.
3. Use a large gauge needle (25) for nerve blocks to reduce the extent of deflection and provide more reliable aspiration.

Don't:

1. Insert needles more than two-thirds of their length into tissue.

---

the United States are designed to hold a 1.8 ml glass cartridge. At the other end of the syringe is the finger grip, thumb ring, and piston. Attached to the piston should be a metallic harpoon which embeds in the rubber stopper of the cartridge, allowing for aspiration to be attempted. Non-aspirating type syringes, which do not contain harpoons, are also available, but ought not be used for any local anesthetic procedure. Recently, a self-aspirating syringe has become available in Europe and Canada.[16] Where the harpoon type aspirating syringe requires the operator to pull the piston rod back to obtain the required negative pressure for aspiration (frequently moving the needle tip with it), the self-aspirating syringe obtains this same pressure by utilizing the elasticity of the rubber diaphragm of the anesthetic cartridge. The diaphragm which is pierced by the needle rests on a small metal projection directing the needle into the cartridge. Pressure acting directly on the cartridge through the thumb disc stretches the rubber diaphragm. Upon release of pressure, sufficient negative pressure is induced within the cartridge to achieve aspiration. In clinical practice any slight movement of the needle tip either by the operator or the patient may lead to intravascular injection and would require a second aspiration attempt. The advantage of the self-aspirating syringe is the ease with which aspiration may be accomplished. Needles may be moved within the tissues and aspiration achieved whenever the injection pressure is released. Another type of syringe available for local anesthetic administration is the sterile, disposable, needle-syringe-barrel combination, and a reusable plastic, barbed piston section.

DIRECTIONS FOR USE: When local anesthetics are to be administered, it is important to prevent intravascular injection by attempting to aspirate blood before injecting the solution. While aspiration of blood into a cartridge does not always indicate that the needle tip is within a blood vessel, local anesthetic injection should not be continued.[17] The needle should be repositioned and aspiration carried out until a negative result is obtained. If the cartridge becomes completely filled with blood (as might occur if an artery is entered) then the cartridge should be replaced prior to reinjection. However, it is much more common for only a trace of blood to enter the cartridge and remain in the region of the rubber diaphragm, the remainder of the cartridge remaining clear. In this situation, the cartridge need not be replaced but the needle should be repositioned and aspiration performed in the new position; if negative, the solution can then be injected.

After each use, the syringe should be washed and rinsed free of any anesthetic solution, saliva or other foreign matter and then autoclaved in the same manner as surgical instruments. After every five autoclavings, the syringe should be dismantled and lightly lubricated at all threaded joints, and where the piston contacts the thumb ring and guide bearing.

LIMITATIONS OF USE: There are a few significant problems related to the use of metallic side loading syringes in dentistry. Probably the most annoying difficulty encountered with this sy-

ringe is the disengagement of the harpoon from the rubber plunger during aspiration. This most commonly is produced by the operator applying too much force on the thumb ring during aspiration. For proper aspiration, only a smooth, gentle, backward motion is required. After repeated use and sterilization the aspirating harpoon may become dulled, therefore leading to the problem of disengagement. Replacement parts can be purchased to remedy this problem.

A second problem noted on occasion is the inability of operators with small hands to aspirate effectively when a full cartridge is in the syringe. It is imperative to remove enough anesthetic solution from the cartridge prior to inserting the needle into the tissue so that effective aspiration can take place.

EVALUATION PROGRAM: The Council on Dental Materials, Instruments and Equipment has an Acceptance Program for dental anesthetic syringe devices.

SYRINGES

Do:

1. Use either metal or non-metal syringes provided they have the ability to aspirate and can be properly sterilized.

Don't:

1. Use syringes without harpoons or other devices for aspiration when administering local anesthetics.

CARTRIDGES

COMPONENTS: The glass local anesthetic cartridge employed in the United States is a cylindrical tube which has the capacity to hold 2.0 ml of solution. However, following manufacture and insertion of the rubber plunger, the volume of local anesthetic solution becomes 1.8 ml. Dental cartridges used in some countries contain 2.2 ml of solution when filled. The dental cartridge virtually ensures sterility and uniformity of concentration. At one end of the cartridge is a thin, permeable rubber diaphragm sealed by an aluminum cap. This diaphragm is pierced by the needle. The opposite end of the cartridge has a rubber plunger which is forced into the cartridge by the piston during injection. The harpoon is embedded within the plunger, and aspiration is performed by the plunger being pulled backwards, creating a negative pressure within the cartridge. The rubber plunger should be indented slightly below the rim of the glass cartridge.

The local anesthetic cartridge contains several different ingredients. They are 1) the local anesthetic drug or drugs, 2) the vasopressor (if included), 3) sodium bisulfate, a preservative for the vasopressor (only present if vasopressor is included) 4) methyl paraben, a preservative and bacteriostatic agent, found in all multidose vials of local anesthetics and in most glass cartridges (Carbocaine does not contain methyl paraben), 5) distilled water, and 6) sodium chloride, to make the solution isotonic.

Following manufacture the cartridges are placed in quarantine for a period of time after which random samples are selected and tested for sterility. Cartridges are placed in vacuum containers holding fifty cartridges. The shelf life of cartridges without vasoconstrictor is 48 months, while those containing vasoconstrictors have an 18 month shelf life.

DIRECTIONS FOR USE: Cartridges may be stored in the container in which they are supplied. Many offices, however, use a cartridge dispenser, a plastic dish with three rows for storage of cartridges. Cartridges stored in the original container should have the rubber diaphragm wiped off with 91 percent isopropyl alcohol or 70 percent ethyl alcohol just prior to use.

If a cartridge dispenser is used, the following procedure is recommended: a dry 2 in x 2 in gauze is placed in the bottom of the central plastic core. Alcohol, either 91 percent isopropyl or 70 percent ethyl, is used to moisten the gauze wipe. One day's supply of cartridges is placed in the outer two rows of the dispenser (approximately ten). Just prior to loading into the syringe, the diaphragm end of the cartridge should be rubbed over the alcohol moistened pad. The pad should be replaced frequently to maintain hygiene and lessen the likelihood of contamination.

LIMITATIONS OF USE: Many problems with dental cartridges are reported by the dental profession. The overwhelming majority of these, however, are of iatrogenic origin, produced through improper care and handling of cartridges.

Breakage: Breakage is a potentially hazardous complication, yet it is one which need not occur. The most common cause of cartridge breakage is improper handling of containers during shipment. Dented anesthetic tins almost always contain one or more broken cartridges. Of greater importance, however, are those with minute cracks which remain full of solution. With the application of pressure in the cartridge, the glass shatters. Common areas for minor cracks are around the rubber plunger and around the neck of the cartridge. These areas should be examined routinely. Another common cause of "exploding" cartridges is the sequence in which the armamentarium is prepared. Under no circumstances should the thumb ring be "hit" to force the aspirating harpoon into the rubber plunger. When prepared properly, gentle finger pressure effectively embeds the harpoon in the plunger. Other causes of breakage include badly worn syringes, aspirating syringes with bent harpoons, the use of syringes not designed to take 1.8 ml cartridges, bent needles, and the use of cartridges with extruded plungers.

Bubbles: Small bubbles, 1 to 2 mm in diameter, may be formed during the manufacturing process by the trapping of nitrogen gas within the cartridge. Large bubbles, with or without plungers that extend beyond the end of the cartridge, are caused by freezing. These should not be used, rather they should be returned to the supplier for replacement.

Extruded Plungers: An extruded plunger which is accompanied by a large bubble indicates that the cartridge has been frozen. An extruded plunger with no bubble means that the cartridge has been left in the chemical disinfecting solution too long, and that the disinfecting solution has passed through the rubber diaphragm into the cartridge. Cartridges with extruded plungers should not be used because in either situation the solution within the cartridge has been altered.

Corroded Caps: Corrosion of aluminum caps usually indicates that the cartridge was immersed in a chemical disinfecting solution that contains nitrite antirust materials. Cartridges with corroded caps should not be used. Corrosion, which is a white deposit, may be distinguished readily from rust which is reddish in color. Rust will form inside the container should a cartridge crack. Rust spotted cartridges should not be used.

Leakage: Leakage during injection of local anesthetic solution into the patient's mouth usually occurs whenever the needle has not perforated the rubber diaphragm in the center. An off-center perforation produces an ovoid hole around the needle which permits anesthetic solution to leak out and into the patient's mouth. Proper sequence of syringe loading can prevent this occurrence.

CARTRIDGES

Do:

1. Store anesthetic cartridges either in their original containers or in a cartridge dispenser.
2. Store cartridge containers at room temperature or slightly colder and out of bright light. Bright lights and elevated temperatures hasten the deterioration of chemicals, particularly vasoconstrictors.
3. Disinfect the diaphragm end of the cartridge with either 91 percent isopropyl alcohol or 70 percent ethyl alcohol prior to use.

Don't:

1. Autoclave dental cartridges as the seals cannot withstand autoclaving temperatures and pressures. In addition, epinephrine is rapidly broken down by excessive heat.
2. Store anesthetic cartridges in quaternary ammonium salts, such as benzalkonium chloride, as they are electrolytically incompatible with aluminum.
3. Use antirust tablets in disinfectant solutions as they contain sodium nitrite or other agents which may release metal ions and produce swelling and edema following injection.

AVAILABLE PRODUCTS

Aspirating Syringe, Healthco, Inc.
ASTRA ASPIRATING SYRINGE, Astra Pharmaceutical Products, Inc.
Autoclavable 3-way Syringe Tips, North Pacific Dental, Inc.
CARPULE ASPIRATOR SYRINGE, Cook-Waite Laboratories, Inc.
Carpule Needles, Cook-Waite Laboratories, Inc.
C-R Syringe, Centrix/Clev-Dent
Delta Standard Syringe, MDT Corp.
Disposable Mixing-Ejecting Syringe, Teledyne Dental Products
Disposable Needles, Healthco, Inc.

Disposable Needles, Mizzy, Inc.
400 Dental Needles—Plastic Hub, Monoject
401 Dental Needles—Aluminum Hub, Monoject
418 Dental Injector, Monoject
503 Dental Syringe with Needle, Monoject Corp.
160 Multi-Purpose Syringe, Monoject Corp.
Hypodermic Needles, Monoject
PCA Pressure Syringe, Pulpdent Corp. of America
Reusable Needles, Mizzy, Inc.
Slide Pak Reusable Needles, Mizzy, Inc.

STEREX ASPIRATING SYRINGE, Sterex Corp.
Syrijet, Mizzy, Inc.
Syrijet Mark II, Mizzy Inc.
Syringes, Zirc Dental Products
Syringes with Luer Tips, Monoject Corp.

LITERATURE REFERENCES

1. Bennett, C. R. Conscious sedation in dental practice. St. Louis, C. V. Mosby Co., 1974.
2. Treiger, N. Pain control. Berlin, Quintessence Books, 1974.
3. Malamed, S. F. USC School of Dentistry, Guidelines for the control of pain and anxiety. Anes. Prog. 21:99, 1974.
4. Jones, T. W., and Greenfield, W. Position paper of the ADA Ad Hoc Committee on trace anesthetics as a potential health hazard in dentistry. JADA 95:751, 1977.
5. Council on Dental Education, American Dental Association. Guidelines for teaching the comprehensive control of pain and anxiety in dentistry. J. Dent. Educ. 36:62, 1972.
6. Aldous, J. A. Needle deflection: a factor in the administration of local anesthetics. JADA 77:602, 1968.
7. Malamed, S. F. Survey of local anesthetic practices among dentists. Unpublished data.

8. Wittrock, J. W., and Fischer, W. E. The aspiration of blood through small gauge needles. JADA 76:79, 1968.
9. Gregory, G. T. Infections in the infratemporal fossa. J. Oral Surg. 2:19, 1944.
10. Council on Dental Materials and Devices. Guide to dental materials and devices, ed. 8, Chicago, American Dental Association, 1976.
11. Fitzpatrick, B. The broken dental needle. Aust. Dent. J. 12:243, 1967.
12. Crouse, V. L. Migration of a broken anesthetic needle; report of a case. S. C. Dent. J. 28:16, 1970.
13. Dudani, I. C. Broken needles following mandibular injections. J. Indiana Dent. Assoc. 43:14, 1971.
14. Kennett, S.; Curran, J. B.; and Jenkens, G. R. Management of a broken hypodermic needle; report of a case. J. Can. Dent. Assoc. 38:414, 1972.
15. Bremer, G. Measurements of special significance in connection with anesthesia of the inferior alveolar nerve. Oral Surg. 5:966, 1952.
16. Persson, G.; Keskitalo, E.; and Evers, H. Clinical experiences in oral surgery using a new self-aspirating injection system. Int. J. Oral Surg. 3:428, 1974.
17. Watson, J. E., and Colman, R. S. Interpretation of aspiration tests in local anesthetic injections. J. Oral Surg. 34:1069, 1976.

PERIODONTAL INSTRUMENTS

HAND SCALERS, CURETS AND ROOT PLANING INSTRUMENTS

All instruments used for calculus removal and root planing are generally referred to as scalers.[1,2] Scaling and root planing procedures are the primary method of treating periodontal inflammation. In early conditions, thorough scaling and root planing by the dentist in addition to teaching effective oral hygiene procedures to the patient may result in complete resolution of the inflammation. In more extensive cases, scaling and root planing results in resolution of inflammation when followed by surgical procedures. In very advanced cases and in the presence of some systemic diseases, scaling and root planing may be the only feasible method of treatment and may prolong the useful life of dentition for many years. During maintenance after active treatment, regular root planing in combination with the patient's effective oral hygiene help to keep the periodontium healthy.

TYPES AND USES: Hand scaling instruments may be classified in five groups: the chisel, hoe and sickle which are employed to remove large deposits of calculus, and curets and files which are intended for the removal of small flecks of calculus and the final smoothing of root surfaces to the bottom of pockets.[3]

The chisel is used to remove large, supragingival calculus deposits, especially those in the anterior mandibular area. It is used with a push stroke to dislodge gross deposits. Hoe-shaped instruments are used to remove gross accumulations of accessible calculus. They are used with a pull stroke and are introduced subgingivally only when the gingiva is easily displaced. Some sickle scalers have a thin rectangular blade and can be used with a push or pull stroke to remove calcified deposits. Sickle scalers with triangular shaped blades are used only with a pull stroke. Jaquette type sickle scalers having a double contra-angled blade are useful for removing calcified deposits in the premolar and molar areas. Curets are spoon-shaped, quite similar to the spoon excavators used in operative dentistry. They have two cutting edges and as the one edge planes the root surface, the other edge removes ulcerated epithelium and granulomatous tissue from the soft tissue wall of the pocket. Curets are designed as push or pull instruments; the face of push instruments have a tool angle of about 40 degrees while the face of pull curets have a tool angle of about 80 degrees. Small files are useful for calculus removal in deep narrow pockets and in tortuous pockets.

DIRECTIONS FOR USE: The instruments should be held in a pen grasp with a finger rest on the tooth being treated or on an adjacent tooth. All pull instruments should be activated with the working edge held securely against the tooth surface apical to the calculus or roughened root surface. Push instruments are used for final root preparation and are activated by short controlled push strokes.

Clinicians differ in their systems of scaling and root planing. Some carry out a gross calculus removal from the entire dentition at the first treatment appointment and at subsequent appointments root plane the individual quadrants. Others prefer to carry out gross scaling and root planing at the same appointment.

LIMITATIONS OF USE: Scaling and root planing procedures are more difficult to carry out effectively in deep pockets, when furcation areas are involved with periodontal disease; in the presence of deep grooves on tooth roots; and on posterior, more inaccessible teeth. It is sometimes necessary to treat areas more than once, as resolution of inflammation after the initial scaling results in shrinkage of the gingiva and a decrease in depth of the pockets making them more accessible for complete calculus removal.

AVAILABLE PRODUCTS

American Dental Periodontal Curettes, American Dental Mfg. Co.

American Dental Periodontal Knives, American Dental Mfg. Co.

Ferrolite Hand Scalers and Curettes, J. R. Rand Specialty Co., Inc.

Hand Scalers, Curettes and Root Planes, E. A. Beck & Co..

Hand Scalers and Curettes, Miltex Instruments Co.

Mastersonics Dental Scalers-Electro 20 Handpieces, Mastersonics

Nurlite Perio Curettes, J. R. Rand Specialty Co., Inc.

Nurlite Perio Knives, J. R. Rand Specialty Co., Inc.

Nurlite Scalers and Margin Trimmers, J. R. Rand Specialty Co., Inc.

Periodontal Curettes, E. A. Beck & Co.

Periodontal Curettes, Miltex Instruments Co.

Periodontal Knives, E. A. Beck & Co.

R & R Gracey Curettes, Ransom and Randolph Company

R & R McCall's Periodontal Scalers, Ransom and Randolph Company

R & R Morse Scalers, Ransom and Randolph Co.

Unitek Double Ended Scaler, Unitek Corp.

ULTRASONIC SCALERS

One type of ultrasonic handpiece contains a nickel-magnetostrictive stack which, when placed in an electro-magnetic field energized by an alternating current, shortens and lengthens approximately 0.001 inch. The mechanical shortening and lengthening of the magnetic stack are transmitted to the attached instrument tip, driving it back and forth with a frequency of approximately 25,000 cycles per second. The working tips vary in shape; many resemble the McCall type hand scaler, and others resemble chisel type or Jaquette scalers. Water continually bathes the working tip to cool it and prevent overheating of the teeth being treated. Ultrasonic scalers can remove calculus and other accretions from crown and root surfaces and curet the crevicular tissue. To date there is no clear-cut evidence that ultrasonic scaling is superior to hand scaling for removal of calculus.[4,5] Conclusive evidence is not yet available as to which method of scaling results in a smoother root surface.[6,7]

DIRECTIONS FOR USE: In general the lowest power setting that is effective should be employed. The instrument tip is applied with a continual light back-and-forth brush stroke. An adequate water supply should be used, particularly during subgingival scaling where the water flow at the instrument tip may be impeded. Tooth and root surfaces should be explored frequently with a suitable instrument to determine the degree of calculus removal and root smoothing.

LIMITATIONS OF USE: Ultrasonic scaling has many of the same limitations as hand scaling. Its effectiveness is reduced in deep pockets, in furcation areas involved with periodontal disease, and on root surfaces with deep grooves. There is general agreement that it is most useful for removing heavy supragingival calculus. Most periodontists believe that final root planing is carried out most effectively with hand instruments. Ultrasonic scaling is of limited value for removing coronal stains. There have been a few reports of pain with its use and tooth sensitivity after repeated use. Care is required in the presence of porcelain jacket crowns of inlays as the vibration could result in fracture of the porcelain.

AVAILABLE PRODUCTS: See product listing following the section on Sonic Scalers.

SONIC SCALERS

A mechanical scaler which produces nonrotary orbital motion of a scaler tip is also available. It is a handpiece-sized device which attaches to the air source of a conventional turbine handpiece. The vibration is produced by a shaft set into motion by an air driven turbine. The sonic frequency of the instrument tip is approximately 2,000 cycles per second. The frictional heat of a two thousand cycle vibratory motion is sufficient to warrant the use of a water spray. The instrument tips are shaped much the same as those for ultrasonic scalers.

EVALUATION PROGRAM: The Council on Dental Materials, Instruments, and Equipment has a

Classification or Acceptance Program for scaling devices: Type A, ultrasonic scaling devices and Type B, sonic (mechanical) scaling devices. The packaging of accepted products may carry the following statement:

"_____ Scaling Device is *Acceptable* (Provisionally Acceptable) for use in scaling and cleaning surfaces of teeth in conjunction with other suitable prophylactic measures."

ULTRASONIC AND SONIC SCALERS

Do:

1. Use the lowest effective power setting for removal of calculus, cement, etc.
2. Use an adequate supply of water to avoid overheating of the instrument and tooth surfaces.
3. Keep the tip continually in motion.
4. Remove any roughness on the instrument tips to prevent scratching of the tooth surface.

Don't:

1. Apply pressure with the instrument tip against the tooth. It will not increase the effectiveness of calculus removal and can damage tooth and root surfaces.

AVAILABLE PRODUCTS

TYPE A: ULTRASONIC SCALING DEVICES

Airc Ultrasonic Scaler Unit, Zirc Dental Products
Amdent, A-dec
DENTSPLY-CAVITRON MODELS 76; 1010; POWERMATIC, Dentsply International, Inc.
GIRARD ULTRASONIC SCALER MODELS 800; 800A, Girard, Inc.
LITTON LT-200 ULTRASONIC SCALER, Litton Dental Products
Odontoson 3, MDT Corp.
System S, Den-Tal-Ez Mfg. Co.

TYPE B: SONIC SCALING DEVICES

Sonic Automatic, Sonic Plus, Sonic Piezo-Electric, Uni-Sonic, Spartan Ultrasonics, Inc.
Steele's Orbison, Columbus Dental
Titan S, Star Dental
Unitek 2000 Ultrasonic Scaler, Unitek Corp.

ROTARY SCALERS

A rotary tapered instrument which fits into a high speed contra-angle handpiece in the same fashion as a bur is used for scaling. The instrument has six sides or working fins on a tapered working surface and is used with a water spray. The inventor states that when rotating under maximum speed, the instrument produces 10,000 to 20,000 vibrations per second and that this frequency is beyond the perception of the patient, who feels neither the rotation nor the vibrations.[8]

DIRECTIONS FOR USE: The lower third of the instrument is held parallel to the tooth being scaled and is moved rapidly and lightly over the tooth. High or maximum handpiece speed should be employed in conjunction with the light pressure. The working tip should be continually bathed with water to prevent a build-up of heat in the treated tooth and to wash away dislodged calculus and accretions.

LIMITATIONS OF USE: Access into subgingival areas is difficult with the rotary scaler and can result in considerable trauma to the soft tissues. Studies have shown that use of the rotary air turbine instrument causes the greatest defects on tooth and root surfaces and results in grooved and some ledged surfaces.[9,10]

AVAILABLE PRODUCTS

PCA SPEE-DEE Polishers, Pulpdent Corp. of America

ROTARY SCALERS

Do:
1. Hold the lower third of the rotary tapered instrument parallel to the tooth being scaled.
2. Use a high speed with the air turbine handpiece.
3. Keep the instrument tip moving lightly and rapidly over the surfaces being treated.
4. Use an adequate water supply.

LITERATURE REFERENCES

1. McCall, J. O. The evaluation of the scaler and its influence on the development of periodontia. J. Periodontol. 10:69, 1939.

2. Waerhaug, J.; Arno, A.; and Lovdal, A. The dimensions of instruments for removal of subgingival calculus. J. Periodontol. 25:281, 1954.

3. Barnes, J. E., and Schaffer, E. M. Subgingival root planing—a comparison using files, hoes, and curettes. J. Periodontol. 31:300, 1960.

4. Stewart, J. M. High speed dental prophylaxis. J. Florida Dent. Assoc. 33:19 Fall 1962.

5. Stende, F. W., and Schaffer, E. M. Comparison of ultrasonic and hand scaling. J. Periodontol. 32:312 Oct. 1961.

6. Pameijer, C. H.; Stallard, R. E.; and Heip, N. Surface characteristics of teeth following periodontal instrumentation: A scanning electron microscope study. J. Periodontol. 43:628, 1975.

7. Wilkerson, R. F., and Maybury, J. E. Scanning electron microscopy of the root surface following instrumentation. J. Periodontol. 44:559, 1973.

8. Ellman, I. Safe high-speed periodontal instrument. Dent. Survey 36:759 June 1960.

9. Allen, E. F., and Rhodes, R. H. Effects of high speed periodontal instruments on tooth surface. J. Periodontol. 34:352 July 1963.

10. Stewart, J. L., et al. Relative calculus and tooth structure loss with use of power-driven scaling instrument. JADA 83:840 Oct. 1971.

Equipment

RADIOGRAPHIC EQUIPMENT

X-RAY GENERATORS

X-ray generators are instruments which generate non-luminous electromagnetic rays of extremely short wave lengths by bombardment of a target with a focused electron beam within a vacuum tube. The electron beam is usually produced from a tungsten filament. The target material is also usually tungsten.

USES: Dental x-ray generators are used as an x-ray source for the projection of radiographic images. The generators are used in virtually all aspects of dentistry where radiographic information is desired for diagnosis, treatment planning, and the carrying out of treatment procedures. X-ray generators for x-ray therapy are not ordinarily used within the context of dental practice and will be excluded from consideration here.

TYPES: The most common types of dental x-ray generators are those for periapical, bitewing, and occlusal radiography; those for panoramic, curved surface tomography; and those for skull-view radiography. For periapical, bitewing and occlusal radiography, the x-ray source is positioned extraorally, and the image receptor is positioned intraorally for a stationary projection. For curved surface tomography, the x-ray source and the image receptor rotate extraorally about the patient's head to create a tomographic projection of the oral-facial region. For skull-view radiography, the x-ray source and the image receptor are positioned extraorally for a stationary projection. This type of projection may include the complete skull or may only image a limited region of interest. An x-ray generator may be designed to perform more than one of the basic types of dental radiography.

Another type of x-ray generator is that designed specifically for intraoral source radiography. This type of x-ray generator is characterized by location of the target at the end of a rod-like structure. The rod-like source is positioned intraorally and the image receptor is positioned extraorally for a stationary projection. Some clinicians use this type of x-ray generator routinely; however, its overall use has been very limited.

Some types of x-ray generators intended primarily for medical radiography are also used for dental radiography. This is especially true for skull-view radiography and special purpose tomographic radiography.

PROPERTIES AND COMPONENTS: There are many technical factors which collectively influence the performance of an x-ray generator.

Beam Quality: The radiation produced by an x-ray generator is polychromatic.[1] The x-ray spectrum or intensity wave length distribution, also known as beam quality, is a very important property of an x-ray generator. A radiation beam with a relatively large proportion of long wave lengths is referred to as a soft beam. A beam with a relatively large proportion of short wave lengths is referred to as a hard beam. Photon energy is inversely proportional to wave length such that long wave lengths correspond to low photon energies, and short wave lengths corresond to high photon energies. If the majority of wave lengths are sufficiently long, then most of the photons are absorbed in the subject without contributing to formation of a useful image. If the majority of the wave lengths are sufficiently short, then most of the photons pass through the subject without formation of a useful image. Between these two extremes, there is a useful range of wave lengths for the projection of radiographic images. Within the useful spectrum, soft beams tend to produce higher subject contrast than hard beams.[1] Hard beams tend to produce more secondary scatter radiation than soft beams.[2] Soft beams create a higher entrance tissue exposure than hard beams, but hard beams tend to produce a higher dose to deep tissues than soft beams.[3,4]

The beam quality is determined primarily by the tube potential, the waveform, and the filtration.

1. Tube Potential: The tube potential is the difference of electrical potential between the filament and the target. The filament is negative

with respect to the target, and accordingly, the filament is the cathode and the target is the anode of the x-ray tube. The electrons produced at the filament, or cathode, are attracted to the target, or anode. The difference of potential between the filament and the target is typically between 50 and 110 kilovolts for dental x-ray generators.

The greater the tube potential, the greater is the kinetic energy of the electrons as they bombard the target, and accordingly, the more the polychromatic spectrum is shifted toward shorter wave lengths.[1] Increases in tube potential also result in an increase in the intensity of the x-ray beam for a given tube current.[1]

2. Wave Form: The manner in which the tube potential varies with time is known as the wave form. Most dental x-ray generators use alternating current (a.c.), such that the tube potential varies from zero up to the kilovoltage peak (kVp), and back down to zero with each cycle of the alternating current. These x-ray generators are often referred to as a.c. generators. The a.c. generators produce x-radiation in discrete bursts corresponding to the a.c. cycles. For one-half of the a.c. cycle the tube potential is reversed so that electrons are not attracted to the target and therefore x-radiation is produced only during the other one-half of the a.c. cycle. Most a.c. generators operate at the frequency of the a.c. supply current, however, some generators increase the frequency of the a.c. supply. High frequency has the potential advantages of an increase in the efficiency of the high voltage transformer and enhancement of timer accuracy.

Some dental x-ray generators transform the a.c. supply into direct current (d.c.) so that the tube potential is maintained at a constant kilovoltage (kV). These x-ray generators are often referred to as d.c. generators or as constant potential (c.p.) generators.

It should be emphasized that an a.c. generator does not produce the same x-ray spectrum as a d.c. generator. An a.c. generator set, for example, at 70 kVp, varies continuously between a tube potential of 0 kV and 70 kVp. A d.c. generator set at 70 kVp maintains essentially a constant tube potential at 70 kV. The spectrum of a.c. generators can be made to approach that of d.c. generators if the a.c. waveform is electronically altered to be more like square waves than the sinusoidal waves of a.c. supply currents. Also, high frequency generators may approach the spectrum of d.c. generators if the capacitance keeps the tube potential near the peak potential.

3. Filtration: Filtration also affects the spectrum produced by x-ray generators. Basically, filtration is intended to block preferentially the lower energy part of the spectrum which would otherwise be almost totally absorbed by the patient, thereby adding to the patient radiational dose without contributing to formation of an image. Usually aluminum and sometimes copper have been the traditional materials for filtration.

Another use of filtration is to block preferentially both the low and high energy parts of the spectrum to create an optimum energy band for imaging. Because of special absorption properties, samarium is used as a filter material for this purpose.

The tube potential, the waveform and the filtration all interact to determine the x-ray spectrum produced by an x-ray generator. In general, high tube potentials, increases in filtration, and d.c. waveforms tend toward hard beams. Low tube potentials, low filtration, and sinusoidal a.c. waveforms tend toward soft beams.

Ordinarily, the wave form of a particular x-ray generator is fixed by its design and cannot be altered by the user. The filtration of an x-ray unit can usually be altered by the user, but care should be exercised not to violate government regulations regarding minimum levels of filtration, and not to reduce the radiation output rate of the x-ray generator excessively by over-filtration. For some x-ray generators, the kVp of a.c. generators or the kV of d.c. generators cannot be altered; however, others provide for adjustments over a range of 50 kV.

Tube Current: The tube current of an x-ray generator is the flux of electrons between the filament and the target. The tube current is di-

rectly related to the intensity of the x-ray beam, but the tube current does not directly affect the spectrum of the x-ray beam. The tube currents of dental x-ray generators usually range from about 5 to 20 milliamperes (mA). Some x-ray generators have a fixed tube current and others provide for selection of two or more tube current levels.

Timer: The timer of an x-ray unit controls the length of the overall time interval during which x-radiation is produced.

X-ray generators for curved surface tomography generally have the interval of x-ray generation coordinated with the length of time of the panoramic scan. In this case, the optical density produced on the image receptor is controlled by the tube potential or the tube current. The use of tube potential to control x-ray output also alters the beam quality. The other types of x-ray generators provide for timer adjustment to control the optical density on the image receptor. Typical timer adjustments range from 1/60 of a second to several seconds. The a.c. generators often express times of less than one second in terms of pulses of the a.c. supply currents. In the United States, one pulse corresponds to 1/60 of a second since a.c. supply currents operate at 60 Hz. The a.c. generators that operate at higher frequencies than 60 Hz arbitrarily express times as though the frequency was 60 Hz.

Time-Intensity: Exposure time and tube current may be multiplied together to give an indication of total x-ray output in terms of milliampere seconds (mAs). Due to a number of technical factors, many x-ray generators are not consistent in output at very short timer settings; however, high speed image receptors may require short times. If the desired results cannot be achieved by timer settings, then distance or tube current can be used to achieve practical exposure times.

For a given total x-ray exposure, relatively low exposure time, and relatively high exposure intensity are desired. Short exposure times help to reduce motion blur. Also, some image receptors, especially screen-film combinations, exhibit an optimum efficiency at a particular time and intensity due to time-intensity reciprocity failure.[5] The optimum is usually in the short time, high intensity region.

Focal Spot: The focal spot is the region of the target actually bombarded by electrons, and hence the region of the target from which x-rays are effectively produced. The smaller the focal spot size, the higher is the resolution of the projected image.[1,2,5] However, to reduce the focal spot size, the intensity and the total output of an x-ray tube must be restricted to avoid overheating the target. If a given electron beam bombarding the target is focused into a sufficiently small region for a long time, the target can melt. Some dental x-ray generators have rotating targets so that, from one instant to the next, the electron beam is not bombarding the same region of the target.

For any given x-ray generator, the intensity of the electron beam, the length of time of exposure, the focal spot size, and the time interval between exposure must be coordinated to prevent damage to the target. The sum of permissible "on" times during a given time interval is known as the duty cycle.

In some situations, the focal spot may be made effectively smaller by increasing the distance at which it is used. For periapical and bitewing radiography, the trend has been to use a source-subject distance of 40 cm or greater. On the other hand, the opportunity to use small focal spots, low exposure outputs, and short source-subject distances may be advantageous in many situations. If short distances and radiographic magnification are desired, then a small focal spot size becomes a very important factor.[6]

Collimation: The collimation of an x-ray generator restricts the cross-section of an x-ray beam to coincide as closely as possible to the size and shape of the image receptor. Collimation helps to reduce some aspects of patient radiational dose and presumably enhances image quality by reducing the amount of scatter radiation that reaches the image receptor.[7]

For curved surface tomography and most forms of skull-view radiography, the image receptor and the beam cross-section can be closely aligned.

For periapical, bitewing, and occlusal radiography, the beam cross-section has traditionally been collimated in a manner to allow for some uncertainty in the alignment of the beam and the image receptor. Now, a number of auxiliary instruments are available to align and closely collimate the beam to the image receptor.[8]

For periapical and bitewing radiography, the collimation is usually incorporated into a cylindrical position indicating device (PID). The PID serves as a guide in establishing the source-subject distance and also as a guide in aligning the x-ray beam, the subject, and the image receptor.

For curved surface tomography, collimation of the x-ray beam to a narrow slit is an intrinsic part of the geometry of projection rather than a dose reduction measure as such. In general, the more narrow the slit, the greater is the thickness of the zone in focus for a tomographic projection.

Shielding: In addition to collimation, the housing of an x-ray tube is shielded to prevent radiation from being emitted in any direction other than the direction of the primary beam. Shielding is a means of protecting patients and clinicians from unnecessary exposure to radiation.

Mechanical Adjustments: A number of mechanical features are important to optimal performance of dental x-ray generators.

For periapical, bitewing and occlusal view radiography, the tube heads are generally mounted in an articulating arm. It is important to properly adjust the arm mechanism to prevent motion of the tube head after it is positioned. The range of motion in a horizontal and a vertical plane are considerations to achieve desired clinical projections. Associated with range of motion is the location and method of mounting the tube head. The basic types of mounting are wall, floor, or ceiling.

For curved surface tomography, alignment of the patient head positioner with the rotational motion of the tube head is important. It is usually essential to have the instrument properly leveled and plumbed. Another important mechanical adjustment is alignment of the narrow slit-like primary beam with the slit-like opening in the front of the cassette holder.

For skull view radiography, especially cephalometric radiography, alignment of the headholder, the primary beam, and the image receptor is the important mechanical consideration.

EVALUATION PROGRAM: Many of the technical features of x-ray generators are regulated by the Performance Standards of the Bureau of Radiological Health, Food and Drug Administration, Rockville, Maryland. These standards are oriented towards regulation of the introduction of x-ray generators into commerce by manufacturers.

Regulations of individual state governments are generally oriented towards the users of x-ray generators.

American Dental Association Specifications No. 26 and 31 delineate important features for x-ray generators used for periapical, bitewing, and occlusal radiography. These specifications are used in conjunction with the Acceptance Program of the Council on Dental Materials, Instruments and Equipment.

X-RAY GENERATORS

Do:

1. Select the type of x-ray best suited to the clinical task.
2. Adjust the beam quality to optimize the relationship between the visual task and the patient radiational dose.
3. Adjust the time:intensity relationship within the duty cycle limitations of the x-ray generator to optimize the efficiency of screen-film image receptors and to minimize motion blur.
4. Select an x-ray generator with a focal spot size commensurate with the geometry of projection and image receptor desired.
5. Use proper collimation for the geometry of projection desired.
6. Make periodic examinations of the mechanical adjustments of the x-ray generator.

AVAILABLE PRODUCTS

ABACUS 9022 DENTAL X-RAY MACHINE, The Abacus Group, Inc.
BELMONT DENTAL X-RAY UNIT 065, Belmont Equipment Co.
GE-700 CENTURY II INTRA-ORAL X-RAY SYSTEM, General Electric Co.
GE-700 INTRA ORAL X-RAY SYSTEM, General Electric Co.
GE-1000 INTRA ORAL X-RAY SYSTEM, General Electric Co.
GEX INTRA ORAL X-RAY SYSTEM, General Electric Co.
HELIODENT 2 WITH DOSIMATIC, Siemens Corp.
HELIODENT 70 WITH DENTOTIME, Siemens Corp.
INTRA-ORAL 90 X-RAY UNIT, Universal X-Ray Products
ORALIX 65, Philips Medical Systems
Ortho-Ceph, Siemens Corp.
Orthopantomograph OPSE, Siemens Corp.

PANPAS-E X-RAY MACHINE, Vacudent/md.
PERIAPICAL DENTAL X-RAY EQUIPMENT, S. S. White Dental Products International
RITTER EXPLORER P-3 X-RAY SYSTEM, Ritter Co., Div. of Sybron Corp.
RITTER METEOR II MODEL R-1A, Ritter Co., Div. of Sybron Corp.
SANKO DENTAL EXPLORER MODELS 55, 70 KVP, Sanko Distributing Co.

FILM HOLDERS

Film holders are instruments that hold and position radiographic film intraorally for periapical and bitewing radiography. These instruments also may perform some or all of the additional functions of aligning the film with the primary beam, collimating the primary beam closely to the size and shape of the film, and blocking a major part of the primary beam behind the plane of the film.[8,9] Holding instruments can also be used for non-film receptors such as xeroradiographic cassettes.[10] The holders are generally designed to be used either with the "parallel" technique or the "bisecting angle" technique.[1] Holding instruments may help avoid retakes and may improve some aspects of image quality by achieving consistency, accuracy, and convenience in film placement. In addition, substantial reductions in some aspects of patient dose may be achieved by the holders that also collimate the primary beam and block the beam beyond the receptor plane.[11,12] The ability to sterilize, or at least disinfect, film holders between use from one patient to the next, is an important consideration for these instruments.

AVAILABLE PRODUCTS

Adamounts—Dental X-Ray Film Holders, ADA Products, Inc.

Dr. Eggen's X-Ray Film Holder Set, American Dental Mfg. Co.

Intraoral Film Holder, Pulpdent Corp. of America

Kodak X-Ray Exposure Holders, Eastman Kodak Co.

Shure-Shot Disposable X-Ray Film Holder, Pulpdent Corp. of America

Twix 2-way Disposable X-Ray Film Holder, Pulpdent Corp. of America

LEADED PROTECTIVE APRONS

Leaded protective aprons are aprons intended to shield patients from some of the unnecessary radiational exposure that may occur during a radiographic examination. The traditional primary purpose is to shield the genital region, although some aprons include a collar to shield the cervical (thyroid) region. Cervical shields may be used separately from aprons. There is

apparently greater rationale for the use of cervical shielding than genital shielding because the radiational dose in the cervical region is relatively higher than that in the genital region.[13,14] Furthermore, the genetically significant dose from dental radiography has been considered to be negligible.[15] (See the chapter on "Safety in the Dental Office" for radiational hygiene suggestions.)

PERSONAL RADIATION MONITORING DEVICES

Radiation monitoring badges are detecting devices intended to monitor the occupational radiation exposure of individuals. The badges are generally designed to clamp onto the clothing of the individual being monitored. Typically, the badges contain a combination of thermoluminescent and film dosimeters. Services are commercially available which provide exposure readings from the dosimeters and a replacement badge at regular intervals in time. Although radiation monitoring badges are widely accepted for personnel dosimetry monitoring, there are some uncertainties regarding the levels of accuracy.[16]

Devices using the ionization technique are also used to monitor the radiation received by a person. These may require an auxiliary reading device or the reading devices may be incorporated within each unit. Commercial models of the size of a large fountain pen are available that measure X and gamma rays of low electron energy and neutrons. One advantage of such devices over photographic emulsion is that calibration is less dependent upon the energy of the incident photon.

AVAILABLE PRODUCTS

Replacement Identification Tabs, Eastman Kodak Company

RADIOGRAPHIC ILLUMINATORS

Radiographic illuminators are instruments intended for viewing radiographic film by means of transmitted light. Important characteristics of radiographic illuminators are the level of light intensity and the uniformity of the light intensity across the viewing surface. For some illuminators the level of light intensity can be varied by the operator. An important consideration is to block out extraneous light by masking around a film being viewed.[1,17] It is also considered advisable to turn off the room lights while viewing films. Elimination of all sources of extraneous light increases the visual perception of the viewer.

It is sometimes helpful to have a spot type illuminator of about one inch in diameter with a variable intensity control. A spot illuminator may be a separate unit or part of a conventional viewing unit. Such a device permits a particular region of interest to be viewed at the proper intensity of illumination without extraneous light from other parts of the image. Illuminators are available in a variety of sizes to accommodate different size films.

Available Products

ADA Viewers, ADA Products, Inc.
ADA Viewer/Enlarger/Projector, ADA Products, Inc.
X-Ray Viewer, Time Motion System Company

RADIOGRAPHIC DUPLICATORS

Radiographic duplicators are instruments for use with radiographic duplicating film to make copies of original radiographs. The duplicators should establish direct contact between the original and the duplicating film; provide uniform light intensity across the illuminated surface; and have an accurate timer controlling the light source. An ultraviolet light source is recommended to achieve contrast in the copy similar to that in the original.[18] Direct visualization of the ultraviolet light should be avoided to prevent possible eye injury. (See the chapter on "Safety in the Dental Office" regarding further information on ultraviolet light safety.)

AUTOMATED PROCESSORS

Automated processors are instruments for processing radiographic and duplicating film whereby the films are mechanically transported through the developing, fixing, washing, and drying stages of processing. Most automated processors use a roller system to transport the film; however, some processors use special film holders. Most processors are limited with respect to both the maximum and minimum size of films that can be accommodated.

The processing chemicals used in automated processors are designed specifically for that purpose. Some processors can be equipped with automatic replenishers for the developer and fixer solutions. Loading chambers are available for some processors that permit the processor to be located in a daylight or roomlight environment. The suitability of the filter in the loading chamber should be confirmed for each type of film to be processed. Many automated processors perform film washing in a reservoir of water that is subject to contamination from previous washing cycles; some processors provide a fresh water washing cycle. Most processors function at a fixed processing rate and a fixed processing temperature. Some processors provide for variation of the processing time and temperature. The accuracy of the temperature control in the processing solutions, and the consistency and reliability with which films are transported through the different stages of processing are very important features of automated processors.[19,20] Proper routine maintenance and cleaning is generally essential for successful processor operation. A processing quality control procedure should be conducted routinely to monitor the status of the overall processing performance.[21,22]

It is especially important to determine the suitability of any particular type of film for the type of automated processing to be used. For example, some emulsions require the squeezing action of transport rollers, and other emulsions cannot tolerate rollers. Some films may be processed by either automated or manual methods. In general, the films must be compatible with the time and temperature of each phase of the processing.

For films that may be processed either automatically or manually, automated processing may require substantially greater patient exposures than manual processing to achieve equivalent image densities.[23]

Available Products

ALL-PRO AUTOMATIC X-RAY FILM PROCESSOR, Air Techniques, Inc.
DENTL-D-VELOPER, General Electric Co.
MODEL P-4, P-6, P-10 AUTOMATIC DENTAL X-RAY FILM PROCESSORS, Xonics Medical Systems
PHILIPS 810 AUTOMATIC FILM PROCESSOR, Philips Dental Systems
PERI-PRO, Air Techniques, Inc.
Phocomat, Siemens Corp.
X-Ray Automatic Processor Developer, Healthco, Inc.

Other Available Products

ACCESSORY DEVICES FOR X-RAY MACHINES

BAI (BISECTING ANGLE INSTRUMENT), Rinn Corporation
Bite Wing Loops, Healthco, Inc.
Bite Wing Loops, J. R. Rand Specialty Co., Inc.
Cush-N-Tab Bitewing Holder, Greene Dental Products, Inc.
Darcview Mounts, Greene Dental Products, Inc.
Kodak Dental Film Clips, Eastman Kodak Co.
Mastic F Series Mounts, Greene Dental Products, Inc.
PID (POSITION INDICATING DEVICE), Rinn Corporation
Poly Bite Wing Tabs, Pulpdent Corp. of America
PRECISION X-RAY DEVICE, Isaac Masel Company

Pressure Sensitive Bite Wing Tabs, Healthco Inc.
Prolastic X-Ray Radiation Detector, Prolastic Co., Inc.
PV-20 SAF-T-STOR Pages System, Franklin Distributing Corporation
Regular Bitewing Holders, Greene Dental Products, Inc.
Spec-Dec Halo X-Ray Mounts, Pulpdent Corp. of America
Periapical Film Holder Stabe, Greene Dental Products, Inc.
Sta-Put Bite Wing Tabs, Teledyne Dental Products
Transview Mounts, Greene Dental Products, Inc.
Wing-Master, Innovators, Inc.
XCP (EXTENSION-CONE-PARALLELING INSTRUMENT), Rinn Corporation
X-Ray Angulators, Premier Dental Products Co.
X-Ray Film Mounts, Healthco, Inc.
X-Ray and/or Slide Storage Sleeves, Franklin Distributors Corporation

DARKROOM INSTRUMENTS

Kodak Achromatic Magnifier, 5x, Eastman Kodak Co.
Kodak Adjustable Safelight Lamp, Model B, Eastman Kodak Co.
Kodak Darkroom Lamp, Eastman Kodak Co.
Kodak Dental Film Dispenser, Model O., Eastman Kodak Co.
Kodak Dental Film Dispenser, Model 2, Eastman Kodak Co.
Kodak Dental Film Receptacle, Eastman Kodak Co.
Kodak Dental Processing Hanger, Eastman Kodak Co.
Kodak Dental Processing Tank, 12 oz., Eastman Kodak Co.
Kodak Flashed Opal Glass, Eastman Kodak Co.
Kodak Process Thermometer, Eastman Kodak Co.
Kodak Safelight Filters, No. 6B (Brown) for Extraoral X-Ray Films, Type ML-2 (Light Orange) for Intraoral X-Ray Films, Eastman Kodak Co.
Kodak Tank and Tray Thermometer, Eastman Kodak Co.
Kodak 2-Way Safelamp, Model A, Eastman Kodak Co.
Kodak Utility Safelight Lamp, Model D, Eastman Kodak Co.
Kodak X-omatic Cassette C-2, windowless, Eastman Kodak Co.

Kodak X-omatic regular intensifying screen, Eastman Kodak Co.

Kodak X-Ray Film Identification Printer, Model B, Eastman Kodak Co.

Kodak X-Ray Processing Hanger, Eastman Kodak Co.

Rand X-Ray Room Timers, J. R. Rand Specialty Co., Inc.

X-Ray Developer Replenisher, Healthco, Inc.

X-Ray Timer Extension Cord, J. R. Rand Specialty Co., Inc.

LITERATURE REFERENCES

1. X-rays in dentistry. Rochester, New York, Eastman Kodak Co.

2. Ter-Pogossion, M. M. The physical aspects of diagnostic radiography. New York, Hoeber, 1976.

3. BRH Bulletin, XI (21):1. Rockville, Maryland, Bureau of Radiological Health, Nov. 7, 1977.

4. Richards, A. G., and Webber, R. L. Dental x-ray exposure of sites within the head and neck. Oral Surg., Oral Med. Oral Path. 18:752 Dec. 1964.

5. Johns, H. E., and Cunningham, J. R. The physics of radiology. Springfield, Illinois, Charles C. Thomas, 1974.

6. Rao, G. U. V. Do high detail screens always yield better resolution than high speed screens? Am. J. Roentgenol. 112:812 Aug. 1971.

7. Winkler, K. G. Influence of rectangular collimation and intraoral shielding dose in dental radiography. JADA 77:95 July 1968.

8. Preliminary report on radiographic holding, paralleling, and shielding devices. Council on Dental Materials and Devices, American Dental Association. JADA 77:884 Oct. 1968.

9. Thunthy, K. H. Evaluation of X-ray instruments. Dent. Hygiene 50:455 Oct. 1976.

10. White, S. C., and Gratt, B. M. Clinical trials of intra-oral dental xeroradiography. JADA 99:810 Nov. 1979.

11. Winkler, K. G. Influence of rectangular collimation and intraoral shielding on radiation dose in dental radiography. JADA 77:96 July 1968.

12. White, S. C., and Rose, T. C. Absorbed bone marrow dose in certain dental radiographic techniques. JADA 98:553 Apr. 1979.

13. Block, A. J.; Goepp, R. A.; and Mason, E. W. Thyroid radiation dose during panoramic and cephalometric dental X-ray examinations. Angle Orthodontist 47:17 Jan. 1977.

14. Whitcher, B. L.; Gratt, B. M.; and Sickles, E. A. Leaded shields for thyroid dose reduction in intraoral dental radiography. Oral Surg., Oral Med., Oral Path. 48:567 Dec. 1979.

15. The effects on populations of exposure to low levels of ionizing radiation, (BEIR Report), National Academy of Sciences, Washington, D. C. Ch. V, 1972.

16. Advance notice of rulemaking on certification of personnel dosimetry processors. Fed. Register 45:20493 March 28, 1980.

17. Wuehrmann, A. H. Radiation hygiene and its practice in dentistry as related to film viewing procedures and radiographic interpretation. JADA 30:346 Feb. 1970.

18. Allen, M. J., and Silha, R. E. New copiers for dental radiograph duplicating film. Dent. Radiogr. Photogr. 49:14, 1976.

19. Alcox, R. W., and Waggener, D. T. Status report on rapid processing devices for dental radiographic film. JADA 83:330 Dec. 1971.

20. Anderson, G. K., and Johnston, G. J. Effect of development temperature changes in an automatic processor. Application of Optical Instrumentation in Medicine IV 70:26, 1975.

21. Gray, J. E. Photographic quality assurance in diagnostic radiology, nuclear medicine, and radiation therapy. HEW Publication (FDA) 76-8043, U. S. Dept. of Health, Education and Welfare, 1976.

22. Film processing (Supplement to Radiography in modern industry). Rochester, New York, Eastman Kodak Co.

23. Moore, B. K., et al. Techniques for comparing automatic and manual dental X-ray film processing. J. Dent. Res. 56(B):B175 June 1977.

OPERATORY EQUIPMENT

DENTAL CHAIRS

TYPES: Dental chairs are sturdy, padded chairs allowing various types of adjustment to facilitate oral therapy. The types of chairs that are available currently from manufacturers include the following.

Full Fixed: The contour of the chair is fixed into one position. When the patient is tipped backwards, the entire body must be tipped.

Contour Chairs With One Movable Joint: The lower portion of the chair is separate from the upper portion and can hinge in the location of the patient's lower back. These chairs usually have a flat headrest, or they may have a typical two pad headrest if desired for certain aspects of dentistry. On certain models, the headrest portion is hinged also. The headrest portion can often be removed, shortening the chair, to allow easier treatment of children.

Contour Chairs With Two Movable Joints: Another design similar to the model hinged at the lower back region also allows movement by way of a hinge at the patient's knees. Some patients prefer this type of chair because their feet are not as high.

Contour Chairs With Rotating Seat Portion: Certain chairs allow the patient to rotate 90° horizontally from the normal position of the chair, and assume a normal sitting position while talking to the dentist, or entering or exiting from the chair. When rotated back to the normal position, the chair allows the patient to be in a supine position during treatment.

Contour Pedodontic Chairs: These are smaller versions of the designs described previously.

Conventional Dental Chairs: Some dentists prefer to operate standing up, and others require strong patient head support while operating. Such dentists usually prefer the conventional dental chair.

DIRECTIONS FOR USE: Chairs range from simple pump operation, with hand operated levers to move the back and headrest, to totally automated chairs that move to a pre-determined position with the movement of only one control.

DENTAL CHAIRS

Do:

1. Select a chair that meets your needs relative to standing, sitting, size of patients treated, and the discipline of dentistry most commonly practiced.
2. Observe the thickness of the back of the chair. While sitting, does it allow easy access of your legs when operating with the patient in a supine position?
3. Select a chair with the type of covering material that meets your needs.
4. Make certain that electrical switches for the chair are in a convenient location for your style of operating.
5. Check the location of the patient's arms while in a supine position. Are they held by a sling or other support? If not, the chair may be uncomfortable for long appointment periods.
6. Expect to have occasional maintenance on motorized and automatic chairs.
7. Clean the surfaces of the chairs routinely. Most of the covering materials can be kept attractive if cleaned often. However, infrequent cleaning may cause irreparable discoloration.

Don't:

1. Attempt to perform sit down dentistry in a conventional dental chair.
2. Allow sharp objects to penetrate vinyl surfaces of chairs. Although some new vinyl materials have relatively "rip" free backings, certain materials will rip when penetrated by sharp objects.
3. Allow ball point pens to mark vinyl surfaces. Many vinyl coverings do not afford easy cleaning of ball point pen marks, and they remain on the surface until worn off.
4. Allow articulating paper or ribbon to drop on the chair. Some papers or ribbons will make nearly indelible markings on the vinyl or fabric.
5. Allow patients to exert force on the arms of chairs when exiting. Some of the current contour chair arms will break when excessive force is applied to them.
6. Select a chair without very careful examination of several models. Contemporary contour chairs vary considerably in cost, options offered, durability, serviceability and acceptability for "sit down" dentistry.

LIMITATIONS OF USE: Many chairs intended for "stand-up" dentistry do not adapt easily or well to "sit down" concepts. As the older chairs are reclined to place the patient in a supine position, the patient's arms tend to slide backwards off the chair. Additionally, the thickness of the chair usually interferes with the operator's legs when the patient is placed in a fully supine position with the operator sitting close enough to the chair for comfort and adequate vision.

EVALUATION PROGRAM: Specifications for dental chairs are currently under development by ANSC MD156 based on an existing ISO Standard.

AVAILABLE PRODUCTS

Chairman Regular Dental Chair, Pelton and Crane
Chairs, Dental Corporation of America
Del-Tube Motorized Chair, Del-Tube Corporation
Dentsply Classic Chair, Dentsply International, Inc.
Elegán Patient Chair, Den-Tal-Ez Mfg. Co.
JS & VS Series Patient Chairs, Den-Tal-Ez Mfg. Co.
PM 2000 Automatic Patient Chair, Planmecca Oy (Distributed by Time Motion System Company)
Relaxadent Chair, MDT Corporation

"Reliance" Coronet I and IIB Examination Chairs, F & F Koenigkramer

"Reliance" 475 FB and FB2 Chairs, F & F Koenigkramer

"Reliance" 660 Examination and Treatment Chair, F & F Koenigkramer

Series 3 Patient Chair, Den-Tal-Ez Mfg. Co.

SL 3 Patient Chair, Siemens Corporation Dental Division

Unitek/Metalcraft Dental Chair, Unitek Corp.

Veeco Dental Chair, Veeco Mfg.

DENTAL UNITS

TYPES: Dental units provide the dentist and auxiliary with compressed air, water, suction, electricity, table top or bracket table surfaces, and occasionally an operating light, cuspidor and gas. They can be divided into the following categories.

Fixed Floor Mounted Units: This traditional type of equipment is located at the left of the patient. It has a flushing cuspidor, the usual utilities, and a bracket table which swings over the patient and may or may not be adjustable in height. The operating light is usually connected to the unit. Many new forms of units use the basic design described with various modifications such as: smaller cuspidors, disappearing cuspidors, streamlined bracket tables, bracket tables that contain the utilities and handpieces, and other features.

Two Mobile-Cart System: This concept uses two mobile carts, one for the dentist and one for the dental assistant. The dentist's cart is located at the dentist's right side near the right side of the patient, while the assistant's cart is located on the patient's left, near the head of the patient. Both dentist and auxiliary sit to operate. Usually the patient is treated in a supine position. Utilities in the dentist's cart include air, water, electricity, and handpieces. The assistant's cart includes air, water and suction. Operating lights must be connected to the dental chair or the ceiling.

DENTAL UNITS

Do:
1. Select a unit concept that meets your needs and desires.
2. Observe dentists working with a given concept before deciding to adopt it yourself.
3. Expect routine maintenance on every unit.
4. Consider sit down dentistry if it meets your needs.
5. Consider eliminating the cuspidor if you elect to change to sit down, four handed dentistry.

Don't:
1. Adopt a concept because others say it is right. Only you can decide what is right for *you*.
2. Expect to use low speed, belt driven handpieces with a cart concept. The cart concept usually requires low speed, air driven handpieces.
3. Be concerned about changing to another concept. Most dentists adapt well to changing to another operating concept.

One Mobile-Cart System: In this unit, the assistant has one mobile cart, containing the utility needs—suction, air, water and electricity, while the dentist's handpieces and utilities are usually chair mounted and are available over the patient's chest. The operating light must be connected to the chair or ceiling.

Rear Instrument Delivery: All utility, handpiece, and table top requirements are behind the patient in this unit. Lights are attached to the chair or ceiling. As the patient is reclined into a supine position, the utilities, handpieces, and table top space may or may not slide closer to the patient. All equipment and supplies are out of the patient's sight. Handpieces and utilities come from behind the patient, make a 180° turn, and turn back into the mouth.

DIRECTIONS FOR USE: Each unit has its specific and detailed directions; no single set of general directions applies to all units.

LIMITATIONS OF USE: Dental units without close proximity of instruments to operator do not adapt well to "sit down, four handed" dentistry. Many cart systems do not adapt well to stand up dentistry. Certain systems do not adapt well to oral surgery or removable prosthodontics.

EVALUATION PROGRAM: Portions of the dental unit are covered by specifications or recommendations by various agencies, such as Underwriters Laboratories, and IEC Technical Committee 62. Specifications are also under development by ANSC MD 156.

AVAILABLE PRODUCTS

ADS (Accessory Delivery System), MDT Corporation

Anti-Retraction Valve/Vacuum Breaker Automatic Control Units, Zirc Dental Products

Basic 4 Delivery System, MDT Corporation

Basic HO Delivery System, MDT Corporation

Den-Tal-Ez Turbine, Den-Tal-Ez Custom Vac

Dental Units, Dental Corporation of America

Dental Units Models 360, 500, Cart Mover, Proma

Dentassist Liberty, Health Science Products, Inc.

Dentsply Spectrum I, Dentsply International

Dentsply Spectrum II, Dentsply International

Dentsply Spectrum III, Dentsply International

Dispos-a-Screens, Zirc Dental Products

Duo-Vac, The Lorvic Corporation

Executive; Exec-Aire and Ranger, Pelton and Crane

Flex-O-Jet Saliva Ejector, The Lorvic Corporation

443 Single-Use Oral Evacuator, Monoject

444 Single-Use Surgical Aspirator Tip, Monoject

Hygoformic Saliva Ejectors, North Pacific Dental, Inc.

Iso-Shield Saliva Absorbers, 3M Company

Johnson's Single Use Saliva Ejectors, Johnson and Johnson Dental Products Company

Lactona Angulated Aspirator Tips, Lactona Corporation

Lactona Vacu-Rinse Kit, Lactona Corporation

Micro-Cart Dental Unit, A-Dec, Inc.

Mobile Carts, Zirc Dental Products

Oral Evacuation Pump, Den-Tal-Ez Custom Vac

Oral Evacuator Safe-Guard, North Pacific Dental, Inc.

PCA Speejecter, Pulpdent Corporation of America

Plastip Evacuation Tubes, J. R. Rand Specialty Co., Inc.

Rackson Hantrol Dental Units, Hantrol Corporation

Roto-Vac High Volume Aspirator Tip, Lorvic Corporation

Saliva Ejectors, Healthco, Inc.

Signature Delivery System, Den-Tal-Ez Mfg. Co.

Siro 3 Cuspidor, Siemens Corporation

Sirona-S-4, S-5 Units, Siemens Corporation

Super Sof-ti, Spee-Dee, and Super Spec-Dee Saliva Ejectors, Pulpdent Corporation of America

Super Sof-ti-tips, Pulpdent Corporation of America

Total Concept Dental Environment, Time Motion System Co.

Uni-Chair Dental Unit, A-Dec, Inc.

Unitek/Metalcraft Dental Equipment, Unitek Corp.

Unitek/Metalcraft Dental Unit, Unitek Corp.

Unitrac Instrument Delivery System, MDT Corporation

Vent-O-Vac Aspirator, The Lorvic Corporation

Vent-O-Vac Tips, Lorvic Corporation

Wind Mill, Pelton and Crane

MISCELLANEOUS ACCESSORIES

Accessory Cabinets, Dental Corporation of America

Alabama Mobile Cabinet, Health Science Products, Inc.

"Associate Group" and "Team Center" Wall Cabinets, Health Science Products, Inc.

Cabinet Trays, Plastic, Zirc Dental Products

Cox Chairside System, Cox Systems Limited

Cox Open Operatory, Cox Systems Limited

Dental Cabinets, Dental/Medical, Inc.

Dentsply Spectrum, Dentsply International, Inc.

Instrument Mats, Zirc Dental products

Set Up Trays and Racks, Zirc Dental Products

Sink Cabinets, Health Science Products, Inc.

DENTAL OPERATING LIGHTS

TYPES: Lights specifically designed for dentistry deliver intense focused lighting to the operating site. Most types of operating lights may be connected to either the dental unit, dental chair, or a ceiling track. Dentists should consider the advantages of each location before selecting operatory lights.

a. Fixed floor mounted unit lights have the disadvantage of being in the way of the assistant; however, compensation for this problem can be overcome easily.

b. Chair mounted lights have a genuine advantage in that they remain in the correct position when the chair is raised or lowered. However, because of the difficulty encountered when stabilizing the light to a movable chair, such light posts have observable lack of stability which may be objectionable.

c. Ceiling mounted lights offer the advantage of being out of the way and are especially well suited for x-ray rooms. Such lights are very stable, but they require the placement of a track in the ceiling which is usually an additional expense. They have a further advantage of elimination of the light pole, but they must be readjusted as the chair is raised or lowered.

Less used forms of dental operating lights include head mounted lights commonly used by oral surgeons, and fiber optic lights which provide intense well directed light from a small source.

USES: Dental operating lights are used to illuminate the field of oral operation or any other site where other work is accomplished in the operating environment.

DIRECTIONS FOR USE: Manufacturers have specific directions for installation of each type of light. Such devices have need for little maintenance after installation.

LIMITATIONS OF USE: Most brands of dental operating lights are satisfactory. However, some have varying ability to focus, intensity of light delivered, and esthetic appeal. Handles may be a source of bacterial cross contamination.

EVALUATION PROGRAM: There are recommendations for dental operating lights available from IEES. The ISO Standard for Dental Operating Lights is under development.

DENTAL OPERATING LIGHTS

Do:

1. Clean the light cover frequently to remove dust, dried blood, and other debris. Such debris is in direct view of patients.
2. Cover the light source with the manufacturer approved and provided cover. Some light bulbs can shatter and cause possible harm to patients.
3. Maintain a supply of spare bulbs.

Don't:

1. Use a light if a protective shield is broken or cracked. Shields provide filtration of ultraviolet radiation which may be emitted from the operating light.
2. Touch the light bulb when it is in use. They are very hot and can easily cause injury!
3. Use the light at an improper focus distance. Each manufacturer describes the approximate correct distance at which the light should be located from the operating field.
4. Leave the light on when not in use.

AVAILABLE PRODUCTS

Alger-Lite, Alger Equipment Co., Inc.
Daray Operating Light, Den-Tal-Ez Mfg. Co.
Fiber Optic Devices, Cameron-Miller, Inc.
Rolux Light, MDT Corporation
Sirolux Dental Light, Siemens Corporation Dental Div.

DENTAL STOOLS

Operator and assistant stools are designed to be used during the performance of dental therapy. The accepted level of stools for dentists allows the operator to sit with knees bent at a right angle and the feet flat on the floor. Many stools also provide an adjustable back support for dentists. Dental assistant stools are several inches higher than stools for dentists. The dental assistant sits with the knees bent at a right angle, and the feet supported by a ring or platform on the stool several inches above the floor. The extra height for dental assistants affords a better view of the operating field and more access for introduction of instruments into the operating field. Many assistant stools also have an arm that extends in front of the chair and on which the assistant leans for support.

There are various types of stool coverings ranging from vinyl to fabrics. The stools are raised and lowered by different activating mechanisms. The stools that can be raised and lowered by using the feet are more acceptable than the hand operated stools, because they avoid the necessity of contaminating the hands when the stool height needs to be adjusted.

USES: Those dentists and assistants practicing sit down dentistry require some form of operating stool. Because of the design and cost of some of these stools, they are usually used during operating times only, and not as laboratory or utility stools.

DIRECTIONS FOR USE: Proper adjustment of the stools should be made to ensure optimum acceptability. Suggestions relative to height have been made in a previous section.

LIMITATIONS OF USE: Sitting down all of the time can become as tiring as standing all of the time. Most practitioners have accepted a combination of sit down and stand up times to break the strain of being in either position all of the time. Generally, the cost of stools is related directly to their comfort and longevity.

EVALUATION PROGRAM: There are no specifications for dental operating stools for dentists and assistants nor do they appear necessary.

AVAILABLE PRODUCTS

Del-Tube Assistants' Stool, Del-Tube Corporation

Del-Tube Doctors' Stool, Del-Tube Corporation

DENTAL STOOLS

Do:

1. Try to adapt to sit down operating positions at least some of the time.
2. Be sure the stools allow the dentist to sit flat on the seat, with knees bent at a right angle, and feet flat on the floor.
3. Be sure that dental assistant chairs have provisions to allow the assistant to sit several inches higher than the dentist and to place the feet on a ring or platform above the floor.
4. Select stools with casters that will accommodate to your flooring. Certain carpets will not allow easy rolling of the stools and these carpets will wear excessively.

Don't:

1. Locate sharp cornered objects near the area where operating stools will be used. Some stools rip or puncture easily.
2. Operate with stools adjusted too high.

Dental Stools, Time Motion Systems Company

Dentsply Classic Dental Stool, Dentsply International, Inc.

Front-Row Seat, Pelton and Crane

Operator and Assistant Stools, Dental Corporation of America

Operator and Assistant Stools, Brandt Industries

Relaxadent Stools, MDT Corporation

"Reliance" 348 Pneumatic; 456 Adjustable; and 556 Hydraulic Stools, F&F Koenigkramer

Sirona Stool, Siemens Corporation Dental Division

Series 3 Operating Stool, Den-Tal-Ez Mfg. Co.

Team Mate Operating Seating, Series 5 & 9, Den-Tal-Ez Mfg. Co.

Unitek/Metalcraft Ergo Dental Seating, Unitek Corp.

ULTRAVIOLET LIGHT DEVICES

Ultraviolet light sources accomplish polymerization of various types of resins used in operative dentistry, fixed prosthodontics, orthodontics, and pedodontics. They are available in the form of hand held "guns," lights, light emitting cords, or other types.

The safety of ultraviolet light devices has been debated vigorously for the past few years. Guidelines have been established, and are published in the section of this book on Safety in the Dental Office. If care is used with an approved device, there appears to be no danger for the operator or patient.

USES: Ultraviolet light devices are used for the polymerization of resins for restoring pieces of teeth, building contour on teeth, splinting teeth, placing pontics between teeth, veneering teeth, placing orthodontic brackets, placing wire space maintainers between teeth, pit and fissure sealants and other uses. Each of these tasks can also be accomplished using chemically cured resins; however, ultraviolet light is advantageous in that it allows resin material to be shaped and contoured more easily before polymerization and brackets may be polymerized en masse after positioning.

DIRECTIONS FOR USE: The safety precautions described in the section of this book on Safety in the Dental Office should be followed. Some devices can be turned on and kept active at will, unless they overheat and turn off automatically. Others have timed activity and will turn off automatically at the end of a prescribed period of time. Dentists and auxiliaries are advised to determine the activity of their device by conducting a simple "out of the mouth" test to determine how deep the light will polymerize resin when turned on for a given period of time. This period of time should be used clinically. Excessive exposure to ultraviolet light is contraindicated.

LIMITATIONS OF USE: A common error in the use of these devices is placing the resin too thickly before polymerization and expecting to polymerize deeper than the capability of the specific device. Soft spots in the resin occur, and the potential result is failure of the technique. Certain devices overheat and can turn off at inopportune times. Some ultraviolet producing lights can lose their polymerization effectiveness and yet still produce light. Periodic checking is advised to avoid such problems.

EVALUATION PROGRAM: The Council on Dental Materials, Instruments and Equipment has guidelines for the acceptance of ultraviolet devices as used in dentistry. In addition, a specification is under development in ANSC MD156.

AVAILABLE PRODUCTS

MODEL 80C QUICK-LITE, Cavitron Corp.
MODEL 80S QUICK-LITE, Cavitron Corp.
NUVA-LITE PHOTO CURE UNIT, Dentsply
   International, Inc.

ULTRAVIOLET LIGHT DEVICES

Do:
1. Survey the market carefully to select the best device for your needs.
2. Test your device carefully so that you know its capabilities.
3. Check the polymerizing potential of the device periodically to assure optimum polymerization capability.
4. Use a rubber dam if possible to cut down ultraviolet light contact with the soft tissues.

Don't:
1. Allow the device to overheat.
2. Use the light more than necessary on a given date.
3. Touch the tip of the polymerization device to the resin. Small amounts will attach to the device.
4. Place large portions of resin to be polymerized.

COMPRESSORS

These devices provide compressed air of sufficient pressure and volume to air outlets and air propelled devices. Many dental offices obtain a supply of compressed air from a central source in the building. This central source often serves several dentists. However, other offices require compressed air of a sufficient quantity to satisfy the needs of only a few operatories. Compressors are often located in the basement, laboratory, or other remote places to lessen the noise of the device in the operating environment. The size of the device is directly related to the needs of the dentist. Dentists should determine the maximum air usage if all air using devices are operating at one time and purchase a quality device that satisfies these air pressure and volume needs. Usually a compressor creates pressure far in excess of the needs of dentists. Most air rotors use 30 psi at the handpiece, however, because of the differing volumes of air consumed by specific handpieces, air pressure at the *unit* is usually much higher than at the *handpiece*. Dentists should have air pressures checked at the *handpiece* with a special device that most suppliers have for routine use. Each brand of handpiece consumes a different quantity of air.

USES: Compressors are used to create air pressure for the operation of dental handpieces, air syringes, periodontal scalers, condensors, laboratory equipment, and other devices. They operate with little maintenance or observation. Some dentists turn the devices off at night, while others leave them on all of the time.

A dryer should be connected to the air line, since moist air can easily ruin the bearings of most handpieces. Compressor tanks should be drained routinely as rust-contaminated water collects at the bottom of these tanks. Periodic tightening and maintenance is required of most devices.

DIRECTIONS FOR USE: Compressors do not require very much maintenance. They should be drained, oiled, and tightened according to manufacturers' specifications.

LIMITATIONS OF USE: If the dentist has selected a compressor and dryer which is adequate for the needs of the office, there are no limitations with today's technology.

EVALUATION PROGRAM: There are no dental specifications for compressors, but they should be capable of providing an adequate volume of dry air at optimum pressure. Most dental suppliers are competent and helpful in determining optimum capacities for all operatory needs. General electrical standards of Underwriters Laboratories and of IEC Technical Committee 62 apply.

COMPRESSORS

Do:

1. Select a compressor that provides adequate air pressure and an adequate volume of air with all possible devices in the office in operation.
2. Connect an air dryer in the line to assure that handpieces are not damaged.
3. Check air pressure at the *handpiece* with a special pressure gauge from the supplier. Most handpieces operate at 30 psi.
4. Drain the compressor tank according to the manufacturer's directions.
5. Because of the vibration of the device, tighten all moving parts periodically.
6. Place the compressor a distance away from the patient area to limit the noise.

Don't:

1. Purchase a compressor too small for your needs.
2. Locate the compressor near operating areas.

AVAILABLE PRODUCTS

Air Compressor, Air Techniques, Inc.
Air Compressors: 420-C; 840-C; Hustler I; Hustler II; Hustler I-10, Pelton and Crane
Blue Ox, Narco/McKesson
Deaquavator, Pelton and Crane
Den-Tal-Ez Compressor, Den-Tal-Ez Mfg. Co.
Jun-Air Compressor, Great Lakes Orthodontic Products
McKesson Compressed Air Systems, Narco/McKesson
Quick Care-High Speed Air Turbine, Siemens Corporation Dental Division

EVACUATORS

TYPES: Evacuating devices are suction systems located either locally at the dental unit or remotely to serve several operatories. Evacuator systems are usually one of the following types.

a. Canisters located on the dental unit that evacuate debris from the operating site and collect it in a reservoir in the cannister.

b. Mobile carts operating on the same basis as canisters and intended for general or surgical use.

c. Venturi systems connected to the air supply which create a negative pressure in a collecting tube. The debris is deposited down the drain.

d. Central suction devices, located remotely from the operating area. These devices usually serve several operatories and deposit debris down the drain.

USES: The major use of evacuating devices is to remove water and debris from the operating site. The increased use of "washed field" operation initiated in the 1950's has made these devices almost mandatory. Evacuation devices are used also for saliva ejectors. Various different tips and suction intensity controls are needed to adapt these devices to the described different uses.

DIRECTIONS FOR USE: Although evacuation devices are an essential part of dental operatory equipment, they require frequent cleaning to remain functional and sanitary. The tank type evacuators require at least daily cleaning, or the debris in the collection reservoir becomes extremely foul smelling. The hoses of all types of evacuators should be flushed with disinfectant solution daily to lessen the potential of microbiologic contamination and subsequent odor formation. Central suction systems usually have clean out locations that should be cleaned according to the specific manufacturer's directions. Care should be taken to perform maintenance on all evacuators according to the manufacturer's directions. Most types of evacuators can be flooded if large quantities of water or

---

EVACUATORS

Do:

1. Select an evacuation system that fits your needs. Older buildings may demand local units. New construction can certainly be adapted for central evacuation systems.
2. Carry out maintenance daily!
3. Clean out the hoses daily by running a disinfectant through them.
4. Plan the volume of a central suction system on the basis of the *total* potential volume need at one time.
5. Use disposable or easily sterilizable evacuator tips.

Don't:

1. Plan for too little volume of evacuation. A strong system can be controlled. A weak system is a continuing problem.
2. Forget to service local and/or central clean out points according to the manufacturer's directions.
3. Run large quantities of cleaner through the system. It may flood and cause problems.

cleaner are forced through them. Flooding can cause mechanical problems. It is suggested that disposal or easily sterilizable tips be used with evacuators.

LIMITATIONS OF USE: Some evacuators intended mainly for surgical use evacuate too little volume of air for general use; however, most general use evacuators can be controlled for use in surgery.

EVALUATION PROGRAM: There are no existing specifications for evacuation devices. Evacuation devices will be included in the specifications for dental units under development in ANSC MD156.

AVAILABLE PRODUCTS

See product listing following the section on Dental Units.

STERILIZERS AND STERILIZATION DEVICES

Sterilizers and sterilization devices are intended for use in dental practice for sterilization of dental instruments, materials and equipment. They must be capable of destroying all forms of living organisms especially all microbial forms, including viruses and spores.

There are four basic types of sterilization devices practical for use in dentistry. These include the steam autoclave, dry heat oven, formaldehyde-alcohol vapor pressure sterilizer, and ethylene oxide chamber. They come the closest to assuring penetration of heat and/or chemical activity to destroy all microbes in crevices and adherent debris.

STEAM AUTOCLAVE STERILIZERS

The word "autoclave" means self-locking. The term is reserved for an apparatus that sterilizes by the use of steam under pressure. This is at a prescribed temperature, pressure and time that will destroy bacterial spores. Early autoclaves had an internal door that was automatically held in place against the opening by steam pressure, which may explain the term "self-locking."

All office autoclaves operate on the same principle as a pressure cooker; boiling water produces steam pressure and expels air that would interfere with sterilization. Moist heat devices that do not use steam under pressure are not autoclaves.

Time is a critical factor in recycling instruments which are in short supply. The fact that moderate loads of unwrapped instruments can be sterilized in steam autoclaves in only 3 minutes and wrapped instruments in 7 minutes *after* they reach 134°C (270°F) can provide a great savings of time. Some of the least expensive autoclaves with a good record of service can provide total cycles of 11 to 16 minutes. (See Table I)

A number of factors are involved in selecting an autoclave, including price, chamber size to

Table I.
Autoclaves

Company	Model No.	Chamber size in inches	Total time for a cycle; instruments unwrapped 250	270	Timer function	Special features
Pelton & Crane	Sentry model	5⅞ x 14	25 min.	14 min.	sounds alarm	plastic door cover protects hands
	Omniclave model OCM	6 x 7 x 13	25 min.	14 min.	sounds alarm	has a separate dry heat cycle
	Omniclave model OCR	8 x 9 x 17½	29 min.	19 min.	sounds alarm	has a separate dry heat cycle
	Omniclave model OCR +	8 x 9 x 17½	29 min.	19 min.	sounds alarm	has separate dry heat cycle— ASME approved
NAPCO	704-7000	12 x 5⅞	30 min.	16 min.	electronically automated	tap water accepted; continuous pressure purge feature
	704-9000-D	18 x 9	40 min.	26 min.	electronically automated	tap water accepted; continuous pressure purge
Ritter Co.	No. 7 Speedclave	14½ x 7½	18-20 min.	8-11 min.	turns off sterilizer	choice of colors
AMSCO	613-R	6 x 13	22 min.	11 min.	turns off sterilizer	—
	8816-M	8 x 8 x 16	27 min.	15-16 min.	turns off sterilizer	—
	8816-A	8 x 8 x 16	27 min.	15-16 min.	turns off sterilizer	ASME approved;
Spectronics	Spectroline 750	7½ x 14½	23 min.	14 min.	turns off sterilizer	automatic air vent & steam bleeding; patented door for easy operation
Vernitron	V8000	8 x 8 x 16	22 min.	11 min.	timer starts automatically when temperature is reached & turns off sterilizer	uses tap water

meet office needs, efficiency, timing features and other convenience of operation features. These are reviewed in Table I for most small American autoclaves suitable for office use. Larger models are available for larger clinics.

COMPONENTS AND FEATURES: Autoclaves must have a temperature gauge to assure that the sterilization temperature is reached.[1] Most sterilizers have a safety feature that shuts off or warns the operator if the chamber runs dry or overheats. Both a shutoff device and warning light are preferred.

Timers: Many autoclaves are equipped with timers, which can have different important functions. The simplest timer just sounds an alarm at the end of the time for which it was set. The sterilizer must be turned off manually and the pressure allowed to drop before the door can be opened but this assures that packs are still hot and will dry rapidly. Many sterilizers have a timer that cuts off the power and sounds an alarm, but the door must be opened soon after to dry the instruments while they are still hot.

Both cutoff and simple timers can be set to alert the operator when sufficient time has elapsed for sterilization temperatures to be reached. Then the temperature must be checked and the timer reset for the sterilization cycle.

Timing the entire cycle once the sterilizer is loaded is usually not considered to be a reliable procedure unless carefully controlled with time and temperature sensitive indicators.

In automatic sterilizers, the timer is triggered when the sterilization temperature is reached. Electronically automated sterilizers shut off the sterilizer and vent it at the end of the cycle as well. Internal tests or indicators are needed to verify adequate heating.

Drying Cycle: Some steam autoclaves have a drying cycle; some do not. Most surgical packs dry fairly well if at the end of the cycle while the chamber is still warm the door is opened about a half an inch for a few minutes. Experience reveals how long to allow packs to dry, depending on the load size used. Automatic models vent themselves at the end of the cycle, which may or may not completely dry packs unless the door is opened immediately.

DIRECTIONS FOR USE: Autoclaving is the most efficient sterilization process. Autoclaves can be operated at two ranges: a) 121°C (250°F) at 15 lbs pressure for 15 minutes, and b) 134°C (270°F) at 30 lbs pressure for a minimum of 3 minutes. These are conditions for moderate loads of unwrapped instruments. For lightly wrapped instruments 5 minutes must be added to both time periods. For heavily wrapped well separated surgical packs, 20 minutes remains sufficient at 121°C, but 10 minutes is required at 134°C. Despite use of these accepted sterili-

zation conditions, sterilization must be frequently verified by indicators and spore tests to assure proper functioning.

What Instruments to Autoclave: All high quality stainless steel instruments can be steam autoclaved without damage. Non-stainless instruments and low quality stainless steel found especially in imported orthodontic pliers may rust and corrode extensively unless carefully protected.

Autoclavable handpieces are gradually becoming available from most American dental manufacturers. However, some can be autoclaved more often than others without reduced life.

Some dental mirrors tend to cloud in the autoclave.

Most metal prophylaxis angles and contra-angle attachments can be autoclaved. If not, they can be sterilized by dry heat or by chemical vapor pressure. Cleaning the instrument before autoclaving and lubrication afterward is important and lengthens the life of the angle.

Rubber gloves can be cleaned, powdered, wrapped with muslin and autoclaved. Cloth goods are best autoclaved.

Anesthetic ampules should not be autoclaved. Their surfaces are clean and some are sterile when received in the cannister. The label should be consulted. They should be stored dry and just wiped with alcohol before use. Individually packaged sterile ampules are available for surgical use if desired. Anesthetic ampules should never be reused.

Most glass slabs, dishes, and stones can be autoclaved. Stones should be dry; wet stones may rupture under steam sterilization.

Large plastic suction tips that can be autoclaved can be obtained commercially but most small disposable plastic saliva ejector tips cannot be autoclaved and are best discarded. Some rubber polishing tips and cups cannot withstand autoclaving and should be discarded following use. Low melting plastics and rubber cups can be sterilized with ethylene oxide if necessary.

Needles should be disposable and not reused. If needles must be reused, autoclaving is the optimal sterilization technique, provided the needles are thoroughly cleaned.

Protection of Instruments: Most manufacturers do not specify a method for protecting carbon steel instruments from rust. Several manufacturers recommend autoclaving only for high quality stainless steel instruments. Some indicate that non-stainless instruments should be sterilized by dry heat.

At least one manufacturer recommends use of a nontoxic nonsilicone oil emulsion for treating rustable instruments prior to wrapping and autoclaving. This tends to prevent or reduce rust and lubricates instruments without leaving a noticeable oily or sticky film. These emulsions do not impair sterilization. Placing a vial containing about 10 ml of fresh household ammonia solution into the chamber with each load to neutralize corrosive carbon dioxide is sometimes necessary to prevent rust in addition to using the emulsion dip.[2]

Dipping instruments in a bath of 1 percent sodium nitrite before sterilization has also been recommended as an alternative to emulsion dips.[3] Other chemicals, especially amine compounds have been recommended in *Accepted Dental Therapeutics.*[4]

Water Used in Autoclaves: Distilled or deionized water is recommended by most manufacturers. Whenever tap water is allowed, some cleaning is eventually required to remove scale deposits.

LIMITATIONS OF USE: In general, despite methods to protect curets, burs and other non-stainless instruments from rust, autoclaving appears to be the least desirable method for the frequent sterilization of large numbers of non-stainless instruments. If time permits, dry heat is the simplest and cheapest method for sterilizing nonstainless instruments. The formaldehyde vapor pressure sterilizer is the most rapid method for safely sterilizing such instruments. However, the life of carbide burs may be shortened by vapor pressure sterilization, according to personal communication with one bur manufacturer. Burs may also be sterilized in a hot salt

endodontic sterilizer in 15 to 20 seconds at 475°F.[5]

EVALUATION PROGRAM: Federal standards for autoclave sterilization have not been established but are forthcoming. Autoclaves should be demonstrated to sterilize spores in prescribed times. This control should be run routinely at least on a weekly basis. Indicator tape or strips should be included in each cycle.

AVAILABLE PRODUCTS

AMSCO 613-R, American Sterilizer Co.
AMSCO 8816-A, American Sterilizer Co.
AMSCO 8816-M, American Sterilizer Co.
Autoclave Indicator Tape, The Lorvic Corp.
NAPCO 704-7000, National Appliances Co.
NAPCO 704-9000-D, National Appliances Co.
Omniclave, Pelton and Crane Co.
Omniclave OCR, Pelton and Crane Co.
Sentry, Pelton and Crane Co.
Spectroline 750, Spectronics Co.
Speedclave, Ritter Co., Div. of Sybron Corp.
Three-M Brand Autoclave System Indicator Tape, 3M Company
Vapor Phase Rust Inhibitor, The Lorvic Corp.
Vernitron V8000, Vernitron Medical Products

DRY HEAT STERILIZERS

Dry heat, used properly, is an accepted and effective means of instrument sterilization and is safe for all mirrors and dry metal instruments with the exception of some handpieces. Bare, moderate loads of instruments placed in an efficient oven at 320 to 340°F (160 to 170°C) should be reliably sterilized in one hour.[2,6,7] Ovens are preferably set at 330°F (165°C) with no more than an 8°C variation. A variation of only ±2°C is preferred.

TYPES: Suitable ovens are manufactured specifically for medical and dental use. A number of commercial, home, laboratory and industrial ovens will also serve the purpose. Mechanical convection (forced air) ovens provide more rapid heating and better heat distribution than gravity convection ovens of the same wattage, but they tend to cost more as well.

Efficiency of dry heat ovens depends mainly on the number of watts provided per cubic foot of chamber space. Most dry heat gravity convection sterilizers made for office use provide over 1000 watts per cubic foot of chamber space. It should provide at least 550 watts per cubic foot in order to reach sterilizing temperatures in 30 minutes after loading.

Any oven not designed specifically for instrument sterilization should be carefully tested and calibrated. Low cost biscuit ovens, small broilers and other small home appliances are usually too poorly designed for clinic use. They often have wide temperature swings during a cycle and hot spots can damage instruments. Home ovens and dry heat ovens designed for clinical use can provide a sterilization cycle of an hour for an average load of unwrapped dental instruments placed in a preheated oven.[6]

Claims of half hour sterilization cycles have not been justified. In tests made for the Council on Dental Therapeutics,[8] forty-five minutes were required for sterilization of spore test strips placed together with light loads of twenty unwrapped hand instruments. Loads of eighty restorative instruments could be sterilized in an hour in these efficient gravity ovens if the instruments were not wrapped. Wrapping light and heavy loads with paper or foil increased the time required to reach sterilizing temperatures to 45 and 60 minutes.

This confirms the concept that dry heat sterilization needs to be tested under actual use conditions and monitored with spore strips or equivalent time temperature indicators in addition to a chamber thermometer. This is also important when using covered trays or pans. A relatively low cost pyrometer and thermocouple wire can be purchased for this purpose.

DIRECTIONS FOR USE: The time required for dry heat sterilization is often misunderstood. It increases with the size of the load or wrap of instrument packs, according to the ability of heat to reach all of the instruments. Ordinary packs of not more than ten dental hand instruments can be wrapped in two thicknesses of paper or aluminum foil and arranged at least ½ in. apart on shelves in a suitable oven. These will usually reach 320°F (160°C) in a preheated oven in 45 to 60 minutes and be sterilized in 30 minutes more, making the total time 1¼ to 1½ hours. Thirty minutes is roughly twice the time required to destroy clean, dry bacterial test spores at 160°C and provides a 50 percent safety factor. Spores found in organic debris or in moisture take longer to be destroyed by dry heat, so instruments must be clean and dry. Muslin wrapping can increase the time to 2 hours. Some means of internally monitoring performance should always be used.

What Instruments to Dry Heat: At temperatures of 320 to 335°F (160 to 168°C) all dry metal hand instruments, including mirrors and burs (but not handpieces), can be dry heat sterilized without damage or rust. Above 345°F (174°C) solder used in some instruments melts. Solder in some impression trays appears to melt even at or near 340°F (171°C). Most other instruments withstand up to 345°F (174°C) safely.

Autoclavable handpieces cannot be sterilized by dry heat. Dry heat is not quite as suitable for cloth goods and paper items as autoclaving because it oxidizes and browns the materials. Dry heat is not suitable for liquids, rubber goods and most plastics, but it is preferred for oils.

Testing and Verifying Dry Heat Sterilization: Since instrument numbers, pack sizes, and ovens vary, a thermocouple wire and pyrometer should be used to verify that instruments do indeed reach sterilization temperatures when deciding upon instrument packaging, loads and times. Spore tests or chemical time temperature tests should also be run on a weekly basis to verify sterilization. A heat sensitive indicator should be included in each load to show that temperatures were reached.

AVAILABLE PRODUCTS

Dri-Clave Sterilizer, Dri-Clave
Omniclave OCR, OCM, Pelton and Crane Co.

Premier Hot Bead Sterilizer, Premier Dental Products Co.
PCA Glass Bead Sterilizer, Pulpdent Corporation of America
Steri-Dent, Steri-Dent Corporation

FORMALDEHYDE-ALCOHOL VAPOR PRESSURE STERILIZERS

The heated chemical vapor pressure process offers three main advantages: a relatively short total cycle of about 25 minutes at sterilization temperature; instruments do not rust and fabrics do not char; and instruments are dry at the end of the cycle. It does require adequate ventilation which is not a problem with steam or dry heat. This process uses a vapor created by heating a deodorized alcohol-formaldehyde solution, obtainable only from the manufacturer, to 270°F (132°C) at 20 to 40 lbs pressure for 20 minutes. An indicator light for temperature, a pressure indicator and semi-automated controls make sterilizer operation simple.

DIRECTIONS FOR USE: Unlike autoclaves, all chemical vapor sterilizers must be preheated before use with the vapor reservoir sealed. Clean dry instruments are placed in the sterilizer tray, preferably unwrapped. The door is sealed and the preheated vapor is released into the chamber where it must condense on the instruments. The cycle is completed in about 30 minutes. At the end of the cycle, vapors are discharged through an air-cooled coil into a container beneath the sterilizer and cannot be reused.

What Instruments to Vapor Pressure Sterilize: The formaldehyde-alcohol vapor pressure technique lends itself well to office sterilization of orthodontic pliers, carbon steel and diamond burs, as well as all other metal hand instruments, files, wire and bands and metal crowns.

Testing and Verifying Sterilization: Instrument bags are available which have a color indicator that only indicates *exposure* to the sterilization vapor and *not* that sterilization conditions have been maintained throughout processing. Spore tests must be used to determine sterilization and to evaluate wrapping and loading procedures. Large loads of heavy paper or muslin wrapped instruments may extend sterilization time significantly and must be monitored with sporicidal tests. If metal trays are used, they must be perforated or uncovered. Nylon and plastic bags are not recommended.

LIMITATIONS OF USE: Whenever the chamber is opened at the end of a cycle, some formaldehyde vapor is emitted necessitating good ventilation.

According to the American Conference of Govenmental and Industrial Hygienists Report of 1977,[9] 2 ppm of formaldehyde is the maximum safe limit for repeated short term exposures or peak exposures.

This method may not be useful for sterilizing autoclavable handpieces that contain temperature sensitive plastics. This should be checked with the manufacturer of any handpiece in question. The process does not lend itself to sterilizing most heat sensitive plastic materials, liquids or heavy loads of cloth goods.

AVAILABLE PRODUCTS

Chemiclave 5000; 6000; MDT Corporation

ETHYLENE OXIDE STERILIZERS

Almost any material, including any handpiece, can be sterilized with ethylene oxide. The cycles of 2 to 8 hours are long for routine use but it serves as a good backup sterilization process for items used infrequently and instruments used to treat hepatitis carriers.

Ethylene oxide sterilization utilizes a gas that is toxic for all viruses and bacteria. At room temperature, an 8 to 10 hour exposure period is required to kill all microorganisms. The gas acts more rapidly at elevated temperatures. An inexpensive room temperature system consists only of a metal container, a small ampule of condensed ethylene oxide and a plastic bag in which to place the instruments and ampule.

Much more expensive sterilizers that provide a 90 minute cycle are available from dental supply companies. These require regular maintenance every few months to assure proper functioning of the pump and optimal protection for dental personnel.

DIRECTIONS FOR USE: The ethylene oxide ampule is enclosed in a small protective bag of its own to avoid direct skin contact with the gas. The ampule is broken and placed at the bottom of the large plastic bag. Instruments are then added and the bag is inserted into the metal container. The ethylene oxide sterilizer must be operated outside or where air is evacuated to the outside and not recirculated. This is important during use when the cannister and bag are opened.

All gas devices require that adequate humidity be added to the chamber or sterilization will not occur. This makes the use of indicators and routine testing important. Again, spore test strips are used to verify sterilization.

LIMITATIONS OF USE: There are some limitations to using this method of sterilization. Some plastics are degraded on repeated exposure. Large quantities of wrapped goods or towels are more reliably sterilized by steam.

EVALUATION PROGRAM: The Environmental Protection Agency has challenged the registration of ethylene oxide for medical use because of possible direct skin toxicity, and mutagenic or carcinogenic effects. The medical need for ethylene oxide appears to far outweigh its risks and it will probably be approved for controlled use, but with much closer regulations and safeguards. Local safety standards and Occupational Safety and Health Administration standards should be consulted and monitoring should be requested to assure adequate venting and safe handling procedures.

AVAILABLE PRODUCTS

Anprolene Model AN70, Anderson Products Inc.
Steri-Dome System, Boekel Corporation
Steri-Vac, 3M Company

OTHER PHYSICAL METHODS OF INSTRUMENT STERILIZATION

While other physical methods such as irradiation and radio waves of certain wave lengths can have germicidal properties, the effectiveness and safety of such methods to sterilize batches of dental instruments on a reliable and yet practical basis have not been evaluated and verified. Consultation with manufacturers of industrial and home style microwave ovens indicated lack of effectiveness of such ovens to sterilize metal instruments. One indicated that attempts to do so would void the warranty on the oven, although it may have germicidal activity for liquids and foods not containing metal.

SELECTING A STERILIZATION SYSTEM

Practices vary as to kinds and inventories of instruments in use. Therefore, no simple recommendation can be made. Table II lists some possibilities.

Choosing a process for sterilization involves making a careful inventory of the kinds of instruments to be sterilized, determining whether they need to be packaged and deciding how this will be done. For example, will surgery packs (best sterilized by steam) be used, or will small tray set-ups, individual bags or unwrapped instruments be used permitting a wider choice? Does the process need to be rapid to meet a large patient and instrument load? Are large tray assemblies planned that require a large chamber? Or, are large instruments in short supply to be sterilized rapidly in small numbers, such as autoclave handpieces, requiring an efficient sterilizer with a small capacity and rapid warm-up time?

If the office has a large inventory of instruments that are processed just one or two times a day, a slower process such as dry heat sterilization using a large built-in home oven may be preferred. If many instruments are not made of stainless steel, a system that avoids rust may be

Table II.
Suitable Methods of Sterilization or Treatment

Items	Steam Autoclave	Dry Heat Oven	Formaldehyde Vapor Pressure	Ethylene Oxide	Cold Disinfection	Discard
Stainless instruments (loose), restorative, burs	++*	++	++	+	−	−
Instruments in packs	++	+ small packs	±	+ small packs	−	−
Instrument tray setups, surgical or restorative	+ size limit	++	+ size limit	+ size limit	−	−
Rustable instruments	only with chemical protection	++	++	+	−	−
Handpiece (autoclavable)	++	−	−	+	−	−
Handpiece (non-autoclavable)	−		−	+	+ (iodophore scrub)	−
Angle attachments	+ confirm	+ confirm	+	+	−	−
Rubber items, prophy cups	++	−	−	++	−	+
Low melting plastics, saliva evacuator tips, ejectors	−	−	−	+	±**	+
Disposable needles	−	−	−	−	−	++
Rag wheels	++	+	+	+	−	−
Removable prosthetics	−	−	−	−	+‡	−
Heat resistant plastic evacuators	++	+	+	+	−	−
Time required per cycle	15-30 min.	1-1½ hr.	30 min.	10 hrs. at room temp.	**	

* ++ = the most convenient or preferred method

** Cold disinfectants are not recommended for sterilization of any items used in the mouth. When they must be used for lack of other suitable procedures, thoroughly cleaned plastics may be disinfected for 10 hours in a glutaraldehyde disinfectant or for 20 minutes in 1:10 dilution of household 5 to 6 percent sodium hypochlorite bleach solution.

‡ Rinse well, immerse in 1:10 household 5 to 6 percent sodium hypochlorite bleaching solution for 5 min., rinse well and perform laboratory procedures. Repeat disinfection procedure before returning prosthetic to patient.

preferred such as dry heat or formaldehyde vapor pressure sterilization.

Most offices require more than one system but careful planning can provide efficient sterilization with a minimum of problems.

INSTRUMENT CLEANING AND STERILIZATION SEQUENCE

Efforts must be made to avoid direct contact of bare hands with used instruments. Auxiliaries are often injured this way and exposed to hepatitis B infection.

A heavy plastic film or bib napkin towel with plastic backing can be placed open as a drape over the instrument tray and bracket table before operative treatments. The white paper tray cover placed on top of the drape provides a smooth surface. Used instruments can be easily bundled up in this wrap and carried to the cleanup area, avoiding the necessity of direct contact with the instruments.

If an infected patient has been treated, the loosely bundled package of instruments should be placed directly into a steam autoclave or ethylene oxide sterilizer or inserted in a formaldehyde vapor sterilizer, before washing and handling the instruments. If a formaldehyde vapor sterilizer is used, the bundle must be well opened.

It is recommended practice to wear heavy rubber work gloves whenever handling instruments used for treatment. Gloves made for household cleaning will do. Instruments should be scrubbed with a brush reserved just for that purpose, or placed directly into a perforated ultrasonic pan, cleaned with a hard spray of water and then inserted into an ultrasonic device, equipped with a timer, for about 5 minutes.

A cleaning solution of household automatic-dishwasher detergent is effective or special solutions to dissolve alginate and other materials may be obtained from distributors. The device should always be covered to avoid contamination from splatter.

The instrument tray is then removed and the instruments hosed off. Any individual dirty instrument should be inspected and cleaned by hand. Gloves should be worn while cleaning. Instruments are dipped in 90 to 100 percent isopropyl alcohol for drying purposes and sorted according to the type of packaging or sterilization required. Preferably paper or plastic covers are placed over work areas where non-sterile instruments are sorted.

Instruments that are not to be wrapped can be placed into the sterilizer in the perforated pan. (A tray containing rustable instruments can be dipped into a protective oil emulsion before autoclaving.)

After handling instruments and loading the sterilizer, gloved hands should be washed with an iodine surgical scrub before the gloves are removed; then the sterilizer can be closed and the adjustments set. If the sterilizer door handle or controls are contaminated, an iodine surgical scrub should be used to wipe the surfaces.

Cautions: The ultrasonic solution should always be covered and changed daily unless an expensive germicide is used in it. One part of iodine scrub can be added to each 100 parts of the water to provide some antibacterial activity if instruments are never exposed more than a few minutes; phenolic disinfectant can be used to help reduce contamination and prevent rust during longer exposures.

Crowns, splints, dentures and other dental devices that are disinfected or cleaned should be placed into a glass container or plastic self-sealing bag containing hypochlorite, iodine scrub, or cleaning solution in order to avoid cross contamination, if the same ultrasonic bath is used.

BAGGING AND WRAPPING OF DENTAL INSTRUMENTS

Standards for dental surgical packs are identical to those for hospital surgical packs and trays. Muslin or paper are used. Improved paper wrapping materials made especially for this purpose are available from hospital supply companies.

Nylon bags have also been used for dental surgical instruments if they are heat sealed or taped rather than stapled. These can only be autoclaved.

The objective of sterilizing non-surgical dental instruments is to break the chain of cross contamination and prevent spread of bacteria and viruses from one patient to the next. Therefore, non-surgical items and instruments need not be packaged but must be stored clean.

Although it may be difficult, unwrapped restorative instruments and items must be stored away from aerosols and dust. Drawers and shelves must be disinfected weekly or more often. Instruments and items must not be removed with saliva contaminated fingers that will contaminate other items. Items that are not used often must be packaged.

Nylon bags or bags made with one side paper and one side plastic to allow steam passage are ideal for autoclaving instruments. Bags can often be reused several times.

Sharp points of many dental hand instruments poke through most paper or even nylon bags unless tips are covered with gauze or heavy paper. A small pouch made by cutting a coin envelope or x-ray envelope in two provides an adequate means for bagging sharp instruments. Kraft paper such as the heavy paper used for hardware bags provides useful wrapping or bagging material.

Covered metal trays are offered by several manufacturers. These and wrappings such as paper, muslin or aluminum foil can greatly extend the time required for sterilization in a dry heat oven, especially if two or more are sterilized at the same time.

In summary, operative instruments can be sterilized unwrapped and stored under clean conditions. Packaging suited to sterilization is as follows:

Autoclaves: muslin, paper of any kind, nylon or other steam permeable materials, open trays, uncovered tubes or other vessels tipped on their side; no closed containers.

Formaldehyde vapor pressure sterilization: Unwrapped instruments preferred or wrapped in light weight paper bags; no closed containers.

Ethylene oxide: Any plastic wrap, light paper, or light cloth wrap, no closed glass or metal containers.

Dry heat: Paper, aluminum foil, or metal or glass containers. No plastics but certain nylon bags may be used. Cloth may char slightly. Heavy wraps and large tight containers extend sterilization time. Instruments must be dry before packaging to avoid rust.

MONITORING STERILIZATION

Accepted means of indicating instrument sterilization include the following. a) Simple color change tape placed on a few instruments in unwrapped loads or on the outside of packs and trays verifies processing. b) Other color change indicator labels or strips are sensitive to both time and temperature or other sterilization conditions. These are used to indicate that sterilization conditions reached the center of loads, trays or packs. c) Weekly sporicidal tests provide biological verification and control of the sterilization process.

Controls of instrument sterilization are required in hospitals, and may become federal or state regulated requirements for sterilization in all health care facilities.

Materials for monitoring sterilization are commercially available. Indicators and bags for use in alcohol-formaldehyde vapor pressure sterilizers are available from the manufacturer. Detailed information on sterilization procedures, monitoring, testing and record keeping can be obtained from several companies.

Test strips containing harmless bacterial spores are commercially available. Strips containing *Bacillus stearothermophilis* are used for autoclaves; strips with *Bacillus subtilis* var. niger are designated for use in dry heat and ethylene oxide sterilizers.

Only plain spore strips of *Bacillus subtilis* var. niger can be used to test dry heat ovens. After a test strip is used it is removed from its envelope using forceps heated over a flame. The strip is then placed in a tube of endodontic culture medium or other suitable nutrient broth, incubated for 48 hours, and examined for cloudy growth.

Weekly spore tests are the only accurate biological test for sterilization but results are not obtainable for several days. Indicator strips or labels fill the immediate need to verify that instruments have been processed and exposed to sterilization conditions.

AVAILABLE PRODUCTS

Attest Brand Biological Monitoring System, 3M Company

Glassine Envelopes, Pulpdent Corporation of America

Instrument Cold Sterilizing System, Time Motion Company

Nyclave, The Lorvic Corporation

Nyclave Heat Sealer, The Lorvic Corporation

Steri-Bur, Zirc Dental Products

Steri-Instrument Containers, Zirc Dental Products

LITERATURE REFERENCES

1. Block, S. S. Disinfection, sterilization and preservation. Philadelphia, Lea and Febiger, 1977, p. 494.

2. Crawford, J. J. in Block, S. S. (ed.) Disinfection, sterilization and preservation. ed. 2, Philadelphia, Lea and Febiger, 1977, p. 688.

3. Hurst, V. Reducing the risk of transmitting viral hepatitis via dental instruments. IADR Program and Abstracts of Papers, Abstract 408, 1972.

4. Council on Dental Therapeutics. Accepted dental therapeutics. ed. 38, Chicago, American Dental Association, 1979.

5. Dayoub, C. M., and Devine, M. J. Endodontic dry heat sterilizers effectiveness. J. Endod. 2:343 Nov. 1976.

6. Rabin, A. N., and Crawford, J. J. Use of a home oven in a dental office for instrument sterilization. N.C. Dent. J. 57:12 Jan. 1974.

7. Perkins, J. J. Principles and methods of sterilization in health sciences. ed. 2, Springfield, Charles C. Thomas, 1969, pp. 286-295.

8. Crawford, J. J. (unpublished data)

9. Obtainable from Secretary-Treasurer of ACGIH, P. O. Box 1937, Cincinnati, Ohio 45201.

DENTAL ELECTROSURGICAL EQUIPMENT

Solid state circuitry miniaturization and other sophisticated advances in electronics have contributed materially to the numerous changes featured in present day dental electrosurgical devices.

"Solid state" circuitry, substitutes transistors for the traditional deForest radio vacuum tube power generator. In conjunction with the marked reduction in size and weight of coils and other bulky circuit components significant reduction in the size and weight of most of the present day dental devices has been possible.

THE CUTTING CURRENTS

Spark gap generators and partially rectified electronic devices no longer are factors in dental electrosurgery. All present day devices produce fully rectified (RF) cutting current, and/or fully rectified and filtered continuous wave (CWRF) cutting current.[1]

RF Current

RF current is produced by radio vacuum tube power generators. This current, due to its wave-form, is slightly oscillating and modulated. At each half-cycle constriction there is a slight drop in power output. This drop produces an accompanying slight coagulation along the surface of the tissue as it is cut. When the RF current is used properly this coagulation is so superficial it is imperceptible clinically and histologically; nevertheless, it provides effective capillary hemostasis when the tissues are not engorged.

CWRF Current

This current is produced primarily by solid state circuits. The filtration eliminates the constrictions at the half-cycles producing a non-oscillating, unmodulated current. As there is no drop in power output at the half-cycles there is no accompanying coagulation. The result is a slightly "purer" surgical incision. However, since this current is incapable of providing hemostasis when it is used properly, the cutting is accompanied by free bleeding.

Hemostasis is one of the most valuable advantages electrosurgery offers dentistry. Since CWRF current used properly does not provide hemostasis there is a temptation to obtain the hemostasis by deviating somewhat from optimal use. Theoretically it may seem feasible to obtain the hemostasis by applying the current to the tissues a little more slowly, or by reducing power output, but this has not borne out clinically. When both currents are used properly the difference in their respective surgical "purity" is negligible; when they are used improperly both produce comparable extraneous tissue destruction that cannot be consistently or effectively controlled or limited. Deviation from optimal instrumentation and power output to attempt to obtain hemostasis with CWRF current is unreliable and unrealistic.

AUTOMATIC AND MULTIPLE CUTTING CURRENT DEVICES

TYPES: Some cutting current devices are being advertised as "automatic" devices that are supposed to eliminate need for manual operator control of power output to meet varying power needs. The term "automatic" needs clarification. If the device includes in its circuit an electronic sensor that will instantly increase or decrease power output in response to changes in the size and shape of the electrodes, thickness and density of the tissues, and depth of incision, this constitutes a genuine automatic device. If however, the device merely has in its circuit a broad voltage band that permits wider latitude within which acceptable albeit not optimal cutting can be performed for many procedures, it is not an automatic device, but at best is a semi-automatic device. Most competent electrosurgeons have found that even with these devices they obtain the best results when they regulate the power output manually, but the greater latitude in power output setting can be helpful to the novice.

Most dental devices provide either RF or CWRF current, but some provide both cutting currents. Some also produce a simulated fulgurating sparking current that offers several advantages for dentistry over the true Oudin fulgurating current.

DIRECTIONS FOR USE: Watt output capability is measured by passing the current through measured resistances. A standard drafted by a committee of ADA/ANSI (American National Standards Institute) specifies that all dental devices shall provide power output capability equal to but not less than 50 watts, nor more than 100 watts. It also specifies that all watt power output ratings shall be made by identical tests, passing the current through identical amounts of ohm resistance.

At present, however, watt output ratings are not necessarily based on identical ohm resistance measurements. As a result, if the manufacturers base their watt output ratings on different ohm resistances, the watt output determinations become an unreliable index of power output.

An electrical phenomenon called internal impedance further complicates the reliability of the watt ratings. Internal impedance affects all electric circuits to varying degrees, causing loss of power output capability that is comparable to the reduction in efficiency of mechanical devices due to friction. The impedance factor varies from circuit to circuit, and the resultant amount of power output loss varies. Devices that produce identical watt power output capability at their power source therefore may produce different watt power input into the tissues. Inasmuch as all watt power output ratings are determined at the power source of the devices and not at the site of power input into the tissues, the watt power output ratings are not as reliable an index of power efficiency as clinical testing of power input into a beefsteak. Since all the power output into the tissues is potentiated at the tip of the electrode the fine needle electrode maximizes the cutting effect and is therefore not suitable for clinical evaluations, since they produce little difference. To arrive at a meaningful determination it is advisable to use a large round loop electrode, preferably 10 to 12 mm in diameter, and excise a section of tissue to a depth of 4 to 5 mm in a direction parallel to the long axis of the muscle fibers. If the loop electrode can excise the tissue cleanly and efficiently and there remains a reserve of power output, the device will be able to provide adequate cutting power to meet any conditions it might encounter in the oral cavity. Watt power output ratings will be disregarded in this evaluation, since this clinical evaluation provides a much more reliable index of the circuit's power output capability.

LIMITATIONS OF USE: Early electrosurgical devices used radio vacuum tube generators. Radio vacuum tube generators are subject to breakage and their filaments are occasionally damaged during shipment. They require a warm-up period before activation, especially after they have been moved around. Transistors, on the other hand, are not subject to breakage. However, with the exception of an expensive heat-resistant variety, all are highly vulnerable to heat deterioration. A protective shield called a heat sink must be incorporated into the circuit for protection from the heat generated within the circuit. Blower fans also are installed wherever possible to help cool the transistors.

Miniaturization, with its resultant reduction in size and weight of the device greatly simplifies transporting from operatory to operatory, or from office to hospital. It also simplifies the problem of where to place it in the operatory, and minimizes storage space needs. However, the small size of the housing of the device creates a lack of air space and lack of room in which to place the heat sink. Blower fans are used in the large hospital size medical devices, but are not used in the dental devices. Hence, the burden of protection against heat deterioration falls on the heat sinks. It is difficult to provide adequate heat sinks in the small devices, and some miniaturized devices with inadequate heat sinks tend to break down during lengthy clinical procedures.

It is regrettable that in their desire to keep the devices small and inexpensive most of the manufacturers have eliminated the fulgurating circuits. Fulguration has many unique invaluable uses in dental therapy that cannot be duplicated with coagulating current or use of cutting current powerful enough to cause sparking and charring of the tissues.

Fulguration is the least frequently used therapeutic electrosurgical current, but like the spare tire in the automobile, when it is needed it is indispensible and should be available. Ideally, dental devices should make available to the clinician all the useful therapeutic currents.

EVALUATION PROGRAM: The American Dental Association Council on Dental Materials, Instruments and Equipment has drafted a list of manufacturing guidelines to minimize the hazard of accidental electric shock to the patient due to circuit malfunctions, and to reduce the danger of accidental RF burns to the patient or attending personnel.[2] The Council is also co-sponsoring with the American National Standards Institute (ANSI) a Standard for Dental Electrosurgical Devices and Attachments that is very comprehensive and includes many additional specifications that will help to assure maximum safety and efficiency for all dental devices.[3] Conformation to the specifications of the Council's certification requirements and to the specifications of the Standard will not mean all the devices will perform the same. Each will still offer its own unique clinical and circuit features; they will only conform in the matter of safety and minimum performance requirements of the circuits.

AVAILABLE PRODUCTS

CAMERON-MILLER MODELS 26-230, 26-240R, Cameron Miller, Inc.
COLES MODEL TR-5, Cavitron Corp.
DENTO-SURG 70, 90 FFP, AND AUTOMATIC ELECTROSURGICAL DEVICE, Ellman Dental Mfg. Co.
MACAN ELECTROSURGICAL UNIT, Macan Engineering Co.
PARKELL SENSIMATIC MODEL 300 SE, Parkell Products, Inc.
STROBEX MARK II, Whaledent International, Div. of Ipco Hospital Supply Corp.
STROBEX MARK III, Whaledent International, Div. of Ipco Hospital Supply Corp.

Literature References

1. Oringer, M.J. Electrosurgery in dentistry. ed. 2, Philadelphia, W. B. Saunders Co., 1975, pp. 10-82.

2. Council on Dental Materials, Instruments and Equipment. American Dental Association, Revised guidelines for dental electrosurgical devices.

3. Standard for dental electrosurgical devices and attachments. ADA/ANSI (American National Standards Institute) Subcommittee 44, Committee MD 156, Feb. 1979.

INHALATION SEDATION EQUIPMENT

Nitrous oxide was the first anesthetic introduced into clinical practice. Discovered in 1772 by Joseph Priestly, its pain relieving properties were first noted by Sir Humphrey Davy in 1795. Unfortunately, these went unnoticed until the 1840's when a Connecticut dentist, Horace Wells, realizing its potential clinical applications, allowed the agent to be administered to himself as he underwent extraction of a tooth. Nitrous oxide quickly became a very popular anesthetic agent, being administered as 100 percent nitrous oxide. It was used in this manner until 1868 when Edmund Andrews combined oxygen with the nitrous oxide. Nitrous oxide remains the most commonly used general anesthetic in the world today. It has been estimated that approximately 35 percent of the dentists in the United States have nitrous oxide and oxygen at their disposal.[1]

Nitrous oxide has experienced several resurgences of interest over the past century, usually being followed by a period of decreasing popularity. At the present time, nitrous oxide and oxygen inhalation sedation is undergoing a prolonged period of interest which can be attributed primarily to a change of philosophy in the use of the technique, and a continuing upgrading of the safety standards for inhalation sedation units.

Nitrous oxide mixed with oxygen has been used in dentistry as a general anesthetic agent, as an analgesic (obtunding pain), and as a sedative. With the development of newer, more effective local anesthetics for the management of pain, the use of nitrous oxide as a general anesthetic and as an analgesic has decreased. In contemporary dental practice nitrous oxide and oxygen inhalation sedation is primarily used for psychosedation. Its goals include the elimination of fear and anxiety in a conscious patient. One of the many benefits observed when nitrous oxide and oxygen are used for psychosedation is a reduction in the concentration of nitrous oxide required to achieve a desired clinical effect. Approximately 85 to 90 percent of patients receiving nitrous oxide and oxygen are well sedated with less than 40 percent nitrous oxide. At these levels, and if the procedure of administering the drug is properly executed, adverse side effects such as nausea and vomitting are virtually eliminated.

Education must be mentioned as the most

important reason behind the incredible safety record of nitrous oxide and oxygen. The Guidelines for Teaching the Comprehensive Control of Pain and Anxiety in Dentistry, adopted by the American Dental Association's Council on Dental Education in 1971 have upgraded the quality of both undergraduate and continuing education programs in inhalation sedation, as well as other sedation modalities.[2] The contemporary dentist has a better basic understanding of the philosophy and techniques involved in the rational use of conscious sedation in dentistry. For this reason it is expected that the current enthusiasm with inhalation sedation will remain at its present level.

Another important advance in the use of nitrous oxide and oxygen in dentistry has been the continuing development of newer and safer inhalation sedation machines. In fact, a wide range of such devices are currently available. Indeed, the doctor seeking to purchase an inhalation sedation unit faces a situation akin to the purchase of a new automobile: a large number of devices, basically similar in design yet different enough in appearance and cost to confuse the potential buyer thoroughly.

INHALATION SEDATION UNITS

TYPES: There have been two basic types of inhalation sedation units: the demand (or intermittent) flow, and the continuous flow. In the early demand flow machines the flow of a predetermined mixture of gases was activated either by self administration, by the squeezing of a hand held bulb, or by a demand valve activated by the negative pressure of inspiration. Demand flow machines work against the basic physical principle of administration of a relatively insoluble agent such as nitrous oxide. Computer studies of the uptake and distribution of nitrous oxide indicate that nitrous oxide and oxygen should be given in continuous flow rather than intermittent flow. With the finding that many demand flow machines were highly in-

accurate as to the percentage of gas flowing through them, their use became less popular. In 1977 the last of the manufacturers producing demand flow units terminated their production. The only benefit to the use of the demand flow machine was that of economics; the patient only received the agents during breathing.

The preferred inhalation sedation units are the continuous flow machines. These deliver a steady flow of gas to the patient while the machine is in operation. While more costly to operate (in reality a minimal expense) than demand flow machines, it provides a far greater degree of accuracy in delivering gases to the patient.

There are two basic types of continuous flow machines used in dental practice. These are the portable units and the central unit. The portable unit is self contained, with the compressed gas cylinders attached to the machine itself. The central system differs in that the compressed gas cylinders are stored at a site distant from the dental operatory. Each compressed gas then flows through pipes into the operatory where it then attaches to the "head" or control panel of the unit. Larger, more economical compressed gas cylinders are employed in central systems. The major advantage of the portable type of inhalation sedation unit is that they are mobile and thus available for use anywhere in the dental office. They also represent a ready source of emergency oxygen. The primary disadvantage to the portable unit is the relative expense involved in its operation. Utilizing smaller compressed gas cylinders increases the cost of operation per unit of time in relation to the large cylinders employed in the central system. Another disadvantage of the portable system is the space required for this unit. In the typical dental operatory this unit occupies a considerable portion of the available space. The portable unit is advantageous in the office of a doctor who is introducing inhalation sedation into a practice and is uncertain as to the extent of its need. Rather than invest in a central system immediately, a trial period with a portable unit is advisable. The portable unit can later be converted to a central system, which is more economical to operate and occupies less operatory space.

COMPONENTS: Basic components of the continuous flow inhalation sedation unit include the following: compressed gas cylinders, reducing valves (pressure regulators), flow meters, reservoir bag, and patient connections (nasal hood, nasal cannula and full face mask). In addition a number of safety features include: color coding, the pin index safety system, oxygen fail safe system, minimal oxygen flow, oxygen flush button and the non-rebreathing valve.

Gas cylinders: The gases utilized in inhalation sedation are supplied in compressed gas cylinders. Compressed gas cylinders come in a variety of sizes which are designated by the letters A,B,C,D,E,F,M,G,H and HH. The cylinder sizes commonly employed in dental practice are the E on portable units, and the H oxygen and G nitrous oxide on central systems. The E cylinder of oxygen contains about 66 liters, while the E nitrous oxide cylinder contains 1,590 liters of compressed gas. These figures equate to a two hour duration for an oxygen cylinder (at 5 liters per minute) and more than 5 hours duration with a nitrous oxide cylinder at the same flow rate.

In clinical practice it is common to use two and a half oxygen cylinders to each cylinder of nitrous oxide. The G cylinder of nitrous oxide contains over 13,000 liters of gas, while the H oxygen cylinder contains 5,300 liters.

Smaller (E) cylinders are attached to the sedation unit by double yokes. A safety feature incorporated into these cylinders is the pin index safety system. There are two pins on the valve surface of the yoke and there are two holes drilled into the corresponding surface of the valve in the cylinders. Each compressed gas has its own combination of pins and holes, the configuration of which is different for each gas. The pin index safety system makes it impossible for the incorrect cylinder of gas to be connected to a yoke that is pin-indexed for a different agent.

Compressed gas cylinders must meet certain strict requirements established by the Department of Transportation. They are fabricated of ⅜ in. steel and must be tested by internal hydrostatic pressure at least once every five years. The cylinder must be marked with the date of the test. In addition, all compressed gas cylinders are color coded with their own distinctive color. Nitrous oxide cylinders are light blue, while oxygen cylinders are coded green. Each compressed gas differs in pressure in a cylinder. Oxygen compressed gas cylinders, when full, have a pressure of approximately 2,000 pounds per square inch (psi), while nitrous oxide has a pressure of approximately 760 to 800 psi. These pressures vary somewhat depending on the temperature of the room in which the cylinders are contained. Higher temperatures increase gas pressure, while colder temperatures decrease cylinder pressure.

GAS CYLINDERS

Do:

1. Open cylinder valves very slowly in a counterclockwise direction. Close all cylinder valves tightly when not in use.
2. Use no grease, oil or lubricant of any kind or type to lubricate cylinder valves, gauges, regulators or other fittings which may come in contact with gases.
3. Store full cylinders in the vertical position.
4. Store cylinders in an area where the temperature does not fluctuate, particularly avoiding heat.
5. Handle cylinders with care and especially avoid dropping.

Reducing Valves: Reducing valves decrease the stored pressures within the compressed gas cylinder to a safe and usable level of between 50 to 60 psi. Gases which have not been reduced in pressure might cause damage to the sensitive control valves of the anesthetic machine. For a very brief time after opening a gas cylinder (especially oxygen, because of its higher initial pressure) the temperature within the tubing near the reducing valve may reach 1,500 to 2,000°F. To prevent the possibility of fires and/or explosions developing at this time, it is recommended that a two stage pressure regulator be installed on the cylinder to reduce the hazards of adiabatic heating, and the low pressure line capable of supporting a pressure of 50 psi should be ducted through the walls to machine connectors; copper alloy pipe is suitable for this purpose.

Installation of central systems must be completed in accordance with local fire codes. The installation must be approved by the local fire marshal and standards rigidly enforced. The local supplier of sedation equipment is best able to perform and supervise the installation.

Flow meters: Flow meters measure the quantity of gas in motion. If the flow of gas is inter-

INSTALLING CENTRAL SYSTEMS WITH REDUCING VALVES

Do:

1. Install central supply systems of oxygen and nitrous oxide in accordance with the rules of the:

   a. U. S. Department of Labor Occupational Safety and Health Administration.

   b. National Fire Protection Association, N.F.P.A. 56F, 1973, Chap. 6, entitled "Small Systems in Non-hospital Based Facilities."

   c. The local fire department (Fire Prevention Bureau). Should a central system be installed without fire department approval, and should a fire occur, either caused by the central system or not, the doctor's fire policy will be cancelled as of 24 hours before the fire.

2. Hire a licensed contractor to install the unit.

3. Insure that a high pressure reducing valve is on the tank or is connected immediately adjacent to the tank by a rigid, solid nonferrous manifold, or a soft temper copper pigtail designed for high pressure use. A flexi-ble stainless steel braided pigtail with a teflon inner liner should never be used.

4. Open all gas cylinders slowly.

5. Make certain that no delivery line containing over 50 psi passes through a wall in an ordinary installation.

6. Install and store full nitrous oxide and oxygen cylinders in a room well ventilated to the exterior of the building.

7. House the tank part of a nitrous oxide-oxygen system in a room totally separated from any open fire and electric switches.

8. Silver solder all gas supply lines.

9. Turn nitrous oxide and oxygen off at the cylinder when not in use.

Don't:

1. Use or store any petroleum products on or about the tank, controls or lines. Oxygen, leaking at 200 psi or more can in the presence of oil produce combustion.

2. Investigate any gas leaks yourself. Contact immediately the gas supplier to check into any pressure drops noted during non-use.

rupted, the flow meter reads zero. Flow meters are actually rather simple devices. Gas enters the base of the flow meter, which is a glass tube with a tapered lumen that grows wider from inlet to outlet and which contains a metering float or ball. The degree of accuracy of these devices should be within ±5 percent. The gas flow is controlled through needle valves at the base of the flow meter; the liter flow is read at the center of the ball. Rotation of the ball, which is held in place by turbulence and friction against the wall of the graduated tube, indicates gas flow. Calibration marks on the flow meters indicate gas flow in liters per minute.

Features recommended by the Council on Dental Materials, Instruments and Equipment for flow meters include: flow meter scales should be standardized, with oxygen on the right; flow meters for each gas should have positive control valves controlling the flow, each complete revolution of the control knob resulting in a one liter increase or decrease of the flow; flow meters should be protected and covered with a safety shield; and flow meters should be color-coded.

Having passed through the flow meters, the gases are mixed and delivered to the patient and the reservoir bag.

Reservoir bag: In sedation techniques, the reservoir bag serves to compensate for variations in the patient's respiratory demands. The bags are available in a variety of sizes ranging from 1 to 8 liters. The 3 and 5 liter sizes are the most commonly used. Reservoir bags are available in either rubber or silicone plastic. Rubber, while most commonly used, deteriorates more rapidly than silicone, especially in areas where there are high levels of atmospheric pollution.

The reservoir bag is of importance should the patient develop any emergency in which oxygen is required. The reservoir bag can be used to provide positive pressure oxygen by squeezing it to assist or control breathing. A non-rebreathing valve is located on the patient's side of the reservoir bag. This valve prevents the patient's exhaled air, high in carbon dioxide content, from accumulating in the reservoir bag

and possibly producing serious respiratory and other physiologic complications.

Patient connections: Three devices are available for the delivery of nitrous oxide and oxygen to patients: nasal hoods, nasal cannulae, and full face masks. The full face mask, covering both the mouth and nose, has no place in routine sedation procedures. It is of use, however, in emergency situations in which positive pressure oxygen is required. Inhalation sedation units have an adapter for an oxygen quick connect. A demand valve device, such as the Elder or Robertshaw valve, can be attached and oxygen delivered to the patient.

The nasal hood (nose piece) is the preferred method of delivering nitrous oxide and oxygen to a patient. It is usually made of a material, such as silastic rubber, which is easily adapted to the contours of the patient's face, creating an airtight fit. The more recently designed nasal hoods are composed entirely of rubber and plastic; there are no metal parts. Because of this radiographs may be taken without having to remove the nasal hood. Nasal hoods are commonly manufactured with two valves. The expiratory or pop-off valve permits gas to flow out of the system only. As pressure builds up within the system (as when the patient exhales) the pop-off valve opens allowing some gas to escape. The expiratory valve must always be kept open and functional. The second valve is the inspiratory or air-dilution valve. If kept open the delivered concentration of anesthetic gases becomes diluted. Hamilton and Eastwood[3] demonstrated that up to a 60 percent dilution may develop when a 15-gauge needle is inserted into a full face mask. It can therefore be expected that even greater air dilution will develop with the use of the air dilution valve. Under ordinary circumstances the air dilution valve is not used. It should be left in the closed position unless a patient's minute volume is extremely large. In this situation opening of the air dilution valve will ease the patient's respiratory discomfort, permitting lower volumes of delivered gas to be used. It must be remembered, however, that a higher concentration of nitrous oxide is required to compensate for the air dilution factor. Some manufacturers of nasal hoods have eliminated the air dilution valve entirely.

Nasal hoods are available in various sizes. It is recommended that two or three nasal hoods of varying sizes be available to allow for differences in facial size and contour. The nasal hood must be thoroughly cleansed following each use.

A third method of delivering nitrous oxide and oxygen to patients is through the nasal cannula. The cannula is primarily employed in hospitals for the administration of oxygen. It is made of soft plastic with two outlets which fit comfortably into the patient's nares. A major disadvantage of the nasal cannula is its wastefulness. Because of the discrepancy in size between the cannula and the nares a large portion of the delivered gases are dissipated into the environment. To overcome this, larger volumes and higher concentrations of nitrous oxide must be delivered. However, even with a full 10 liter flow and 70 percent nitrous oxide concentration, the inspired gases only achieve a 30 percent nitrous oxide concentration. Additionally, the high flow of gases through the nasal cannula causes some patients to complain of irritation to the sensitive nasal mucous membrane. This drying effect may be minimized through the use of a humidifier. The nasal cannula also obviates use of a reservoir bag.

The nasal cannula is useful in patients who have a fear of the nasal hood, and in patients undergoing dental therapy in the maxillary anterior region. Nasal cannulas are disposable, single use items.

Safety features: Many additional features have been added to inhalation sedation devices in recent years to increase their safety. *Color coding* of all oxygen cylinders and supply lines (tubes, flow meters, control dials) green, and nitrous oxide, blue, has prevented many errors in administration. Older equipment not provided with color coding should be discarded. The *pin index safety system* and the *diameter index safety system* have prevented the inadvertent connection of nitrous oxide and oxygen

to the wrong yoke or connector.

An extremely important safety feature is the *oxygen fail safe* device. In this device, a slave regulator is attached to the oxygen source. Should the oxygen line pressure fall to approximately 40 psi or lower, the nitrous oxide gas supply is automatically terminated. There is thus little or no hazard of 100 percent nitrous oxide being administered to a patient. Inhalation sedation units are equipped with a device which limits the *minimal oxygen flow.* In one form, turning on the unit automatically establishes a minimum flow of approximately 2.5 to 3 liters per minute. Some other machines are designed so as to be unable to deliver less than 30 percent oxygen and 70 percent nitrous oxide; or a minimum 50 percent oxygen in nitrous oxide. Other fail safe devices include an audible alarm or a flashing light which indicates that the oxygen delivery pressure is low. An *oxygen flush button* is also required which when activated delivers oxygen in high flows (30 liters per minute minimum) to the patient, bypassing the flow meters. This device is useful in emergencies or whenever large volumes of oxygen are indicated. Two other safety features are the *non-rebreathing valve* and a *lock* for the inhalation sedation unit. The non-rebreathing valve is located on the patient's side of the reservoir bag and was discussed previously. The addition of a lock to the inhalation sedation unit is strongly recommended. Unfortunately, nitrous oxide has become a drug with a significant abuse potential. Non-dental and nonmedical persons, as well as medical and dental personnel, are using nitrous oxide on a recreational basis. Serious consequences may develop through the long-term chronic abuse of this agent. Reports are available of suicides and of accidental deaths with nitrous oxide as well as serious sensory neuropathies in recreational users of this drug.[4,5] The use of nitrous oxide in this manner can only be condemned and must be stopped. Locking of the sedation unit during non-office hours and the securing of compressed gas cylinders may effectively deter the non-dental use of this important drug.

EVALUATION PROGRAM: The American Dental Association has adopted an Acceptance Program for inhalation sedation units which permits the dentist to better evaluate those units being considered for purchase. The primary emphasis in recent years has been the addition of safety features to these units which are aimed at making it quite difficult, if not entirely impossible, to administer less than 20 percent oxygen to a dental patient. To receive a satisfactory classification manufacturers must submit their devices to the Council on Dental Materials, Instruments and Equipment for evaluation. Copies of the guidelines are available upon request to the Council office.

AVAILABLE PRODUCTS

ALPHA III NITROUS OXIDE/OXYGEN SEDATION DEVICE, Accutron, Inc.

ANALOR III SEDATION DEVICE, McKesson Co.

CHEMTRON NITROUS OXIDE/OXYGEN FLOWMETER, Chemtron Dental Products

Dupaco Inhalation Sedation Equipment, Dupaco, Inc.

MINI-3 NITROUS OXIDE/OXYGEN SEDATION UNIT, Star Dental Mfg. Co.

NRC-2 NITROUS OXIDE/OXYGEN SEDATION DEVICE, Veriflow Corp.

PARKELL SEDATRON MODEL P-1, Parkell Products, Inc.

PORTER NITROUS OXIDE SEDATION SYSTEMS, Porter Instrument Co., Inc.

QUANTIFLEX MDM-30, MDM-50, RA, Fraser Sweatman, Inc.

SPICA NITROUS OXIDE/OXYGEN SEDATION DEVICE, Spica, Inc.

NITROUS OXIDE TRACE CONTAMINATION SCAVENGING SYSTEMS

During the past few years concern has developed in both the dental and medical profes-

sions over the long-term effects of breathing minute amounts of exhaled anesthetic gases.[6] This potential problem termed "trace anesthetic contamination" has received much publicity and investigation. Recently, devices known as nitrous oxide scavenging systems have been developed in response to the concern over trace anesthetic contamination.[7] While a wide variety of devices are available, among the more effective is the Brown nitrous oxide scavenging mask. A mask within a mask, this device operates by eliminating the expiratory valve and removing the exhaled gases through the outer mask, which is connected via hoses to the central vacuum system in the office. Fresh anesthetic gases are delivered to the patient through the inner mask.

EVALUATION PROGRAM: The American Dental Association has adopted an Acceptance Program for nitrous oxide/oxygen scavenging and monitoring devices.

AVAILABLE PRODUCTS

BLUE MASK, Health Care Technology, Inc.

BROWN MASK, Summit Services, Inc.

FRASER HARLAKE SCAVENGING NASAL INHALER, Fraser Sweatman, Inc.

Nitrous Oxide Scavenging System, Narco/McKesson

LITERATURE REFERENCES

1. Jones, T.W., and Greenfield, W. Position paper of the ADA Ad Hoc Committee on trace anesthetics as a potential health hazard in dentistry. JADA 95:751, 1977.

2. Council on Dental Education, American Dental Association. Guidelines for teaching the comprehensive control of pain and anxiety in dentistry. J. Dent. Educ. 36:62, 1972.

3. Hamilton, W.K., and Eastwood, D.W. A study of denitrogenation with some inhalation anesthetic systems. Anesthesiology 16:861, 1955.

4. Layzer, R.B., et al. Neuropathy following abuse of nitrous oxide. Neurology 28:504 May 1978.

5. Hershfeld, S; Fifield, P.; and Malamed, S.F. Nitrous oxide neurotoxicity; report of a case. Submitted for publication.

6. Ad Hoc Committee on Trace Anesthetics. Trace inhalation anesthetics in the dental office. JADA 95:749, 1977.

7. Council on Dental Materials, Instruments and Equipment, American Dental Association. Council position on nitrous oxide scavenging and monitoring devices. JADA 101:62 July 1980.

Oral Hygiene Materials and Devices

AIDS TO ORAL HYGIENE
AND ORAL HEALTH

DISCLOSING SOLUTIONS

TYPES AND USES: Disclosing solutions are dyes which permit the patient and the operator to visualize the otherwise nearly invisible plaque.[1,2] Erythrosine (FD&C Red No. 3) in both tablet and liquid form is commonly used for home use. Bismark Brown is frequently used in dental offices but seldom in the home.

A colorless solution of fluorescein sodium (D&C Yellow No. 8) is essentially invisible when applied to plaque.[3] However, when it is viewed under an ultraviolet light source with a wave length of approximately 380 nm, plaque on the teeth becomes clearly discernible.

DIRECTIONS FOR USE: Most disclosing solutions are applied topically after the patient has rinsed thoroughly with water. One exception is the concentrated solution of erythrosine, whereby 6 ml of the concentrate are diluted in 100 ml of water and the patient rinses with the solution. Another exception is the fluorescein sodium; three drops of the solution are placed in the floor of the mouth, and the patient then rinses with the solution for one minute, expectorates and removes the excess solution by rinsing with water for thirty seconds.

LIMITATIONS OF USE: The erythrosine and Bismark Brown solutions do not selectively stain only plaque. They also stain pellicle, the gingiva and the tongue. Some patients find this staining esthetically unacceptable. The sodium fluorescein solution stains plaque on the teeth, tongue and gingiva while plaque-free teeth and pellicle on the teeth do not fluoresce under the ultraviolet light.

AVAILABLE PRODUCTS

Butler Red-Cote Plaque Disclosant, John O. Butler Co.
Dector Crack Disclosing Solution, Den-Mat, Inc.

Disclosing Solution, Healthco, Inc.
Disclosing Tablets, Healthco, Inc.
Dis-Plaque Solution, Pacemaker Corp.
Dis-Plaque Swabs, Pacemaker/Cooper Laboratories
Dis-Plaque Tablets, Pacemaker Corp.
Trace: Dental Disclosing Agent, The Lorvic Corp.
Trace Gel, The Lorvic Corp.
Two Tone Disclosing Solution, The Lorvic Corp.

POWERED TOOTHBRUSHES

TYPES: Powered toothbrushes are available with a variety of brushing motions including: 1) a reciprocating (back-and-forth) motion in the same direction as the long axis of the handle; 2) an arcuate (up-and-down) motion in a direction generally at right angles to the long axis of the handle; 3) a combination of the reciprocating and arcuate motions; and 4) a rotating motion. They are supplied with nylon filament bristles set in various configurations. A review of reports dealing with the effectiveness of the electric versus the hand toothbrush leads to the conclusion that for the average patient they are of equal effectiveness in removing plaque, debris and materia alba and preventing the deposition of supragingival calculus.[4,5] There is evidence that the electric brush is more effective than the hand brush for handicapped children.[6]

DIRECTIONS FOR USE: Each manufacturer supplies written instructions for use of its brush. These instructions are written in general terms and tell how to use the device to remove supragingival irritants without causing damage to the teeth and gingiva. Many dentists are of the opinion that the patient should receive office instructions in use of the powered brush. Office instruction usually concentrates on proper positioning, overlapping of positions and a sequential procedure so that facial, lingual and palatal areas are thoroughly cleansed.

LIMITATIONS OF USE: Powered brushes have the same limitations as hand brushes. They are not effective for interdental plaque removal and their use must be supplemented by some type of interdental cleaning aid. In the presence of crowding, tipping, or overlapping of teeth, their effectiveness is decreased. In a patient with a hyperactive tongue, a small mouth, or unyielding cheeks, their effectiveness is also diminished.

EVALUATION PROGRAM: The Council on Dental Materials, Instruments and Equipment has a classification for these devices. Those products voluntarily submitted to the Council and accepted may carry the following statement.

"_____ is Acceptable (Provisionally Acceptable) as an effective cleansing device for use as part of a program for good oral hygiene to supplement the regular professional care required for oral health.
Council on Dental Materials, Instruments and Equipment, American Dental Association."

AVAILABLE PRODUCTS

BROXODENT AUTOMATIC TOOTHBRUSH, E. R. Squibb & Sons, Inc.
GENERAL ELECTRIC AUTOMATIC TOOTHBRUSH ARCUATE, DUAL, CORDED, General Electric Co.
J. C. PENNEY AUTOMATIC TOOTHBRUSH DUAL, J. C. Penney Co., Inc.
Porta-Pro Tooth Polisher, Porta-Pro Inc.

FLOSS, TAPE AND HOLDERS

Dental floss is supplied in two forms, waxed and unwaxed. At present waxed floss is made up of nylon filaments in a parallel alignment and covered with a soft wax. Unwaxed floss is made up of a smaller number of nylon filaments. One of the more popular brands is said to contain 112 nylon filaments. Dental tape, sometimes referred to as flat floss, is usually made up of nylon filaments, although cotton can be used. In either case the tape is covered by a soft wax. Dental tape differs from waxed dental floss primarily in size. Tapes vary considerably in width; some are less than 2 mm while others exceed 4 mm in width. The use of waxed floss has been advocated by the dental profession for many years, but unwaxed floss has gained considerable popularity over the past 20 years.[7]

A variable diameter floss made of nylon strips of different lengths has recently been introduced. The ends of each floss unit are of approximately the same diameter as conventional unwaxed floss while a segment towards one end, (approximately 4 inches long) is considerably wider and porous.

USES: Floss, both waxed and unwaxed, and dental tape are used to loosen plaque from the proximal surfaces of the teeth and to dislodge materia alba and debris from the interproximal areas. To date there is no convincing evidence that one type of floss is superior to the other or that either form is superior to dental tape.[7,8]

DIRECTIONS FOR USE: Floss: A short length of floss is held firmly between the fingers and inserted into each interdental area by gently sawing it back and forth until it slips through the contact point.[9] It is carried just below the gingival margin and then activated by moving the floss up and down while holding it firmly against the proximal surface to loosen the accumulated bacterial plaque and dislodge any materia alba and debris beneath the contact points.

The variable diameter floss is used by inserting the regular floss portion underneath the contact points of the teeth and then pulling the larger diameter, porous segment back and forth several times.

Floss holders: A number of devices are available which hold dental floss taut while it is passed through the contact point and moved up and down against the proximal tooth surfaces. Essentially they consist of two arms that extend from a plastic handle. The floss is threaded over grooves on the ends of the arms and secured by winding over projections at the base of the arms. The devices are useful especially for physically handicapped patients and other patients with poor manual dexterity.

Several floss-threading devices are available

to assist patients in introducing floss under soldered joints between individual splinted teeth and under fixed partial dentures. Made of thin plastic or wire, they have an eyelet or loop through which the floss is threaded. The tip of the threader is then placed under the solder joint and pushed through to the palatal or lingual surface.

Floss tends to "hang-up" and tear in interproximal areas where there are large accumulations of calculus on the tooth surfaces, or where open carious lesions or overhanging dental restorations are present.

AVAILABLE PRODUCTS

Bit O'Wax Lightly Waxed Dental Floss, John O. Butler Co.

Bridgeaid Dental Floss Threader, Floss Aid Corp.

Caulk Dental Floss, L. D. Caulk Co.

Caulk Flat Ribbon Dental Floss, L. D. Caulk Co.

Dial-O-Floss, Thierman Products, Inc.

Dr. C. C. Bass Right Kind Unwaxed Dental Floss, John O. Butler Co.

Ex-Plac Threader, Preventive Dentistry Products, Inc.

E-Z Dental Flosser, Preventive Dentistry Products, Inc.

E-Z Floss Dental Floss Holder, E-Z Floss Co.

Flossaid, Floss Aid Corporation

Floss Fingers II, Preventive Dentistry Products, Inc.

FlossMate Floss Handle, John O. Butler Co.

Flosspan Holder, Gretacor Devices, Inc./Texell Products Co.

Johnson's Floss. Johnson & Johnson Dental Products Co.

Johnson's Dentotape, Johnson & Johnson Dental Products Co.

#840 Eez-Thru Floss Threader, John O. Butler Co.

Oral-B Litewax, Oral-B/Cooper Labs

Oral-B Unwaxed, Oral-B/Cooper Labs

Pycopay Softex Dental Floss, Block Drug Co., Inc.

Sunny Smiles Floss, Preventive Dentistry Products, Inc.

Super Floss, Educational Health Products, Inc.

Tuff-Spun Unwaxed, John O. Butler Co.

Zon Dental Bridge Cleaners, Johnson & Johnson Dental Products Co.

MISCELLANEOUS INTERDENTAL CLEANING AGENTS

TYPES: Various devices have been proposed for use in cleaning the proximal surfaces of teeth. They include round and triangular toothpicks made of wood or plastic, small cylindrical or tapered brushes consisting of a wire core from which numerous fine bristles emerge in various configurations, and rubber tips of assorted shapes.[10] The toothpick has the distinction of being the first oral hygiene device mentioned in the literature. It in turn may have evolved from the "chew stick" used in ancient times by many populations and still employed today in some underdeveloped or partially developed countries.

USES: Toothpicks, rubber tips and interdental brushes are used to dislodge materia alba and debris from interdental areas and to remove bacterial plaque accumulations from the teeth.

DIRECTIONS FOR USE: Patients are instructed to hold the device firmly on the crest of the gingival papilla and work it in and out along the proximal surface of the tooth. It is gradually moved more occlusally until it is stopped by the contact points of the teeth. Each of the two tooth surfaces in each interdental area should be cleaned separately. According to promotional material accompanying the rubber tip devices, these devices also stimulate the gingival tissue.

LIMITATIONS OF USE: Toothpicks, brushes and rubber tips are of limited value when the papillary tissue fills the interdental area below the contact point, or when the teeth are malposed buccally and lingually, crowded or tilted. Patients with small mouths, inelastic cheeks, or a combination of these factors often experience difficulty in using these devices effectively in the molar interproximal spaces.

AVAILABLE PRODUCTS

Caulk Pumice, L.D. Caulk Co.
Caulk Special Lava Pumice, L.D. Caulk Co.
Denta-Kleen, Premier Dental Products Co.

INTERDENTAL CLEANING AGENTS

Don't:
1. Exert pressure on the tissue—over a period of time it results in recession of the gingiva.
2. Concentrate on the front teeth. Overuse can result in gingival recession and abrasion of proximal root surfaces. At the same time the posterior surfaces may only be partially cleaned or may be entirely neglected.

E-Z Handle w/attachments, E-Z Floss Co.
Lustrex, L.D. Caulk Co.
Plac-Pik, Preventive Dentistry Products, Inc.
Squeak-a-Dent, Silver Mfg. Co.
Surgident Hydroclean, Lactona/Surgident

ORAL IRRIGATING DEVICES

TYPES: Two types of oral irrigating devices are commonly available. One type uses a motor-driven pump to generate a pulsating jet of water. There is provision for regulating the pressure of the water jet and a large reservoir provides a sufficient flow of water. The second type is attached directly to the water faucet. Most devices of this kind provide either a continuous stream of water or a pulsating stream. Oral irrigating devices have been advocated and used both in Europe and in this country since the last century for removing debris around the teeth. To date there is no conclusive evidence that they are effective in reducing plaque or calculus accumulations, or the incidence and severity of gingival and periodontal disease.[11-13]

DIRECTIONS FOR USE: The devices are most effective if used after toothbrushing and interdental cleaning procedures have loosened debris and plaque from the teeth. The tip of the device should be held about one-half inch from the gingival tissue and should be kept in motion and moved over all facial and palatal/lingual surfaces of both the maxillary and mandibular teeth.

LIMITATIONS OF USE: There is no evidence that the devices remove adherent plaque from the teeth or that their use in an average home care situation decreases calculus accumulation or improves gingival and periodontal conditions. They should not be used in the presence of acute gingival diseases such as necrotizing ulcerative gingivitis or herpetic gingival stomatitis or in the presence of a periodontal abscess. Irrigating devices should be used with care by patients with advanced periodontal disease or a predisposition to systemic bacteremia.[14] Particular care should be taken if the patient has a synthetic heart valve or lengths of a synthetic artery or vein.

EVALUATION PROGRAM: The Council on Dental Materials, Instruments and Equipment has a classification or Acceptance Program for Oral Irrigating Devices. The packaging and advertisement of those products voluntarily submitted to the Council and Accepted may carry the following statement:

"_____ Oral Irrigating Device is Acceptable (Provisionally Acceptable) for use as an effective aid to the toothbrush in a program of good oral hygiene to supplement the regular professional care required for good oral health.

Council on Dental Materials, Instruments, and Equipment, American Dental Association"

AVAILABLE PRODUCTS

DENTO-SPRAY, Texell Products Co.
Den-Z-Orb, Professional Disposables, Inc.

ORAL IRRIGATING DEVICES

Do:
1. Brush the teeth and clean the interdental areas first.
2. Use the device at the lowest effective water pressure.
3. Keep the irrigating tip continuously moving and about one-half inch from the gingiva.

Don't:
1. Use the device in place of brushing or interdental cleaning.
2. Use it at high pressures.
3. Use it in the presence of acute inflammatory conditions.

DENTURE ADHERENTS

COMPOSITION: Adherent powders are made from finely powdered vegetable gums such as acacia, karaya or finely ground tragacanth, ethylene oxide polymer, or other agents which assume mucilaginous properties when water is added. The powders are prepared by using these agents individually or by mixing a combination of them. The agent is flavored by adding wintergreen or peppermint oil or similar agents. Antiseptics such as borax or boric acid are sometimes added. Several pastes consisting principally of karaya gum, petroleum (up to 50 percent petroleum jelly), coloring and flavoring agents have become popular in the past several years. Claims have been made that they are more effective than the powder preparations, due to their moisture-resistant properties; to date evidence to support these claims is not available.[15]

USES: A few dentists utilize the preparations to stabilize occlusal rims. They may also be used as an emergency measure to stabilize an ill-fitting denture until the patient can secure an appointment to have a new denture made. In special circumstances, such as for a patient with very flat ridges, an elderly patient, an edentulous cleft palate patient, or a patient with a post cancer prosthesis, the adherent powders or pastes may be prescribed and used safely and effectively provided there is continued professional supervision.

DIRECTIONS FOR USE: Powder: A light even coating is sprinkled on the moistened denture base before it is placed in the mouth. Paste: A thin even coat of the paste is applied to the dry denture base before it is placed in the mouth.

LIMITATIONS FOR USE: It is not possible to apply the same amount of powder or paste in exactly the same place time after time. This means that the denture is always being positioned differently in the mouth, causing a malocclusion and frequently an odd appearance when the anterior teeth are too long or off center due to a thickened layer of denture powder or paste.

There is no evidence in the literature to indicate that either type of denture adherent preparation is effective for making ill-fitting dentures more stable during mastication. Kapur[15] found no significant difference in the adhesive effect of the two types of denture adherent preparations. Neither appreciably improved the masticatory performance of the denture wearers when evaluated by the chewing and sieving techniques.

These products have no therapeutic value and have not been shown to be beneficial to the tissues. Their continuous use encourages the patient to wear dentures which should be adjusted, rebased or reconstructed.[16] Also, by creating a false sense of retention, the use of powder inhibits the development of desirable habits for denture support.

The continual use of adherent powders is often objectionable because the gluey substance formed may become foul when combined with oral secretions, and can act as an irritant when

---

DENTURE ADHERENTS

Do:
1. Use no more than a thin, even coating of the powder or paste.
2. Clean the material from the denture-bearing tissues twice daily and rinse thoroughly.
3. Clean the material out of the denture base with a suitable brush twice daily and then rinse the denture thoroughly.
4. Use the powder or paste only as an emergency short-term measure unless continued use is prescribed by the dentist.

Don't:
1. Add more powder or paste to material already under the denture base. It will further distort the occlusion.
2. Wear the denture during sleep. The material should be cleaned out of the denture base and the denture should be left in water overnight.
3. Use the powder or paste for an extended time period without professional advice. Continued use may make fabrication of a satisfactory denture more difficult.

---

local abrasion is present from an improperly fitting denture.

Many patients report that using denture adherent preparations is unpleasant and messy and that large portions of such materials work out from beneath the dentures, especially the mandibular denture, causing the patient to expectorate or swallow much of the substance. Some patients refrain from using powders in the lower denture because of the difficulty encountered in retaining the substance within the denture.

Continued use of large portions of denture powder accelerates alveolar bone resorption and may make the construction of new dentures most difficult due to the lack of supporting structures.

Atopic coryza, eczema, atopic dermatitis and gastrointestinal distress have been produced in sensitive individuals by karaya gum.[17]

EVALUATION PROGRAM: The Council's program for such products requires that every trade package of an acceptable denture adhesive carry the following statement which indicates acceptance as well as the hazards of the continued wearing of ill-fitting dental appliances.

"_____ is Acceptable (Provisionally Acceptable) as a temporary measure to provide increased retention of dentures. However, an ill-fitting denture may impair your health—consult your dentist for periodic examination.

Council on Dental Materials, Instruments and Equipment, American Dental Association"

AVAILABLE PRODUCTS

BENEFIT DENTURE ADHESIVE, Polymed Laboratories, Inc.

Confident, Block Drug Co., Inc.

CO-RE-GA DENTURE ADHESIVE POWDER, Corega Chemical Co., Inc.

FIRMDENT, Moyco Industries, Inc.

ORAHESIVE, Hoyt Laboratories

PERMA-GRIP DENTURE ADHESIVE POWDER AND CREAM, Lactona Corp., Subsidiary Warner-Lambert Co.

Polident, Block Drug Co., Inc.

Super Poli-Grip, Block Drug Co., Inc.

SUPER WERNET'S DENTURE ADHESIVE POWDER (POLYMER BASED), Wernet Div., Block Drug Co., Inc.

WERNET'S ADHESIVE CREAM (POLYMER BASED), Wernet Div., Block Drug Co., Inc.

WERNET'S POWDER WITH NEOSEAL, Wernet Div., Block Drug Co., Inc.

DENTURE CLEANING AGENTS

A large number of fine abrasives and mild chemical agents have been proposed to assist in cleaning dentures. They include hand soap, bicarbonate of soda, precipitated calcium carbonate, chlorine-containing solutions such as hypochlorite N.F. (half a teaspoon to half a tumbler of water) and denture pastes which are similar in composition to toothpastes. The effectiveness of any of these agents is largely dependent on their thorough application by a brush adapted as closely as possible to the contour of the denture.[18]

USES: Denture cleaning agents are used to remove soft debris from dentures, to prevent staining of dentures, to remove stains before they are firmly adherent to the denture teeth or base, and to prevent the denture from acquiring an unpleasant odor. For optimum effectiveness dentures should be cleaned at least once daily.

DIRECTIONS FOR USE: The denture should first be thoroughly rinsed under running water to remove loosely adherent debris. The cleaning agent is then applied to the moistened brush and all aspects of the denture thoroughly brushed. The denture is then rinsed again to remove any residual cleaning agent.

LIMITATIONS OF USE: None of the cleaning agents prevent the eventual accumulation of stains and in some cases calcified deposits on dentures.[18] Appliances made of cobalt-chromium alloy corrode if allowed to remain in a chlorine containing solution for any length of time. Excessively vigorous and/or misdirected scrubbing with a denture brush can result in abrasion of the denture teeth or base or bending of a metal clasp of a removable partial denture.

AVAILABLE PRODUCTS

Dentu-Creme, Block Drug Co., Inc.

Miller Concentrated Denture Cleaner, Bell Federal Laboratory, Div. of Miller Dental Mfg. Inc.

Polident Effervescent Denture Cleanser Powder & Tablets, Block Drug Co., Inc.

DENTURE CLEANING AGENTS

Do:

1. Rinse the denture thoroughly before applying the cleaning agent.
2. Brush the denture thoroughly but carefully so as not to bend the clasps or abrade the denture.
3. Rinse the denture thoroughly after cleaning and before inserting.
4. Have the denture cleaned by your dentist at least once a year.
5. Because of the chemical nature of these agents, keep the cleaning agent out of the reach of children.

Don't:

1. Neglect cleaning your denture as it will accumulate stains. Calcified deposits can interfere with proper fit of the denture and create an unpleasant odor.
2. Use a harsh abrasive or strong caustic agent to clean your denture as use of these agents can lead to pitting of the denture material and loss of proper fit.
3. Scrub the denture too vigorously. It can result in abrasion of the denture and/or bending or breaking of the clasps of partial dentures.

Prolastic Denture Cleaner, Prolastic Co., Inc.
Prolastic Tartar and Stain Remover, Prolastic Co., Inc.

MECHANICAL DENTURE CLEANERS

A number of mechanical devices operating on ordinary household current and classified as "sonic" or "ultrasonic" are available for cleaning dentures. The word "sonic" refers to audible sound frequencies and "ultrasonic" pertains to high frequency sound waves above the normal hearing range or above 20,000 cycles per second. Ultrasonic devices convert electrical energy into mechanical energy at an ultrasonic frequency.

TYPES: The many mechanical cleaners available can be classified according to their action into basically three types. 1) Devices which are truly ultrasonic use high frequency sound waves to agitate the cleaning solution by means of an electronic transducer. 2) Magnetic stirrers consist of a bar magnet attached to a motor installed in the base of the unit. The rotating magnet in the base interacts with a similar magnet in the reservoir and drives the propeller. 3) A third type of mechanical cleaner includes devices which cause agitation by the vibratory action of a magnetic bar mounted close to but out of contact with the open end of a U-shaped electro-magnet. When the device is energized with a 60 cycle electric current, the bar is attracted toward the magnet and then released twice during each cycle causing vibration of the cleaning solution.

The commercially prepared immersion type denture cleaning solution with such a mechanical denture cleaner is slightly more effective than the soak-type denture cleaning agent.[19] The much more energetic agitation produced by an ultrasonic cleaner provides more efficient cleaning than soaking or sonic agitation at 120 cycles.

USES: The devices are useful for removing soft debris and extrinsic stains from the denture teeth, acrylic base material, partial denture clasps, bars, and rests. Their use helps to prevent the denture from developing an unpleasant odor. For optimum effectiveness dentures should be cleaned at least once daily.

LIMITATIONS OF USE: None of the devices prevent the eventual deposition of extrinsic stains and in some instances calcified deposits on dentures. Tests by the Council with various dental materials and mechanical denture cleaners have shown that none of the mechanical cleaners remove all stain and debris without some brushing with a denture brush.[19] When used with the recommended cleaning solution, the ultrasonic type denture cleaners were the most effective in removing debris and stain; the magnetic stirrer type was the least effective. Leaving a denture in a mechanical denture cleaner for extended periods of time could result in damage.

EVALUATION PROGRAM: The Council of Dental Materials, Instruments and Equipment has an Acceptance Program for mechanical denture cleaners.

MECHANICAL DENTURE CLEANERS

Do:

1. Rinse the denture thoroughly under running water before placing it in the mechanical denture cleaner.
2. Keep out of the reach of children because of the chemical nature of some of the denture cleaner agents.
3. Follow the manufacturer's directions as to how long the denture should be left in the activated mechanical denture cleaner.
4. Supplement mechanical cleaning with brushing to help remove gross deposits.
5. Rinse the denture thoroughly under running water after removing it from the solution.
6. Have the denture cleaned by your dentist when stains or calcified deposits build up on the dentures.

Don't:

1. Substitute a harsh alkaline or caustic solution for the immersion type cleaning agent recommended by the manufacturer. They can discolor and damage the denture, destroying the fit.

AVAILABLE PRODUCTS

K-42 ULTRASONIC CLEANER, Ultrasonic International, Inc.

LITERATURE REFERENCES

1. Accepted dental therapeutics, ed. 38, Chicago, American Dental Association, 1979, p. 309.
2. Arnim, S.S. The use of disclosing solutions for measuring tooth cleanliness. J. Periodontol. 34:227 July 1963.
3. Cohen, D.W., et al. A comparison of bacterial plaque disclosants in periodontal disease. J. Periodontol. 43:333 June 1972.
4. Chilton, N.W.; DiDio, A.; and Rothner, J.T. Comparison of the clinical effectiveness of an electric and a standard toothbrush in normal individuals. JADA 64:777 June 1962.
5. Quigley, G.A., and Hein, J.W. Comparative cleaning efficiency of manual and power brushing. JADA 65:26 July 1962.
6. Smith, J.F., and Blankenship, J. Improving oral hygiene in handicapped children by the use of an electric toothbrush. J. Dent. Child. 31:198, 1964.
7. O'Leary, T.J. Oral hygiene agents and procedures. J. Periodontol. 41:625 Nov. 1970.
8. Hill, H.C.; Levi, P.A.; and Glickman, I. The effects of waxed and unwaxed floss on interdental plaque accumulation and interdental gingival health. J. Periodontol. 44:411 July 1973.
9. O'Leary, T.J., and Nabers, C.L. Instructions to supplement teaching oral hygiene. J. Periodontol. 40:27, 1969.
10. Gjermo, P., and Flotra, L. The effect of different methods of interdental cleaning. J. Periodont. Res. 5:230, 1970.
11. Krajewski, J.J.; Giblin, J.; and Gargiulo, A.W. Evaluation of a water pressure cleaning device as an adjunct to periodontal treatment. Periodontics 2:76, 1964.
12. Krajewski, J.J.; Rubach, W.C.; and Pope, J.W. The effect of water pressure cleaning on the clinically normal gingival crevice. J. South. Calif. Dent. Assoc. 43:452, 1967.
13. Lainson, P.A.; Bergquist, J.J.; and Fraleigh, C.M. Clinical evaluation of Pulsar, a new pulsating water pressure cleaning device. J. Periodontol. 41:401, 1970.
14. Feliz, J.E.; Rosen, S.; and App, G.R. Detec-

tion of bacteremia after the use of an oral irrigating device in subjects with periodontitis. J. Periodontol. 42:785 Dec. 1971.

15. Kapur, K.K. A clinical evaluation of denture adhesives. J. Prosthet. Dent. 17:456, 1967.

16. Woelfel, J.B.; Winter, C.M.; and Curry, R.L. Additives sold over-the-counter dangerously prolong wearing period of ill-fitting dentures. JADA 71:603 Sept. 1965.

17. Figley, K.D. Karaya gum hypersensitivity. JAMA 114:747 Mar. 1940. Correction 114:1091 Mar. 1940.

18. Anthony, D.H., and Gibbons, P. The nature and behavior of denture cleaners. J. Prosthet. Dent. 8:796 Sept.-Oct. 1958.

19. Unpublished investigations conducted by Council on Dental Materials, Instruments and Equipment. 1970-1971.

PUBLICATIONS OF THE COUNCIL ON DENTAL MATERIALS, INSTRUMENTS AND EQUIPMENT

All literature references are to The Journal of the American Dental Association unless otherwise indicated.

1. Certification program for dental materials; List of certified dental materials revised to November 1, 1966. 74:470 Feb. 1967.

2. Provisions for evaluation of dental devices. (As adopted by the House of Delegates, November, 1966). 74:797 March 1967.

3. Irrigating devices. 74:799 March 1967.

4. Radiation hygiene and practice in dentistry. 74:1032 April 1967.

5. New American Dental Association specification no. 19 adopted. 74:1039 April 1967.

6. Specification program for dental materials. 74:1563 June 1967.

7. Council adopts ADA specification no. 8 (dental zinc phosphate cement) and 11 (agar impression material). 74:1565 June 1967.

8. Supplement to the list of certified dental materials. 75:188 July 1967.

9. Radiation hygiene and practice in dentistry. II. 75:1197 Nov. 1967.

10. Standard test methods for direct filling resins. 75:1426 Dec. 1967.

11. Radiation hygiene and practice in dentistry: State regulation of dental X rays. 76:107 Jan. 1968.

12. Supplement to list of certified dental materials. 76:114 Jan. 1968.

13. Radiation hygiene and practice in dentistry. III. 76:115 Jan. 1968.

14. Radiation hygiene and practice in dentistry. IV. 76:363 Feb. 1968.

15. Recommendations of radiation hygiene and practice. 76:365 Feb. 1968.

16. Certification program for dental materials: List of certified dental materials revised to January 1, 1968. 76:366 Feb. 1968.

17. Radiation hygiene and practice in dentistry. V. 76:602 March 1968.

18. New American Dental Association specification no. 20 adopted. 76:604 1968.

19. Myers, G. E. Status report on zinc oxide-eugenol and modified cements. 76:1053 May 1968 (Council-sponsored report).

20. Supplement to the list of certified dental materials. 76:1068 May 1968.

21. Alcox, R. W. Diagnostic radiation exposures and doses in dentistry. 76:1066 May 1968 (Council-sponsored report).

22. Guide to Dental Materials and Devices, ed. 4. Chicago, American Dental Association. 1968-69.

23. Supplement to the list of certified dental materials. 76:1412 June 1968.

24. Supplement to the list of certified dental materials. 77:637 Sept. 1968.

25. Preliminary report on radiographic holding, paralleling, and shielding devices. 77:884 Oct. 1968.

26. Collett, W. K. Diagnostic radiation exposures and doses in dentistry: II. 77:1104 Nov. 1968 (Council-sponsored report).

27. Council adopts American Dental Association specification no.18 (alginate impression material). 77:1354 Dec. 1968.

28. Supplement to the list of certified dental materials. 77:1359 Dec. 1968.

29. Supplement to the list of certified dental materials. 78:136 Jan. 1969.

30. Current status of oral irrigating devices. 78:347 Feb. 1969.

31. Certification program for dental materials: list of certified dental materials revised to January 1, 1969. 78:349 Feb. 1969.

32. Resilient liners: a comment. 78:577 March 1969.

33. New American Dental Association specification no. 21 adopted (dental zinc silico-phosphate cement). 78:577 March 1969.

34. Supplement to the list of certified dental materials. 78:580 March 1969.

35. Ewen, S. J. Devices for calculus removal. 78:795 April 1969 (Council-sponsored report).

36. Oringer, M. J. Evaluation of dental electrosurgical devices. 78:799 April 1969 (Council-sponsored report).

37. Supplement to the list of certified dental materials. 78:1046 May 1969.

38. Water Pik Oral Irrigating Device classified as acceptable. 78:1365 June 1969.

39. Supplement to the list of certified dental materials. 78:1365 June 1969.

40. Supplement to the list of certified dental materials. 79:693 Sept. 1969.

41. Stanford, J. W. Plastics in dentistry. Plastics World, 1969, The Society of the Plastic Industry, Inc.

42. Supplement to the list of certified dental materials. 79:939 Oct. 1969.

43. Stanford, J. W. USA specification and evaluation programs. 50th Anniversary Symposium on Dental Materials Research. Abstract page 115, National Bureau of Standards, Gaithersburg, Maryland, Oct. 1969.

44. American Dental Association specification no. 1 revised. 79:1206 Nov. 1969.

45. Certification program for dental materials: List of certified dental materials revised to January 1, 1970. 80:155 Jan. 1970.

46. Wuehrmann, A. H. Radiation hygiene and its practice in dentistry as related to film viewing procedures and radiographic interpretation. 80:346 Feb. 1970 (Council-sponsored report).

47. Phillips, R. W. Composite restorative resins. 80:357 Feb. 1970 (Council-sponsored report).

48. Supplement to the list of certified oral irrigating devices. 80:359 Feb. 1970.

49. Stanford, J. W. Toxicity evaluations of dental materials. Forum Newsletter 3:1 Feb. 1970. College of Pharmacy, University of Tennessee, Memphis.

50. Supplement to the list of certified dental materials. 80:1066 May 1970.

51. Revised American Dental Association specification no. 22 for intraoral dental radiographic film adopted. 80:1066 May 1970.

52. Supplement to the list of certified dental materials. 80:1069 May 1970.

53. Supplement to the list of certified dental materials. 80:1383 June 1970.

54. Supplement to the list of certified dental materials. 81:187 July 1970.

55. Supplement to the list of classified oral irrigating devices. 81:187 July 1970.

56. Supplement to the list of certified dental materials. 81:431 Aug. 1970.

57. Addition to the list of classified power toothbrushes. 81:431 Aug. 1970.

58. Supplement to the list of certified dental materials. 81:729 Sept. 1970.

59. Supplement to the list of classified oral irrigating devices. 81:729 Sept. 1970.

60. New American Dental Association specification no. 23 for dental excavating burs adopted. 81:961 Oct. 1970.

61. Supplement to the list of certified dental materials. 81:1182 Nov. 1970.

62. Stanford, J. W. The current status of restorative resins. Dent. Clin. N. Am. 15:57 Jan. 1971.

63. Certification program for dental materials: List of certified dental materials revised to January 1, 1971. 82:162 Jan. 1971.

64. List of classified devices revised to January 1, 1971. 82:176 Jan. 1971.

65. Alloys for dental amalgam containing fluoride. 82:399 Feb. 1971.

66. Composite restorative materials: recommended uses. 82:399 Feb. 1971.

67. New American Dental Association specification no. 24 for dental base plate wax adopted. 82:603 March 1971.

68. Supplement to the list of certified dental materials. 82:607 March 1971.

69. Addition to the list of classified powered toothbrushes. 82:607 March 1971.

70. Correction to the list of classified powered toothbrushes. 82:607 March 1971.

71. Bondoc, L.G.; Mujwid, D. and Stanford, J. W. Effect of varying test procedures on physical properties of zinc oxide-eugenol cements. IADR Abstract Papers, No. 453 March 1971.

72. Boaz, D. E., and Stanford, J. W. Deterioration of elastomeric impression materials. IADR Abstract Papers, No. 597 March 1971.

73. Bondoc, L. G., Coe, M. H. and Stanford, J. W. The reciprocating rheometer for evaluation of elastomeric impression materials. IADR Abstract Papers, No. 598 March 1971.

74. Pit and fissure sealants. 82:1101 May 1971.

75. Rupp, N. W., and Paffenbarger, G. C. Review—Significance to health of mercury used in dental practice. 82:1401 June 1971.

76. Supplement to the list of certified dental materials. 82:1408 June 1971.

77. Stanford, J. W. Mechanical aids in oral hygiene. Pharmacy Times, July 1971.

78. Supplement to the list of certified dental materials. 83:174 July 1971.

79. Supplement to the list of certified dental materials. 83:367 Aug. 1971.

80. Addition to the list of classified oral irrigating devices. 83:367 Aug. 1971.

81. Correction to the list of classified powered toothbrushes. 83:367 Aug. 1971.

82. Stanford, J. W. Standardization, self-regulation and acceptance programs for dental materials and devices. Proceedings of Conference on Product Liability Prevention. Newark College of Engineering, Aug. 1971, pp. 33-39.

83. Supplement to the list of certified dental materials. 83:655 Sept. 1971.

84. Correction to the list of certified dental mercuries. 83:655 Sept. 1971.

85. Alcox, R. W., and Waggener, D. T. Status report on rapid processing devices for dental radiographic film. 83:1330 Dec. 1971.

86. Supplement to the list of certified dental materials. 83:1338 Dec. 1971.

87. Certification program for dental materials: List of certified dental materials revised to January 1, 1972. 84:163 Jan. 1972.

88. Standardization program for dental materials and devices. 84:375 Feb. 1972.

89. Recommended standard practices for biological evaluation of dental materials. 84:382 Feb. 1972.

90. Recommended standard practices for clinical evaluation of dental materials and devices. 84:388 Feb. 1972.

91. Expansion of acceptance programs. 84:391 Feb. 1972.

92. Supplement to the list of certified dental materials. 84:395 Feb. 1972.

93. New American Dental Association specification no. 25 for dental gypsum products. 84:640 March 1972.

94. Nitrous oxide-oxygen explosions. 84:645 March 1972.

95. Supplement to the list of certified dental materials. 84:646 March 1972.

96. Baez, R.; Ramsden, E.; Halstead, E. K.; and Stanford, J. W. Development of a single multipurpose dental materials evaluating system. IADR Abstract Papers, No. 866 March 1972.

97. Bondoc, L.; Mujwid, D.; Jagusiak, A.; and Stanford, J. W. Color difference measurements. IADR Abstract Papers, No. 867 March 1972.

98. Supplement to the list of certified dental materials. 84:873 April 1972.

99. Recommendations in radiological practice. 84:1108 May 1972.

100. Nuva-Seal pit and fissure sealant classified as provisionally acceptable. 84:1109 May 1972.

101. Supplement to the list of certified dental materials. 84:1110 May 1972.

102. Guide to Dental Materials and Devices, ed. 6. Chicago, American Dental Association, 1972.

103. Supplement to the list of certified dental materials. 84:1373 June 1972.

104. Natiella, J. R. et al. Current evaluation of dental implants. 84:1358 June 1972 (Council-sponsored report).

105. Stanford, J. W. USA specification and evaluation programs. Nat Bur Stand Special Bulletin 354, p. 221, June 1972, Washington, D.C.

106. Supplement to the list of certified dental materials, 85:180 July 1972.

107. Schram, J. J. Guidelines for electrical

safety in the dental office. 85:365 Aug. 1972 (Council-sponsored report).

108. Precision X-ray device classified as acceptable. 85:372 Aug. 1972.

109. Over-the-counter denture reliners and repair kits. 85:373 Aug. 1972.

110. Going, R. E. Status report on cement bases, cavity liners, varnishes, primers, and cleansers. 85:654 Sept. 1972 (Council-sponsored report).

111. Supplement to the list of certified dental materials. 85:672 Sept. 1972.

112. Stanford, J. W. Proceedings of AAMI/FDA National Conference on Medical Device Standards. JAAMI 6:288 July-Aug. 1972.

113. Supplement to the list of certified dental materials. 85:932 Oct. 1972.

114. Eames, W. B. Status report on amalgamators and mercury/alloy proportioners and disposable capsules. 85:928 Oct. 1972 (Council-sponsored report).

115. Certification program for dental materials: List of certified dental materials revised to January 1, 1973. 86:158 Jan. 1973.

116. List of classified dental materials and devices revised to January 1, 1973. 86:166 Jan. 1973.

117. Additions to the list of classified composite restorative materials. 86:424 Feb. 1973.

118. Visco-Gel treatment reliner material classified as provisionally acceptable. 86:425 Feb. 1973.

119. Supplement to the list of certified dental materials. 86:426 Feb. 1973.

120. Possible electromagnetic interference with cardiac pacemakers from dental induction casting machines and electrosurgical devices. 86:426 Feb. 1973.

121. Supplement to the list of certified dental materials. 86:690 March 1973.

122. Additions to the list of classified composite restorative materials. 86:690 March 1973.

123. Millard, H. D. Electric pulp testers. 86:872 April 1973 (Council-sponsored report).

124. Supplement to the list of certified dental materials. 86:874 April 1973.

125. Norling, B. K.; Stanford, J. W.; and Priest, B. J. Selection of a substrate material for high-speed bur testing. IADR Abstract Papers, No. 784 April 1973.

126. Van Aken, J. Status on panoramic X-ray equipment. 86:1050 May 1973 (Council-sponsored report).

127. Supplement to the list of certified dental materials. 86:1049 May 1973.

128. Hefferren, John J. A review of approaches to the detection of dental caries. 86:1358 June 1973.

129. Mouth protectors: 11 years later. 86:1365 June 1973.

130. Supplement to the list of certified dental materials and devices. 86:1369 June 1973.

131. Federal standard for diagnostic X-ray systems and dental practice. 87:192 July 1973.

132. Complaints regarding the use of dental materials and devices. 87:378 Aug. 1973.

133. Expansion of acceptance program. 87:379 Aug. 1973.

134. Supplement to the list of certified dental materials and devices. 87:300 Aug. 1973.

135. Additions to the list of classified materials and devices. 87:381 Aug. 1973.

136. Supplement to the list of certified dental materials and devices. 87:673 Sept. 1973.

137. Supplement to the list of certified dental materials and devices. 87:1251 Nov. 1973.

138. Supplement to the list of certified dental materials and devices. 87:1450 Dec. 1973.

139. Certification program for dental materials: List of certified dental materials revised to January 1, 1974. 88:146 Jan. 1974.

140. List of classified dental materials and devices revised to January 1, 1974. 88:153 Jan. 1974.

141. List of products evaluated by the Council on Dental Materials and Devices and the Council on Dental Therapeutics, Jan. 1974. 88:231 Jan. 1974.

142. Pit and fissure sealants. 88:390 Feb. 1974.

143. Recommendations in mercury hygiene. 88:391 Feb. 1974.

144. Council statement: Claims related to "adhesion" or to "adhesive" restorative materials. 88:393 Feb. 1974.

145. Current evaluation of dental endosseous implants. 88:394 Feb. 1974.

146. Supplement to the list of classified dental materials and devices. 88:396 Feb. 1974.

147. Additions to the list of classified dental materials and devices. 88:396 Feb. 1974.

148. Nitrous oxide-oxygen sedation machines and devices. 88:611 March 1974.

149. Acceptance program for dental materials and devices. 88:615 March 1974.

150. Additions to the list of classified dental materials and devices. 88:617 March 1974.

151. Additions to the list of classified dental materials and devices. 88:845 April 1974.

152. Supplement to the list of certified dental materials and devices. 88:845 April 1974.

153. Supplement to the list of certified dental materials and devices. 88:1063 May 1974.

154. Supplement to the list of certified dental materials and devices. 88:1367 June 1974.

155. Additions to the list of classified dental materials and devices. 88:1367 June 1974.

156. Supplement to the list of certified dental materials and devices. 89:170 July 1974.

157. Status report on palladium-silver-based crown and bridge alloys. 89:383 Aug. 1974.

158. New American Dental Association specification no. 26 for dental X-ray equipment. 89:386 Aug. 1974.

159. Expansion of the acceptance program. 89:393 Aug. 1974.

160. Supplement to the list of certified dental materials and devices. 89:395 Aug. 1974.

161. Status report on base-metal crown and bridge alloys. 89:652 Sept. 1974.

162. Supplement to the list of certified dental materials and devices. 89:656 Sept. 1974.

163. Additions to the list of classified dental materials and devices. 89:656 Sept. 1974.

164. Mercury surveys in dental offices. 89:900 Oct. 1974.

165. Mercury surveys of the dental offiice: Equipment, methodology, and philosophy. 89:902 Oct. 1974.

166. Recommendations for mercury surveys of dental offices. 89:904 Oct. 1974.

167. Status report on articulators. 89:1158 Nov. 1974.

168. Status report on dental operating handpieces. 89:1162 Nov. 1974.

169. Status report on dental anesthetic needles and syringes. 89:1170 Nov. 1974.

170. Acceptance program for dental anesthetic syringe devices. 89:1177 Nov. 1974.

171. Withdrawal of acceptance of Water Pik Oral Irrigating Device. 89:1178 Nov. 1974.

172. Supplement to the list of certified dental materials and devices. 89:1178 Nov. 1974.

173. Noise control in the dental operatory. 89:1384 Dec. 1974.

174. Polymers used in dentistry: Part 1 cyanoacrylates 89:1386 Dec. 1974.

175. Expansion of the acceptance program for dental materials and devices. 89:1389 Dec. 1974.

176. Supplement to the list of certified dental materials and devices. 89:1391 Dec. 1974.

177. Additions to the list of classified dental materials and devices. 89:1391 Dec. 1974.

178. Recommendations in radiographic practices: January 1975. 90:171 Jan. 1975.

179. Certification program for dental materials: List of certified dental materials and devices revised to Jan. 1, 1975. 90:173 Jan. 1975.

180. List of classified dental materials and devices revised to Jan. 1, 1975. 90:181 Jan. 1975.

181. Revised American Dental Association Specification no. 4 for dental inlay casting wax. 90:447 Feb. 1975.

182. Revised American Dental Association specification no. 12 for denture base polymers. 90:451 Feb. 1975.

183. Revised American Dental Association specification no. 23 for dental excavating burs. 90:459 Feb. 1975.

184. Supplement to the list of certified dental materials and devices. 90:468 Feb. 1975.

185. Partially prefabricated dentures. 90:669 March 1975.

186. Council reaffirms position on dental endosseous implants. 90:670 March 1975.

187. Supplement to the list of certified dental materials and devices. 90:671 March 1975.

188. Additions to the list of classified dental materials and devices. 90:671 March 1975.

189. Polymers used in dentistry: Part II Resins containing BIS-GMA: coating and cementing uses. 90:841 April 1975.

190. Maxillofacial prosthetic materials. 90:844 April 1975.

191. Supplement to the list of certified dental materials and devices. 90:848 April 1975.

192. Supplement to the list of certified dental materials and devices. 90:1027 May 1975.

193. Supplement to the list of certified dental materials and devices. 90:1302 June 1975.

194. Supplement to the list of certified dental materials and devices. 91:153 July 1975.

195. Additions to the list of classified dental materials and devices. 91:153 July 1975.

196. Mercury vapor levels in dental offices: A simple semi-quantitative test. 91:610 Sept. 1975.

197. Acceptance program for rapid processing devices for dental radiographic film. 91:611 Sept. 1975.

198. Pontics in fixed prosthcscs—Status report. 91:613 Sept. 1975.

199. Status report on silver amalgam. 91:618 Sept. 1975.

200. Supplement to the list of certified dental materials and devices. 91:621 Sept. 1975.

201. American Dental Association standard for dental terminology. 91:853 Oct. 1975.

202. Supplement to the list of certified dental materials and devices. 91:856 Oct. 1975.

203. Supplement to the list of certified dental materials and devices. 91:1069 Nov. 1975.

204. Additions to the list of classified dental materials and devices. 91:1069 Nov. 1975.

205. Supplement to the list of certified dental materials and devices. 91:1255 Dec. 1975.

206. Additions to the list of classified dental materials and devices. 91:1255 Dec. 1975.

207. Certification program for dental materials: List of certified dental materials and devices revised to Jan. 1, 1976. 92:163 Jan. 1976.

208. List of classified dental materials and devices revised to Jan. 1, 1976. 92:170 Jan. 1976.

209. Lists of products evaluated by the Council on Dental Materials and Devices and the Council on Dental Therapeutics. 92:254 Jan. 1976.

210. Precious metal scrap: what it is and how to handle it. 92:434 Feb. 1976.

211. Supplement to the list of certified dental materials and devices. 92:436 Feb. 1976.

212. Additions to the list of classified dental materials and devices. 92:436 Feb. 1976.

213. Status report on precision attachments. 92:602 March 1976.

214. Composite restorative materials: some clinical suggestions for their use. 92:606 March 1976.

215. Guidelines on the use of ultraviolet radiation in dentistry. 92:775 April 1976.

216. Hazards of asbestos in dentistry. 92:777 April 1976.

217. Supplement to the list of certified dental materials and devices. 92:779 April 1976.

218. Recommendations in mercury hygiene. 92:121 June 1976.

219. Pit and fissure sealants. 93:134 July 1976.

220. Partially prefabricated dentures. 93:380 Aug. 1976.

221. Supplement to the list of certified dental materials and devices. 93:380 Aug. 1976.

222. New American Dental Association specification no. 28 for endodontic files and reamers. 93:813 Oct. 1976.

223. New American Dental Association specification no. 29 general specification for hand instruments. 93:818 Oct. 1976.

224. Expansion of the acceptance program for dental materials and devices: Alloys for cast dental restorative and prosthetic devices. 93:1188 Dec. 1976.

225. Supplement to the list of certified dental materials and devices. 93:1190 Dec. 1976.

226. Supplement to the list of classified dental materials and devices. 93:1190 Dec. 1976.

227. Certification and classification programs for dental materials and devices. List of certified dental materials and devices revised to Jan. 1, 1977. 94:135 Jan. 1977.

228. Advantages and disadvantages of the use of dental tomographic radiography. 94:147 Jan. 1977.

229. List of products evaluated by the Council on Dental Therapeutics. 94:183 Jan. 1977.

230. Medical device legislation and the FDA Panel on Review of Dental Devices. 94:353 Feb. 1977.

231. Revised American Dental Association specification no. 19 for non-aqueous, elastomeric dental impression materials. 94:733 April 1977.

232. New American Dental Association specification no. 27 for direct filling resins. 94:1191 June 1977.

233. Craig, R. G. Status report on polyether impression materials. 95:126 July 1977 (Council-sponsored report).

234. Cheng, A. S. Mail order merchandise and you, the dentist. 95:326 August 1977 (Council-sponsored report).

235. Revised American Dental Association specification no. 1 for alloy for dental amalgam. 95:614 Sept. 1977.

236. Expansion of the acceptance program for dental materials and devices: ultraviolet radiation–emitting dental devices. 95:618 Sept. 1977.

237. Supplement to the list of certified dental materials and devices. 95:619 Sept. 1977.

238. Supplement to the American Dental Association standard for dental terminology. 95:620 Sept. 1977.

239. How to avoid problems with porcelain-fused-to metal restorations. 95:818 Oct. 1977.

240. Expansion of the acceptance program: nitrous oxide scavenging equipment and nitrous oxide trace gas monitoring equipment. 95:791 Oct. 1977.

241. Johnson, O. N. and Barone, G. J. What the

federal x-ray regulations mean to the dentist. 95:810 Oct. 1977 (Council-sponsored report).

242. New American Dental Association specification no. 30 for dental zinc oxide–eugenol type restorative materials. 95:991 Nov. 1977.

243. New American Dental Association specification no. 32 for orthodontic wires not containing precious metals. 95:1169 Dec. 1977.

244. Supplement to the list of classified dental materials and devices. 95:1172 Dec. 1977.

245. Revised American National Standards Institute/American Dental Association specification no. 8 for zinc phosphate cement. 96:121 Jan. 1978.

246. Certification and classification programs for dental materials and devices. List of certified dental materials and devices, revised to Jan 1, 1978. 96:124 Jan. 1978.

247. Supplement to the list of certified dental materials and devices. 96:310 Feb. 1978.

248. Supplement to the list of classified dental materials and devices. 96:310 Feb. 1978.

249. List of products evaluated by the Council on Dental Materials and Devices and the Council on Dental Therapeutics. 96:354 Feb. 1978.

250. Recommendations in radiographic practices—March 1978. 96:485 March 1978.

251. Recommendations in dental mercury hygiene—March 1978. 96:487 March 1978.

252. Supplement to the list of certified dental materials and devices. 96:489 March 1978.

253. Supplement to the list of classified dental materials and devices. 96:490 March 1978.

254. Supplement to the list of certified dental materials and devices. 96:666 April 1978.

255. Supplement to the list of classified dental materials and devices. 96:667 April 1978.

256. Supplement to the list of certified dental materials and devices. 96:844 May 1978.

257. Supplement to the list of certified dental materials and devices. 96:1058 June 1978.

258. Supplement to the list of classified dental materials and devices. 96:1059 June 1978.

259. Supplement to the list of certified dental materials and devices. 97:89 July 1978.

260. Sarkar, N. K.; Fuys, R. A.; and Stanford, J. W. Corrosion and microstructure of progold. J. Prosthet. Dent. 40:50 July 1978.

261. Nuckles, D. B. Status report on rotary diamond instruments. 97:233 Aug. 1978 (Council-sponsored report).

262. New American National Standards Institute/American Dental Association specification no. 34 for dental aspirating syringes. 97:236 Aug. 1978.

263. Supplement to the list of certified dental materials and devices. 97:238 Aug. 1978.

264. Myers, G. E. Do's and don'ts for three dental luting cements. 97:502 Sept. 1978 (Council-sponsored report).

265. Gwinnett, A. J., Status report on acid etching procedures. 97:505 Sept. 1978 (Council-sponsored report).

266. Supplement to the list of classified dental materials and devices. 97:509 Sept. 1978.

267. Supplement to the list of certified dental materials and devices. 97:509 Sept. 1978.

268. Infection control in the dental office. 97:673 Oct. 1978.

269. Supplement to the list of certified dental materials and devices. 97:693 Oct. 1978.

270. Supplement to the list of classified dental materials and devices. 97:693 Oct. 1978.

271. Supplement to the list of certified dental materials and devices. 97:860 Nov. 1978.

272. Supplement to the list of classified dental materials and devices. 97:860 Nov. 1978.

273. Sarkar, N. K. Creep, corrosion and marginal fracture of dental amalgams. J. Oral Rehab. 5:413 Oct. 1978.

274. Partially prefabricated dentures. 98:268 Feb. 1979.

275. Certification and classification programs for dental materials and devices. List of certified dental materials and devices, revised to Jan. 1, 1979. 98:272 Feb. 1979.

276. Sarkar, N. K.; Fuys, R. A.; and Stanford, J. W. The chloride corrosion of low-gold casting alloys. J. Dent. Res. 58:568 Feb. 1979.

277. Schnitman, P. A., and Shulman, L. B. Recommendations of the consensus development conference on dental implants. 98:373 March 1979.

278. Expansion of the acceptance program for dental materials and devices: rotary-powered devices for removal of plaque or stain. 98:436 March 1979.

279. Supplement to the list of certified dental materials and devices. 98:605 April 1979.

280. Supplement to the list of certified dental materials and devices. 98:758 May 1979.

281. Supplement to the list of classified dental materials and devices. 98:758 May 1979.

282. X-Rays—Council prepares answers to patient questions prompted by Three Mile Island. ADA News May 28, 1979.

283. American National Standards Institute/ American Dental Association specification no. 52 for uranium content in dental porcelain and porcelain teeth. 98:755 May 1979.

284. Supplement to the list of certified dental materials and devices. 98:999 June 1979.

285. Supplement to the list of classified dental materials and devices. 98:999 June 1979.

286. Sarkar, N. K.; Fuys, R. A.; and Stanford, J. W. The chloride corrosion behavior of silver base casting alloys. J. Dent. Res. 58:1572 June 1979.

287. Acceptance program for dental materials and devices. 99:85 July 1979.

288. McLean, J. W. Status report on the glass ionomer cements. 99:221 Aug. 1979 (Council-sponsored report).

289. Supplement to the list of certified dental materials and devices. 99:506 Sept. 1979.

290. Supplement to the list of classified dental materials and devices. 99:507 Sept. 1979.

291. American National Standards Institute/ American Dental Association Document No. 41 for recommended standard practices for biological evaluation of dental materials. 99:697 Oct. 1979.

292. Supplement to the list of certified dental materials and devices. 99:866 Nov. 1979.

293. Supplement to the list of classified dental materials and devices. 99:866 Nov. 1979.

294. Supplement to the list of certified dental materials and devices. 99:866 Nov. 1979.

295. Supplement to the list of classified dental materials and devices. 99:1051 Dec. 1979.

296. Application of electrochemical techniques to characterize the corrosion of dental alloys. Special technical publication 684. American Society for Testing and Materials, Philadelphia, 1979.

297. Expansion of the acceptance program for dental materials and devices: orthodontic brackets. 100:97 Jan. 1980.

298. Supplement to the list of certified dental materials, instruments and equipment. 100:99 Jan. 1980.

299. Gettleman, L. Status report on low-gold-content alloys for fixed prosthesis. 100:237 Feb. 1980 (Council sponsored report).

300. Council reevaluates position on dental endosseous implants. 100:247 Feb. 1980.

301. Addendum to American National Standards Institute/American Dental Association specification no. 1 for alloy for dental amalgam. 100:246 Feb. 1980.

302. Supplement to the list of certified dental materials, instruments and equipment. 100:247 Feb. 1980.

303. Supplement to the list of certified dental materials, instruments and equipment. 100:409 March 1980.

304. American National Standards Institute/ American Dental Association specification no. 44 for dental electrosurgical equipment. 100:410 March 1980.

305. Supplement to the list of certified dental materials, instruments and equipment. 100:577 April 1980.

306. Blatterfein, L. Prevention of problems with removable partial dentures. 100:919 June 1980 (Council-sponsored report).

307. Supplement to the list of certified dental materials, instruments and equipment. 100:925 June 1980.

308. Council position on nitrous oxide scavenging and monitoring devices. 101:62 July 1980.

309. Certification and acceptance programs for dental materials, instruments and equipment. Changes in the list of certified dental materials and devices, since Jan. 1, 1979. 101:68 July 1980.

310. Certification and acceptance programs for dental materials, instruments and equipment. Changes in the list of classified materials and devices since Jan. 1, 1979. 101:70 July 1980.

311. Supplement to the list of certified dental materials, instruments and equipment. 101:306 Aug. 1980.

312. Supplement to the list of classified dental materials, instruments and equipment. 101:306 Aug. 1980.

THE INTERNATIONAL SYSTEM OF UNITS

This system will gradually replace the present U.S. and British customary units. This can be accomplished by mutual agreement of all the major countries of the world. It is the hope that modern metric system (SI) which derives its name from Systeme Internationale d'Unites, will gradually become common knowledge to the U.S.A. readers and help to make all reports and numerical data readily knowledgeable to readers regardless of their origin. In the dental materials area this is especially important because of the fast expanding development of international specifications.

A few basic facts are outlined below to orient and help the reader to visualize the application of the SI to materials. The SI or metric system consists of six base units, two supplementary units, and a series of derived units. Also a series of approved prefixes for formation of multiples and submultiples of these units.

It is suggested that the ASTM Metric Practice Guide, National Bureau of Standards Handbook 102, issued March 10, 1967, price 40 cents, U.S. Government Printing Office, Washington D.C. 20402, gives a concise, useful description of the SI system and how it can be used.

Table I.
The Basic Units

Quantity	Unit	SI Symbol
Length	meter	m
mass	kilogram	Kg
time	second	s
electric current	ampere	A
thermodynamic temperature	degree Kelvin	°K
luminous intensity	candela	cd

Table II.
Multiple and Submultiple Units

Multiplication Factor	Prefix	SI Symbol
10^{12}	tera	T
10^9	giga	G
10^6	mega	M
10^3	kilo	k
10^2	hecto	h
10^1	deka	da
10^{-1}	deci	d
10^{-2}	centi	c
10^{-3}	milli	m
10^{-6}	micro	μ

ABBREVIATIONS

ABBREVIATIONS—terms

ADA	American Dental Association	FDA	Food and Drug Administration
ANSC	American National Standards Committee	FDI	Fédération Dentaire Internationale
		IADR	International Association for Dental Research
ANSI	American National Standards Institute	ISO	International Organization for Standardization
ASTM	American Society for Testing and Materials		
		RHN	Rockwell hardness number
CDMIE	Council on Dental Materials, Instruments and Equipment	SI	The International System of Units
		USP	United States Pharmacopeia
CP	chemically pure	USASI	United States of America Standards Institute
DMG	Dental Materials Group		
EBA	ethoxybenzoic acid		

ABBREVIATIONS—weights, measurements, symbols

A	Angstrom unit, 10^{-8} centimeters	hr	hour
avdp	avoirdupois	in	inch
cm	centimeter	id	inside diameter
cm/cm	centimeter per centimeter	kg	kilogram
cm/min	centimeter per minute	kg/cm²	kilograms per square centimeter
deg	degree	kg/min	kilograms per minute
°C	degree Celsius (centigrade)	max	maximum
°C/min	degree Celsius (centigrade) per minute	m	meter
		μm	micrometer
°F	degree Fahrenheit	μm/cm	micrometers per centimeter
gal	gallon	mg	milligram
g	gram	mg/cm²	milligrams per square centimeter
g/cm²	grams per square centimeter	min	minimum

ml	milliliter	ppm/°C	parts per million per degree Celsius (centigrade)
mm	millimeter		
MN	meganewton	π	pi, 3.1416
MN/m²	meganewton per square meter	psi	pounds per square inch
MPa	megaPascal	R	roentgen
N	newton	rh	relative humidity
N/min	newton per minute	rpm	revolutions per minute
N/m²	newton per square meter	rps	revolutions per second
nm	nanometer	sec	second
oz	ounce	sq	square
od	outside diameter	sq cm	square centimeter
Pa	pascal	wt	weight
ppm	parts per million		

CONVERSION TABLES

Wherever practicable the modern metric system of weights and measures will be used in the *Dentist's Desk Reference*. The following conversion tables will aid the reader in evaluating data in units other than those given in the text.

Additional conversion tables may be found in "Units of Weights and Measure. Definitions and Tables of Equivalents." U.S. Department of Commerce, National Bureau of Standards. Miscellaneous publication M233, 1960.

Table I. Mass

| | | Ounces | | Pounds | | |
| | | Avoirdupois | Troy and apothecary | Avoirdupois | Troy and apothecary | |
Grams	Kilograms	Avoirdupois	apothecary	Avoirdupois	apothecary	Grains
1	0.001	0.03527	0.03215	0.002205	0.002679	15.432
1000	1	35.274	32.151	2.2046	2.679	15432.4
28.349	0.028349	1	0.91146	0.0625	0.07596	437.5
31.103	0.031103	1.0971	1	0.068571	0.08333	480
453.59	0.45359	16	14.583	1	1.2153	7000
373.24	0.37324	13.166	12	0.8229	1	5760
0.06480	0.00006480	0.002285	0.002083	0.0001428	0.0001736	1

Table II. Length

Meter	Millimeter	Inches	Feet
1	1000	39.37	3.28
0.001	1	0.03937	0.00328
0.0254	25.4	1	0.0833
0.3048	304.8	12	1

Table III. Area

Square Meter	Square Millimeter	Square Centimeter	Square Inches
1	1000000	10000	1550
0.000001	1	0.01	0.00155
0.0001	100	1	0.155
0.0006452	645.2	6.45	1

Table IV. Pressure

Meganewtons per square meter	Kilograms per square centimeter	Pounds per square inch
1	10.2	145
0.09807	1	14.223
0.006895	0.0703	1

Table V. Density

Grams per cubic centimeter	Pounds per cubic foot
1	62.428
0.01602	1

Table VI. Capacity—Liquid Measure

Minims	Fluid ounces	Milliliters
1	0.002083	0.06161
480	1	29.5729
16.2311	0.033814	1

Table VII. Thermometer scales

Temperature Fahrenheit (°F.) = (9/5 temperature Celsius) +32°

Temperature Celsius (°C.) = 5/9 (temperature Fahrenheit −32°)

or

(°C. × 1.8) + 32° = °F.

$$\frac{°F. - 32°}{1.8} = °C.$$

Table VIII. SI Units
(Systeme International d'Unites)

to convert	to	multiply by
Kg/cm^2	MN/m^2	0.09807
Kg/mm^2	MN/m^2	9.807
PSI	MN/m^2	0.006895
Kg-force	Newton	9.807
Pound-force	Newton	4.448
Poundal	Newton	0.13826

American Dental Association
Council on Dental Materials, Instruments and Equipment
211 E. Chicago Ave.
Chicago, IL 60611

Complaint Report

1. Specific complaint, defect, or malfunction _____

_____

_____

_____

2. Identification of item _____

_____

_____

_____

3. Source of supply _____

_____

_____

_____

4. Name and address of dentist reporting _____

_____

_____

_____

INDEX TO MANUFACTURERS
AND DISTRIBUTORS

AALBA-DENT, INC.
P.O. Box 5498, Walnut Creek, CA 94596
 dental base metal alloy.

THE ABACUS GROUP, INC.
7441 W. Ridgewood Drive, Parma, OH 44129
 radiographic equipment.

ACCURATE SET, INC.
Dental Manufacturers
10 Mil Street, Paterson, NJ 07501
 dental impression material; denture base resin; denture cold curing repair resin.

ACCUTRON, INC.
2338 West Royal Palm Road, Suite E
Phoenix, AZ 85021
 inhalation sedation equipment.

A-DEC, INC.
P.O. Box 111, 2601 Crestview Drive, Newburg, OR 97321
 dental handpieces; operatory equipment; periodontal instruments.

J. ADERER, INCORPORATED
21-25 - 44th Avenue, Long Island City, NY 11101
 articulators; dental casting gold alloy; dental wrought wire alloy.

AIR TECHNIQUES, INC.
70 Cantiaque Rock Road, Hicksville, NY 11801
 dental operatory equipment; radiographic accessories.

ALGER EQUIPMENT CO., INC.
301 Conroe Drive, P.O. Box 481, Conroe, TX 77301
 dental operatory equipment.

ALLEN DYNAMICS
289 Third Avenue, New York, NY 10010
 dental chromium-cobalt casting alloy.

ALMORE INTERNATIONAL COMPANY
P.O. Box 25214, Portland, OR 97225
 articulators.

AMCO
212 N. 21st Street, Philadelphia, PA 19103
 dental restorative resin.

AMERICAN CONSOLIDATED
MANUFACTURING CO., INC.
212 North 21st Street, Philadelphia, PA 19103
 dental restorative resin.

AMERICAN DENTAL MANUFACTURING
COMPANY
P.O. Box 4546, Missoula, MT 59806
 composite resin instruments; dental amalgam instruments; dental cast restoration instruments; dental restorative instruments; dental surgical instruments; gold foil annealing instruments; periodontal instruments; radiographic accessories.

AMERICAN GOLD CO.
221 N. Westmoreland, Los Angeles, CA 90004
 dental casting gold alloy.

AMERICAN STERILIZER COMPANY
2425 W. 23rd Street, Erie, PA 16512
 dental sterilizers.

AMERICAN TOOTH MANUFACTURING
COMPANY
2623 Saddle Avenue, Oxnard, CA 93030
 acrylic resin teeth.

ANDERSON PRODUCTS, INC.
 dental sterilizers.

ASSOCIATED MERCURY PRODUCTS
9412 Irondale Avenue, Chatsworth, CA 91311
 dental mercury.

ASTRA PHARMACEUTICAL PRODUCTS, INC.
Pleasant Street Connector, P.O. Box 1089
Framingham, MA 01701
  local anesthetic equipment.

ASTRON DENTAL CORPORATION
280 Holbrook Drive, Wheeling, IL 60090
  denture base polymer.

**BAKER DENTAL DIVISION OF ENGELHARD
INDUSTRIES DIVISION OF ENGELHARD
MINERALS AND CHEMICAL CORPORATION**
700 Blair Road, Carteret, NJ 07008
  dental amalgam; dental casting gold alloy; dental
  mercury; dental wrought gold wire alloy.

E. A. BECK & COMPANY
657 W. 19th Street, Costa Mesa, CA 92627
  dental amalgam instruments; dental cast restorative
  instruments; dental plastic instruments; dental restorative instruments; dental surgical instruments; endodontic instruments; gold foil malleting device; orthodontic instruments; periodontal instruments.

**BELL FEDERAL LABORATORY, DIVISION OF
MILLER DENTAL MANUFACTURING, INC.**
34-38 Bell Blvd., Bayside, NY 11361
  denture cleaners.

BELMONT EQUIPMENT COMPANY
One Belmont Drive, Somerset, NJ 08873
  radiographic equipment.

BELMONT METALS
  dental mercury.

BETHLEHEM APPARATUS COMPANY, INC.
  dental mercury.

B & L DENTAL COMPANY, INC.
135-24 Hillside Avenue, Richmond Hill, NY 11418
  dental repair resin; denture base polymer; denture reliner.

BLOCK DRUG COMPANY, INC.
105 Academy Street, Jersey City, NJ 07302
  denture adherents; denture cleaners; oral hygiene
  aids.

BOEKEL CORPORATION
  dental sterilizers.

HARRY J. BOSWORTH COMPANY
7227 North Hamlin Avenue, Skokie, IL 60076
  amalgamators; dental cements; dental impression material.

BRANDT INDUSTRIES
4461 Bronx Blvd., Bronx, NY 10470
  dental operatory equipment.

BRASSELER USA, INC.
800 King George Blvd., Savannah, GA 31405
  dental burs.

BRUNO POZZI DENTAL PRODUCTS
306 Cactus Drive, Oxnard, CA 93030
  acrylic resin teeth.

**BUFFALO DENTAL MANUFACTURING
COMPANY**
2911-23 Atlantic Avenue, Brooklyn, NY 12207
  chromium-cobalt casting alloy; dental impression material.

JOHN O. BUTLER COMPANY
4635 W. Foster, Chicago, IL 60630
  dental mirrors; oral hygiene aids.

W. H. BYRON
Church Street, Kingston, NH 03848
  dental cements; dental restorative resins.

CADCO
8890 Regent Street, Los Angeles, CA 90034
  dental impression material.

CAMERON-MILLER, INC.
3949 S. Racine Avenue, Chicago, IL 60609
  dental electrosurgical equipment; dental operatory
  equipment.

**THE L. D. CAULK COMPANY, DIVISION OF
DENTSPLY INTERNATIONAL, INC.**
P.O. 359, Milford, DE 19963
  cavity liners; composite resin instruments; dental
  amalgam; dental amalgam instruments; dental cements; dental impression materials; dental gypsum
  products; dental mercury; dental preformed crowns;
  dental restorative resin; dental waxes; denture base
  polymer; denture reliners; denture repair resin; endodontic materials; oral hygiene aids; orthodontic appliances; pit and fissure sealant; precision attachments;
  prosthodontic instruments.

CAVITRON CORPORATION
1350 Avenue of the Americas, 18th Floor
New York, NY 10019
  dental electrosurgical equipment; dental operatory
  equipment.

CENTRIX INC.
480 Sniffens Lane, Stratford, CT 06497
  local anesthetic equipment.

CERAMCO, INC.
Division of Johnson & Johnson
20 Lake Drive, East Windsor, NJ 08520
  dental base metal alloy; dental casting gold alloy; dental gypsum products; dental porcelain; dental resins.

CETYLITE INDUSTRIAL, INC.
9051 River Road, Pennsauken, NJ 08110
  cavity varnish.

CHARLES DEVELOPMENT CO.
P.O. Box 23620, 1109 N.E. 34th Court
Oakland Park, FL 33334
  articulators; dental porcelain; dental restorative resin;
  precision attachments.

CHEMTRON DENTAL PRODUCTS
1801 Lilly Avenue, St. Louis, MO 63110
  inhalation sedation equipment.

CHICO DENTAL SPECIALTIES
P.O. Box 1329, Chico, CA 95926
  dental amalgam.

CODESCO, INC.
1234 Market Street, Philadelphia, PA 19107
  dental casting gold alloy; dental impression material;
  denture base resin.

COE LABORATORIES, INC.
3737 West 127th Street, Chicago, IL 60658
  dental duplicating material; dental gypsum products;
  dental impression material; denture base polymer;
  denture cold curing repair resin; denture reliner.

COLUMBIA DENTOFORM CORPORATION
49 E. 21st Street, New York, NY 10010
  precision attachments; prosthodontic instruments.

COLUMBUS DENTAL CO.
634 Wager St., Columbia, OH 43206
  dental flux; dental porcelain; periodontal instruments.

THE COLWELL, INC.
267 Kenyon Rd., Champaign, IL 61820
  dental amalgam.

COOK-WAITE LABORATORIES, INC.
90 Park Avenue, New York, NY 10016
  local anesthetic equipment.

COREGA CHEMICAL COMPANY
  denture adherents.

COX SYSTEMS LIMITED
333 Arvin Avenue
Stoney Creek, Ont., Canada L8E 2M7 3000-3008
  dental operatory equipment.

**CRESCENT DENTAL MANUFACTURING
COMPANY**
7750 W. 47th Street, Lyons, IL 60534
  amalgamator; articulators; crown removers; dental
  amalgam; prosthodontic instruments.

CUTTER LABORATORIES
4th and Parker Streets, Berkeley, CA 94710
  dental impression material.

DARBY DENTAL SUPPLY CO.
100 Banks Avenue, Rockville Centre, NY 11570
  dental amalgam.

DEGUSSA, INC.
181 W. Orangethorpe Avenue Ste. E
Placentia, CA 92670
  dental casting gold alloy.

DEL-TUBE CORPORATION
2360 W. Florist Street, Milwaukee, WI 53209
  dental operatory equipment.

DENAR CORPORATION
1660 S. State College Blvd., Anaheim, CA 92806
  articulators.

DEN-MAT, INC.
P. O. Box 1729, Santa Maria, CA 93456
  dental amalgam instruments; dental cements; dental
  repair resin; dental restorative resin; diamonds; oral
  hygiene aids; orthodontic appliances.

DENSERTS
  dental implants.

DENTAL CORPORATION OF AMERICA
1592 Rockville Pike, Rockville, MD 20852
  dental film duplicator; dental operatory equipment;
  dental x-ray film.

DEN-TAL-EZ MANUFACTURING CO.
1201 S.E. Diehl Avenue, Des Moines, IA 50315
  dental operatory equipment; dental gypsum products;
  denture base polymer; periodontal instruments.

DENTAL/MEDICAL, INC.
  dental operatory equipment.

DENTAL PLASTICS & PRODUCTS CO.
6117 Elm Street, P.O. Box 894
Kansas City, MO 64141
  prosthodontic instruments.

**AMERICAN DENTICON
AMERICAN HOSPITAL SUPPLY CO.**
2020 Ridge, Evanston, IL 60201
  chromium-cobalt casting alloy.

DENTONAMICS CORPORATION
2835 "G" Street, Merced, CA 95340
  articulators.

DENTOOL CO., INC.
224 Sanders Avenue, Somerset, NJ 08873
  endodontic instruments.

DENTORIUM PRODUCTS COMPANY, INC.
153 West 15th Street, New York, NY 10011
  acrylic resin teeth; chromium-cobalt casting alloy.

DENTSPLY INTERNATIONAL, INC.
500 West College Ave., York, PA 17404
  acrylic resin teeth; articulator; dental airator; dental
  base metal alloy; dental base plate wax; dental gypsum products; dental handpiece; dental operatory
  equipment; dental porcelain; dental resin; dental waxes;
  denture base polymer; periodontal instruments.

DIAMOND PRECISION TOOLS, LTD.
4819-13th Ave., Suite 201-2, Brooklyn, NY 11219
  diamonds.

DIRECT DENTAL SALES & SUPPLIES, INC.
2640 Golf Road, Glenview, IL 60025
  dental casting gold alloy.

DORIC CORPORATION
7215 Convoy Court, San Diego,CA 92111
    dental cements; dental impression material; dental mercury.

DRI-CLAVE
DIVISION OF COLUMBUS DENTAL
634 Wager Street, Columbus, OH 43206
    dental sterilizers.

DUPACO, INC.
1740 La Costa Meadow Drive, P.O. Box 98
San Marcos, CA 82069
    inhalation sedation equipment.

EASTERN SMELTING & REFINING CORPORATION
37-39 Bubier Street, Lynn, MA 09103
    dental mercury.

EASTMAN KODAK COMPANY
343 State Street, Rochester, NY 14650
    dental x-ray film; duplicating film; film processing chemicals; radiographic accessories.

EDUCATIONAL HEALTH PRODUCTS, INC.
221 Mill Road, New Canaan, CT 06840
    oral hygiene aids.

ELLMAN DENTAL MANUFACTURING CO.
1135 Railroad Avenue, Hewlett, L.I., NY 11557
    dental electrosurgical equipment.

WALLACE A. ERICKSON
    dental restorative resin.

ESPE DENTAL PRODUCTS CORPORATION
338 Ocean Avenue, Lynnbrook, NY 11596
    dental impression material; dental restorative resin.

E-Z FLOSS CO.
P.O. Box 954, Palm Springs, CA 92262
    oral hygiene aids.

FEDERAL PROSTHETICS, INC.
15 Parkville Avenue, Brooklyn, NY 11230
    chromium-cobalt casting alloy.

FLOSS AID CORPORATION
P.O. Box 624, 365 Mathew Street
Santa Clara, CA 95052
    oral hygiene aids.

FRANKLIN DISTRIBUTING CORPORATION
    radiographic accessories.

G-C INTERNATIONAL CORPORATION
8096 North 85th Way,Scottsville, AZ 85258
    dental cements.

GENERAL ELECTRIC COMPANY
DENTAL SYSTEMS DIVISION
P.O. Box 414, Milwaukee, WI 53201
    powered toothbrush; radiographic equipment and accessories.

GENERAL REFINERIES, INC.
7227 N. Hamlin Avenue, Skokie, IL 60076
    dental amalgam; dental casting gold alloy; dental mercury; dental wrought wire alloy.

GIRARD, INC.
1974 Ohio Street, Lisle, IL 60532
    periodontal instruments.

D. F. GOLDSMITH CHEMICAL & METALS CORPORATION
909 Pitner Avenue, Evanston, IL 60202
    dental mercury.

GREAT LAKES ORTHODONTIC PRODUCTS
1550 Hertel Avenue, Buffalo, NY 14216
    dental handpiece; dental operatory equipment; orthodontic instruments.

GREENE DENTAL PRODUCTS, INC.
90 Park Avenue, New York, NY 10016
    radiographic accessories.

GRETACOR DEVICES, INC./
TEXELL PRODUCTS CO.
1228 N. 1st, El Cajon, CA 92021
    oral hygiene aids.

HAMMOND DENTAL MANUFACTURING COMPANY
4496 Industrial Street, Simi Valley, CA 93063
    dental amalgam; dental mercury.

HANAU ENGINEERING CO.
80 Sonwil Drive, P.O. Box 203, Buffalo, NY 14225
    amalgamator; articulators.

HANTROL CORPORATION
22 Orchard Drive, Woodbury, NY 11797
    dental operatory equipment.

HARPER BUFFING MACHINE CO.
363 Ellington Road, East Hartford, CT 06108
    finishing and polishing instruments

HAUSER & MILLER
4011 Forest Park Boulevard, St. Louis, MO 63108
    dental amalgam.

JAY E. HEALEY COMPANY
688-690 South 16th Street, Newark, NJ 07103
    dental gypsum products; dental impression material.

HEALTH CARE TECHNOLOGY, INC.
3798 Mosswood Drive, Lafayette, CA 94549
    nitrous oxide scavenging equipment.

HEALTHCO, INC.
24 Stuart Street, Boston, MA 02116
    composite resin instruments; dental amalgam; dental amalgam instruments; dental cast restorative instruments; dental cements; dental handpieces; dental mercury; dental operatory equipment; dental restorative instruments; dental restorative resins; dental surgical instruments; denture base resin; endodontic instruments; endodontic materials; local anesthetic equipment; oral hygiene aids; precision attachments; prosthodontic instruments; radiographic accessories.

HEALTH SCIENCE PRODUCTS, INC.
2429 26th Street North, P.O. Box 5545
Birmingham, AL 35207
    dental operatory equipment.

HEREAUS DENTAL GOLD CORPORATION
18 East 16th Street, New York, NY 10003
    dental casting gold alloy.

HIGHLANDER ELECTRICAL SUPPLY
24000 Highlander Road, Canoga Park, CA 91304
    dental mercury.

HOWMEDICA, INC.
DENTAL DIVISION
5101 South Keeler Avenue, Chicago, IL 60632
    chromium-cobalt casting alloy; dental base metal al-
    loy; dental casting gold alloy; dental wrought wire
    alloy; denture base polymer.

HOYT LABORATORIES
633 Highland Avenue, Needham, MA 02194
    dental restorative resin; denture adherent.

HU-FRIEDY
3232 N. Rockwell Street, Chicago IL 60618
    dental amalgam instruments; dental cast restorative
    instruments; dental plastic instruments; dental
    restorative instruments; dental surgical instruments;
    endodontic instruments; periodontal instrument.

THE HYGIENIC DENTAL MANUFACTURING
COMPANY
1245 Home Avenue, Akron, OH 44310
    dental waxes; denture base polymer; denture cold cur-
    ing repair resin.

ILGS
P.O. Box 64, Mount Prospect, IL 60056
    dental casting gold alloy.

IMEX TRADING CO.
    dental amalgam.

INNOVATORS, INC.
2721 Industrial Drive, Jefferson City, MO 65101
    dental surgical instruments; radiographic accessories.

INTERNATIONAL DENTAL PRODUCTS, INC.
P.O. Box 55, Richmond Hill, NY 11418
    dental impression material; denture base polymer;
    denture repair resin.

IVORY EASTERN INSTRUMENTS, INC.
6019 Keystone Street, Philadelphia, PA 19135
    dental amalgam instruments; dental restorative in-
    struments; plastic instruments.

J. F. JELENKO & COMPANY
PENNWALT CORPORATION
99 Business Park Drive, Armonk, NY 10504
    chromium-cobalt casting alloy; dental base metal al-
    loy; dental casting gold alloy; dental gypsum products;
    dental wrought gold wire alloy.

JELINEK ALLOYS DIVISION, I. STERN
PRODUCTS CORPORATION
43-30 22nd Street, Long Island City, NY 11101
    dental amalgam.

JENSEN INDUSTRIES, INC.
417 Washington Avenue, North Haven, CT 06473
    dental casting gold alloy.

JOHNSON & JOHNSON DENTAL
PRODUCTS DIVISION
20 Lake Drive, East Windsor, NJ 08520
    dental amalgam; dental base metal alloy; dental op-
    eratory equipment; dental restorative instruments;
    dental restorative resin; endodontic materials; oral
    hygiene aids; pit and fissure sealant.

H. D. JUSTI COMPANY, DIVISION OF
WILLIAMS GOLD REFINING COMPANY, INC.
32nd and Spring Garden Streets
Philadelphia, PA 19104
    acrylic resin teeth; amalgamators; cavity varnish;
    dental cements; dental impression material; dental
    mercury; dental porcelain; dental resin; finishing and
    polishing instruments; plastic instruments; prostho-
    dontic instruments.

KENSON MANUFACTURING COMPANY
90 Hamilton Street, Cambridge, MA 02139
    acrylic resin teeth; dental porcelain.

KERR MANUFACTURING COMPANY
DIVISION OF SYBRON CORPORATION
28200 Wick Road, P.O.Box 455, Romulus, MI 48174
    amalgamators; cavity liners; dental amalgam; dental
    cast restorative instruments; dental cements; dental
    gypsum products; dental impression material; dental
    restorative instruments; dental restorative resins;
    dental waxes; denture base polymer; denture cold
    curing repair resin; denture reliner; endodontic in-
    struments; endodontic materials; pit and fissure seal-
    ant; prosthodontic instruments.

F & F KOENIGKRAMER
DIVISION OF DENTSPLY INTERNATIONAL
96 Caldwell Drive, Cincinnati, OH 45216
    dental operatory equipment.

LACTONA PRODUCTS DIVISION
WARNER-LAMBERT COMPANY
201 Tabor Road, Morris Plains, NJ 07950
    acrylic resin teeth; dental duplicating material; dental
    gypsum products; dental impression material; dental
    operatory equipment; dental resin; denture adherents;
    matrix bands; oral hygiene aids; preformed crowns;
    prosthodontic instruments.

LANG DENTAL MANUFACTURING
COMPANY
900 N. Franklin St., Chicago, IL 60610
    dental amalgam; dental impression material; denture
    base polymer.

LEE PHARMACEUTICALS
1444 Santa Anita Avenue, P.O. Box 3836
South El Monte, CA 91733
  composite restorative material; dental amalgam; dental forceps; dental impression material; diamonds; orthodontic appliances; pit and fissure sealant.

LEFF DENTAL GOLDS, INC.
70-17 51st Avenue, Woodside, NY 11377
  dental casting gold alloy.

LIBRA GOLD COMPANY
1419 Quaker Lane, Wheeling, IL 60090
  dental casting gold alloy.

LINCOLN DENTAL SUPPLY COMPANY
1617 Wood Street, Philadelphia, PA 19103
  acrylic resin teeth; dental amalgam.

LITTON DENTAL PRODUCTS, INC.
LITTON INDUSTRIES
3035 Moffet Drive, P.O. Box 7266, Toledo, OH 43615
  periodontal instruments.

THE LORVIC CORPORATION
8810 Frost Avenue, St. Louis, MO 63134
  dental cements; dental mirrors; dental operatory equipment; dental restorative resin; dental sterilization equipment; oral hygiene aids.

3M COMPANY
3M Center, St. Paul, MN 55101
  cavity liners; composite placing instruments; composite restorative resin; dental cements; dental operatory equipment; dental restorative resin; dental sterilization equipment; finishing and polishing instruments; orthodontic appliances; pit and fissure sealant; preformed crowns.

MACAN ENGINEERING CO.
1564 North Damen, Chicago, IL 60622
  dental electrosurgical equipment.

MALLINCKRODT CHEMICAL WORKS
Second and Mallinckrodt Streets, St. Louis, MO 63160
  dental mercury.

MASTERSONICS
12877 Industrial Drive, Granger, IN 46530
  periodontal instruments.

ISAAC MAZEL COMPANY
3021 Darnell Road, Philadelphia, PA 19154
  radiographic accessories.

McKESSON CO.
P.O. Box 10668, North Charleston, SC 29411
  inhalation sedation equipment.

MDT CORPORATION
Suite B200, 19401 S. Vermont, Torrance, CA 90502
  dental operatory equipment; dental sterilizers; local anesthetic equipment; periodontal instruments.

MERCURY DISTRIBUTORS, INC.
14028 Almeda Road, P.O. Box 45480, Houston, TX 77045
  dental mercury.

MID-AMERICA DENTAL PRODUCTS
901 West Oakton, Des Plaines, IL 60018
  dental restorative resin.

MID-WEST AMERICAN
901 W. Oakton, Des Plaines, IL 60008
  dental excavating burs; endodontic instruments; endodontic materials.

MILTEX INSTRUMENTS COMPANY
DIVISION OF E. MILTENBERG, INC.
6 Ohio Drive, Lake Success, NY 11042
  composite resin instruments; dental amalgam instruments; dental burs; dental cast restorative instruments; dental handpiece; dental restorative instruments; dental surgical instruments; diamonds; finishing and polishing instruments; orthodontic instruments; periodontal instruments; prosthodontic instruments.

MINIMAX COMPANY
17 West 60th Street, New York, NY 10023
  dental amalgam.

MIRADENT CORPORATION
9 Ungara Drive, New York, NY 10956
  dental impression material.

MIZZY, INC.
P.O. Box 631, Clifton Forge, VA 24422
  cavity liner; dental burs; dental cements; dental impression material; dental waxes; finishing and polishing instruments; local anesthetic equipment.

MODERN MATERIALS MANUFACTURING CO.; DIVISION OF COLUMBUS DENTAL
634 Wagner Street, Columbus, OH 43206
  dental gypsum products; dental impression material; dental waxes; denture base resin; prosthodontic instruments.

MONOJECT
1831 Olive Street, St. Louis, MO 63103
  dental operatory equipment; endodontic syringe; local anesthetic equipment; prosthodontic instruments.

MOSER DENTAL MANUFACTURING COMPANY
P.O. Box 1505, Chico, CA 95926
  dental amalgam; dental mercury.

THE MOTLOID COMPANY
325 West Huron Street, Chicago, IL 60610
  denture base polymer.

W. E. MOWREY COMPANY
1435 University Avenue, St. Paul, MN 55104
  dental casting gold alloy; dental mercury; dental wrought wire alloy.

MOYCO INDUSTRIES, INC.
S.E. Cor. 21st & Clearfield, Philadelphia, PA 19132
cavity liner; dental amalgam; dental cements; dental mercury; dental waxes; denture adherents; denture base resin; denture cold curing repair resin; endodontic materials.

MYERSON TOOTH CORPORATION
90 Hamilton Street, Cambridge, MA 02139
acrylic resin teeth; dental porcelain.

NARCO/McKESSON
7513 Spartan Blvd. East, North Charleston, SC 29411
dental operatory equipment; nitrous oxide scavenging equipment.

NATIONAL APPLIANCES CO.
Portland, OR 97223
dental sterilizers.

NEOLOY PRODUCTS, INC.
14807 McKinley, Posen, IL 60469
chromium-cobalt casting alloy.

THE J. M. NEY COMPANY
Drawer 990, Hartford, CT 06101
dental base metal alloy; dental casting gold alloy; dental gypsum products; dental porcelain; dental wrought wire alloy; finishing and polishing instruments; flux; gold foil; precision attachments; preformed crowns; prosthodontic instruments; solder.

NIRANIUM CORPORATION
34-37 11th Street, Long Island City, NY 11106
chromium-cobalt casting alloy; dental gypsum products.

NOBILIUM PRODUCTS, INC.
221 N. Westmoreland, Los Angeles, CA 90004
chromium-cobalt casting alloy.

NOBLE METALS & ALLOY CO., INC.
310 Argyle Road, Cedarhurst, NY 11516
dental base metal alloy; dental casting gold alloy.

NORTH PACIFIC DENTAL, INC.
13723 100th N.E., P.O. Box 522, Kirkland, WA 98033
dental bur blocks; dental operatory equipment; dental retractors; local anesthetic equipment

NORTHWEST ORTHODONTICS
P.O. Box 7164, Seattle, WA 98133
orthodontic appliances.

NPD DENTAL SYSTEMS, INC.
3 Huntington Quadrangle #2N11, Melville, NJ 11746
endodontic materials; endodontic syringe; irrigating needle.

NU-DENT PORCELAIN STUDIO, INC.
Candler Building, 220 West 42nd Street
New York, NY 10036
dental impression material; dental resin.

OCEANIC CHEMICAL COMPANY, INC.
350 Brannan Street, San Francisco, CA 94107
dental mercury.

ORAL B/COOPER LABS
1259 Rte. 46, Parsippany, NJ 07054
oral hygiene aids.

ORTHOBAND CO.
P.O. Box 278, Barnhart, MO 63012
orthodontic appliances.

ORTHO CRAFT ORTHODONTIC SPECIALTY PRODUCTS
P.O. Box 771, La Jolla, CA 92038
orthodontic instruments.

PACEMAKER CORPORATION
2255 NE 194, Portland, OR 97230
oral hygiene aids.

PARKELL PRODUCTS, INC.
155 Schmitt Blvd., Farmingdale, NY 11735
dental electrosurgical equipment; inhalation sedation equipment.

PELTON & CRANE
200 Clanton Road, Box 3664, Charlotte, NC 28203
dental operatory equipment; dental sterilizers.

J. C. PENNEY COMPANY, INC.
1301 Avenue of the Americas, New York, NY 10019
powered toothbrush.

PENTRON CORPORATION
1260 Old Colony Road, P.O. Box 771
Wallingford, CT 06492
dental amalgam; dental casting gold alloy; dental gypsum products.

PFINGST & COMPANY, INC.
62 Cooper Square, New York, NY 10003
amalgamator; dental amalgam; dental impression material; dental mercury.

PHASEALLOY, INC.
1050 Greenfield Drive, El Cajon, CA 92021
dental amalgam.

PHILIPS MEDICAL SYSTEMS
102 Commerce Road, Stamford, CT 06902
radiographic equipment and accessories.

PLANMECCA OY
dental operatory equipment.

PLASTODENT, INC.
2881 Middletown, Bronx, NY 10461
dental impression material; denture base resin.

POLYMED LABORATORIES, INC.
denture adherent.

PORTA-PRO, INC.
1327 Spruce Street, Boulder, CO 80302
powered toothbrush.

PORTER INSTRUMENTS CO., INC.
P.O. Box 326, Township Line Road, Hatfield, PA 19440
inhalation sedation equipment.

PREMIER DENTAL PRODUCTS COMPANY
Romano Drive, Norristown, PA 19401
dental amalgam instruments; dental burs; dental cast restorative instruments; dental cements; dental hand-piece; dental impression material; dental restorative instruments; dental restorative resin; dental sterili-zers; diamonds; endodontic instruments; endodontic materials; finishing and polishing instruments; oral hygiene aids; prosthodontic instruments; radiographic accessories.

PREVENTIVE DENTISTRY PRODUCTS, INC.
3197-F Airport Loop Drive, Costa Mesa, CA 92626
oral hygiene aids.

PRE-VEST, INC.
23420 Lakeland Blvd., Cleveland, OH 44132
dental gypsum products; dental impression material.

PRODUCT RESEARCH LABORATORIES, INC.
90 Hamilton Street, Cambridge, MA 02139
denture base polymer.

PROFESSIONAL DISPOSABLES, INC.
150 N. MacQuestern Parkway
Mount Vernon, NY 10550
oral irrigator.

PROFESSIONAL PRODUCTS COMPANY
P.O. Box 162, San Diego, CA 92113
dental amalgam; dental impression material; dental mercury.

PROLASTIC CO., INC.
4 Chelmsford Road, Rochester, NY 14618
dental implants; denture cleaners; denture reliner; radiographic accessories.

PROMA
11610 W. Olympic Blvd., Los Angeles, CA 90064
dental operatory equipment.

PULPDENT CORPORATION OF AMERICA
75 Boylston Street, Brookline, MA 02147
cavity liner; dental amalgam instruments; dental cast restorative instruments; dental cements; dental opera-tory equipment; dental restorative instruments; den-tal sterilization equipment; dental surgical instru-ments; endodontic instruments; endodontic materials; local anesthetic equipment; periodontal instruments; prosthodontic instruments; radiographic accessories.

PURE LAB COMPANY OF AMERICA
P.O. Box 191, Norwood, MA 02062
dental amalgam; dental mercury.

QUICKSILVER PRODUCTS, INC.
350 Brannan Street, San Francisco, CA 94107
dental mercury.

J. R. RAND SPECIALTY CO., INC.
683A Glen Cove Avenue, Glen Head, NY 11545
composite resin instruments; dental amalgam instru-ments; dental cast restorative instruments; dental handpieces; dental operatory equipment; dental resto-rative instruments; dental surgical instruments; dia-monds; film processing chemicals; periodontal instru-ments; prosthodontic instruments; radiographic acces-sories.

THE RANSOM & RANDOLPH COMPANY
DIVISION OF DENTSPLY
INTERNATIONAL, INC.
P.O. Box 905, Toledo, OH 43691
chromium-cobalt casting alloy; dental amalgam in-struments; dental burs; dental duplicating material; dental gypsum products; dental impression material; dental restorative instruments; denture reliner; dia-monds; endodontic instruments; endodontic materials; finishing and polishing instruments; periodontal in-struments.

REGAL DENTAL CORPORATION
1130 North Broadway, Massapequa, NY 11758
acrylic resin teeth.

RINN CORPORATION
1212 Abbott Drive, Elgin, IL 60120
radiographic equipment.

RITTER COMPANY
DIVISION OF SYBRON CORPORATION
400 West Avenue, Rochester, NY 14611
dental sterilizers; radiographic equipment and acces-sories.

RUGBY LABORATORIES, INC.
420 Doughty Blvd., Inwood, L.I., NY 11696
dental amalgam.

Rx JENERIC GOLD COMPANY
1260 Old Colony Road, Wallingford, CT 06492
dental base metal alloy; dental burs; dental casting gold alloy; diamonds; flux; solder.

SAFCO DENTAL SUPPLY COMPANY
624 West Adams Street, Chicago, IL 60606
dental amalgam; dental mercury.

SANKO DISTRIBUTING CO.
Rte. 1 Box 80, Irvor, VA 23866
radiographic equipment.

HENRY SCHEIN DENTAL SUPPLY
39-01 170th Street, Flushing, NY 11358
dental amalgam; dental amalgam instruments; dental mercury; diamonds; finishing and polishing instru-ments.

CHARLES B. SCHWED CO.
505 Fifth Avenue, New York, NY 10017
dental cast restorative instruments; dental implants; dental porcelain; endodontic instruments; endodontic materials.

SHOFU DENTAL CORPORATION
4025 Bohannon Drive, Menlo Park, CA 94025
articulators; dental amalgam; dental cement; dental handpiece; dental mercury.

SIEMENS CORPORATION
DENTAL DIVISION
186 Wood Avenue South, Iselin, NJ 08830
dental operatory equipment; radiographic equipment and accessories.

SILVER MANUFACTURING CO.
P.O. Box E, Morton Grove, IL 60053
oral hygiene aids.

SILVERMAN'S DENTAL SUPPLY CO.
5 Apollo Road, Plymouth Meeting, PA 19462
articulators; dental amalgam.

SOLAR DENTAL CO., INC.
P.O. Box 4610, Hialeah, FL 33014
denture base resin.

SPARTAN ULTRASONICS, INC.
519 Rudder Road, Fenton, MO 63026
periodontal instruments.

SPECTRONICS COMPANY
Westbury, NY 11590
dental sterilizers.

SPEYER SMELTING & REFINING COMPANY
213 Medical-Dental Building, Seattle, WA 98101
dental amalgam; dental casting gold alloy; dental mercury.

SPICA, INC.
1171 Sonora Court, Sunnyvale, CA 94086
inhalation sedation equipment.

SQUIBB PRODUCTS COMPANY
E. R. SQUIBB & SONS, INC.
P.O. Box 4000, Princeton, NJ 08540
powered toothbrush.

STAR DENTAL MANUFACTURING CO., INC.
Valley Forge Corporate Center, P. O. Box 896, Valley Forge, PA 19482
dental amalgam; dental mercury; inhalation sedation equipment; periodontal instruments.

STEREX CORPORATION
220 Cushing Street, Stoughton, MA 02072
local anesthetic equipment.

STERI-DENT CORPORATION
37 Reith Street, Copiaque, NY 11726
dental sterilizers.

STERNDENT CORPORATION
320 Washington Street, Mount Vernon, NY 10553
dental casting gold alloy; dental gypsum products; dental impression material; dental wrought wire alloy; diamonds; finishing and polishing instruments; solder.

STERNGOLD, DIVISION OF STERNDENT
60 Viaduct Rd. Extension, Stamford, CT 06907
dental base metal alloy; dental casting gold alloy; dental implants; precision attachments.

STRATFORD-COOKSON COMPANY
2000 Sullivan Road, College Park, GA 30337
dental amalgam; dental cement; dental mercury.

C. E. STUART
Ventura, CA 93001
articulators.

SUMMIT SERVICES, INC.
535 Division Street, Campbell, CA 95008
nitrous oxide scavenging equipment.

SUPERIOR MAGNA CO.
dental gypsum products.

FRASER SWEATMAN, INC.
5490 Broadway, Lancaster, NY 14086
inhalation sedation equipment; nitrous oxide scavenging equipment.

A. SZABO, INC.
17 East 16th Street, New York, NY 10003
dental casting gold alloy.

GEORGE TAUB PRODUCTS, INC.
277 New York Avenue, Jersey City, NJ 07307
cavity liner; dental gypsum products; precision attachments.

TELEDYNE DENTAL PRODUCTS
12901 Saratoga Avenue Ste. 9, Saratoga, CA 95070
cavity liner; dental amalgam instruments; dental cement; dental duplicating material; dental impression material; dental restorative resin; denture base polymer; denture reliner; denture resin; finishing and polishing instruments; local anesthetic equipment; preformed crowns; radiographic accessories.

TEXELL PRODUCTS
3 Asbury Place, Houston, TX 77007
oral irrigator.

THIERMAN PRODUCTS, INC.
oral hygiene aids.

TICONIUM COMPANY, INC.
413 North Pearl Street, Albany, NY 12207
chromium-cobalt casting alloy; dental casting gold alloy; denture base polymer.

TIME MOTION SYSTEM CO.
Box 363 Rt. 5, River Falls, WI 54022
dental operatory equipment; dental sterilization equipment; radiographic accessories.

T-LCR LABORATORY
retainers.

TMJ INSTRUMENTS CO.
3203 W. Pendleton Street, Santa Ana, CA 92704
articulators.

N. UHLER COMPANY
1791 W. Howard Street, Chicago, IL 60626
acrylic resin teeth.

ULTRASONIC INTERNATIONAL, INC.
denture cleaners.

UNITED DENTAL SERVICE
P.O. Box 105002, Atlanta, GA 30348
articulators.

UNITEK CORPORATION
2724 South Peck Road, Monrovia, CA 91016
acrylic-vinyl copolymer denture base resins; alginate;
auxiliary materials; base metal alloys for porcelain
bonding; base metal wrought wire; composite restorative materials; crown and bridge resins; dental amalgam; dental chairs; dental handpieces; dental stools;
dental units; diamond rotary instruments; elastomeric
impression materials; engine driven root canal instruments; excavating burs; extraction forceps; finishing
and polishing instruments; fixed orthodontic appliances; fluxes; hand cutting instruments; hand scales;
instruments and devices for amalgam; instruments
and devices for cast restorations; instruments and devices for composite resins; instruments for examination; jacket crowns; orthodontic auxiliaries; orthodontic instruments; orthodontic materials; phosphate
bonded investments; plaster; porcelain teeth; precious
metal alloys for porcelain bonding; preformed crowns;
removable orthodontic appliances; root canal broaches
and rasps; root canal files and reamers; root canal
filling points; solders; stone; ultrasonic scaler.

UNIVERSAL X-RAY PRODUCTS
4014 West Grand Avenue, Chicago, IL 60651
radiographic equipment.

VACUDENT/md
471 W. 5th Street, Salt Lake City, UT 84101
radiographic equipment.

VAN R DENTAL PRODUCTS, INC.
3780 Selby Avenue, Los Angeles, CA 90034
dental impression material.

VEECO MANUFACTURING
dental operatory equipment.

VERATEX CORPORATION
18610 Fitzpatrick, Detroit, MI 48228
dental mercury.

VERIFLOW CORPORATION
250 Canal Blvd., Richmond, CA 94804
inhalation sedation equipment.

VERNITRON MEDICAL PRODUCTS
dental sterilizers.

VERNON-BENSHOFF COMPANY, INC.
SUBSIDIARY OF CMP INDUSTRIES, INC.
413 N. Pearl Street, Albany, NY 12201
dental impression material; denture base polymer.

VIVADENT
P.O. Box 1400, Buffalo, NY 14214
dental restorative resin.

MARSHALL WEINER COMPANY
1409 Samoa Way, Laguna Beach, CA 92651
dental spatulas.

WERNET DIVISION
BLOCK DRUG COMPANY, INC.
105 Academy Street, Jersey City, NJ 07302
denture adherent.

WHALEDENT INTERNATIONAL
DIVISION OF IPCO HOSPITAL SUPPLY CORP.
236 Fifth Avenue, New York, NY 10001
dental electrosurgical equipment.

WHIP MIX CORPORATION
361 Farmington Avenue, P.O. Box 17183
Louisville, KY 40217
articulators; dental duplicating material; dental gypsum products; dental impression material; dental
waxes; prosthodontic instruments.

S. S. WHITE DIVISION
PENNWALT CORPORATION
Pennwalt Building, 900 First Avenue
Philadelphia, PA 19102
amalgamator; cavity varnish; dental amalgam; dental
cement; dental impression material; dental restorative resin; radiographic equipment.

THE WILKINSON COMPANY
P.O. Box 4558, 31011 Agoura Road
Thousand Oaks, CA 91320
dental base metal alloy; dental casting gold alloy; dental wrought wire alloy; orthodontic material; precision
attachments.

WILLIAMS GOLD REFINING COMPANY, INC.
2978 Main Street, Buffalo, NY 14214
acrylic resin teeth; chromium-cobalt casting alloy;
dental amalgam; dental base metal alloy; dental casting gold alloy; dental gold; dental gypsum products;
dental porcelain; dental wrought wire alloy; denture
base resin; finishing and polishing instruments; gold
matrix foil; orthodontic appliances; precision attachments; preformed crowns; solder.

XONICS MEDICAL SYSTEMS
925 E. Rand Road, Sutie 202, Arlington Heights, IL
60004
radiographic accessories.

YOUNG DENTAL
2418 Northline Industrial Blvd.
Maryland Heights, MO 63043
dental restorative instruments.

ZAHN DENTAL COMPANY, INC.
67 Irving Place, New York, NY 10003
denture base polymer.

ZIRC DENTAL PRODUCTS
6855 Oxford Street, Minneapolis, MN 55426
composite resin instruments; dental cast restorative
instruments; dental handpiece; dental operatory instruments; dental resin; dental restorative instruments; dental sterilization equipment; finishing and
polishing instruments; local anesthetic equipment;
periodontal instruments.

GENERAL INDEX